Oxford Case Histories

Series Editors

Sarah Pendlebury and Peter Rothwell

Published:

Neurological Case Histories (Sarah Pendlebury and Peter Rothwell)

Forthcoming:

Oxford Case Histories in Cardiology (Colin Forfar, Javed Ehtisham, and Rajkumar Rajendram)

Oxford Case Histories in Gastroenterology and Hepatology (Alissa Walsh, Otto Buchel, Jane Collier, and Simon Travis)

Oxford Case Histories in Nephrology (Chris Pugh, Chris O'Callaghan, Aron Chakera, Richard Cornall, and David Mole)

Oxford Case Histories in Respiratory Medicine (John Stradling, Andrew Stanton, Anabell Nickol, Helen Davies, and Najib Rahman)

Oxford Case Histories in Rheumatology (Joel David, Anne Miller, Anushka Soni, and Lyn Williamson)

Oxford Case Histories in Stroke and TIA (Sarah Pendlebury, Ursula Schulz, Aneil Malhotra, and Peter Rothwell)

Oxford Case Histories in Gastroenterology and Hepatology

Alissa J. Walsh
St.Vincent's Hospital Staff Specialist
Sydney, Australia

Otto C. Buchel
Consultant Physician and Fellow in Gastroenterology
Universitas Hospital
Bluemfontein, South Africa

Jane Collier
Consultant Hepatologist
Department of Gastroenterology and Hepatology
John Radcliffe Hospital, Oxford, UK

Simon P.L. Travis
Consultant Gastroenterologist
John Radcliffe Hospital
Fellow of Linacre College
University of Oxford
Oxford, UK

OXFORD
UNIVERSITY PRESS

OXFORD
UNIVERSITY PRESS

Great Clarendon Street, Oxford ox2 6dp

Oxford University Press is a department of the University of Oxford.
It furthers the University's objective of excellence in research, scholarship,
and education by publishing worldwide in

Oxford New York

Athens Auckland Bangkok Bogotá Buenos Aires Cape-Town
Chennai Dar es Salaam Delhi Florence Hong Kong Istanbul Karachi
Kolkata Kuala Lumpur Madrid Melbourne Mexico City Mumbai Nairobi
Paris São Paulo Shanghai Singapore Taipei Tokyo Toronto Warsaw

with associated companies in Berlin Ibadan

Oxford is a registered trade mark of Oxford University Press
in the UK and in certain other countries

Published in the United States
by Oxford University Press Inc., New York

British Library Cataloguing in Publication Data

Data available

Library of Congress Cataloguing in Publication Data

Data available

Typeset in Minion by Glyph International, Bangalore, India
Printed in Great Britain
on acid-free paper by the
MPG Books Group, Bodmin and King's Lynn

ISBN 978–0–19–955789–9

10 9 8 7 6 5 4 3 2

A note from the series editors

Case histories have always had an important role in medical education, but most published material has been directed at undergraduates or residents. The Oxford Case Histories series aims to provide more complex case-based learning for clinicians in specialist training and consultants, with a view to aiding preparation for entry and exit-level specialty examinations or revalidation. Each case book follows the same format with approximately 50 cases, each comprising a brief clinical history and investigations, followed by questions on differential diagnosis and management, and detailed answers with discussion. All cases are peer-reviewed by Oxford consultants in the relevant specialty. At the end of each book, cases are listed by mode of presentation, aetiology and diagnosis.

We are grateful to our colleagues in the various medical specialties for their enthusiasm and hard work in making the series possible.

Sarah Pendlebury and Peter Rothwell

Quotes on the first book in the series – "Neurological Case Histories"

"I recommend this excellent volume highly .... this book will enlighten and entertain consultants, and all readers will learn something."

Lancet Neurology 2007; 6: 951

"This short and well-written text is .... designed to enhance the reader's diagnostic ability and clinical understanding .... A well documented and practical book"

European Journal of Neurology 2007; 14: e19

Preface

This book contains a series of cases that we have encountered in Oxford Gastroenterology practice. One purpose is to assist re-validation. Another is to provide a resource of real cases in preparation for specialist exams. A further purpose is more general, being educational for physicians in general internal or emergency medicine, or indeed gastroenterologists, since the cases are often advanced and sometimes challenging.

All 50 cases include a series of questions, to which we have given detailed, evidence-based answers, although it is the nature of evidence-based practice that clinical judgment is also necessary. We have expressed our views, and hope that you generally agree! We have specifically chosen cases to cover different areas within gastroenterology and hepatology. Included in this selection are acute cases where rapid diagnosis and treatment are crucial, as well as chronic disorders that require strategic thinking, and of course, the management dilemmas of daily practice.

We have used the format of case reports with detailed discussions of differential diagnosis and management, for three reasons. First, we believe that one of the best ways to learn advanced clinical medicine is through the analysis of individual cases. In almost all areas of medicine, it is extremely difficult to illustrate the practical process of diagnosis within the format of a traditional textbook. Second, we strongly believe that it is simply more interesting to consider real cases than to read a text. This allows a clinician to reflect on their own differential diagnosis and treatment. Finally, there is a lack of case series that stretch the abilities of experienced clinicians and specialists: most are aimed at medical students or young doctors doing early postgraduate exams. It is for this reason that the cases and questions are sometimes challenging, although many are simple, since the aim is to educate.

We would like to thank the many colleagues from many disciplines, including those allied to medicine for contributing cases, providing illustrations, or administrative support, and always for making helpful comments on the manuscript as it developed: these include (in alphabetical order and without titles!) Adam Bailey, June Beharry, Helen Bungay, Roger Chapman, Rowan Collinson, Godman Greywoode, Hennie Grundling, Tim James, Christiaan Jansen, Satish Keshav, Siraj Misbah, Juan Piris, Andrew Slater, Helen Small, Alina Stoita, Jan van Zyl, Bryan Warren, and David Williams. Cases 16, 26 and 42 were seen and cared for at the Gastroenterology unit, Universitas Hospital, Bloemfontein, South Africa, which we gratefully acknowledge. We would also like to thank our families for their tolerance, patience, and support for work that occupies evenings, early mornings, and weekends!

Alissa Walsh, Otto Buchel, Jane Collier, Simon Travis
Oxford, August 2009

Contents

Abbreviations

5FU	5-fluorouracil	ECF	epirubicin, cisplatin and 5-fluorouracil combination chemotherapy
5HT	5-hydroxytryptamine		
AGA	American Gastroenterology Association	ECG	electrocardiogram
AFP	α-fetoprotein	ELISA	enzyme-linked immunosorbent assay
ALA	aminolaevulinic acid		
ALF	acute liver failure	EMA	endomysial antibody (for coeliac disease)
ALP	alkaline phosphatase		
ALT	alanine transaminase	ERCP	endoscopic retrograde cholangiopancreatography
AMA	antimitochondrial antibodies		
ANA	antinuclear antigen	ESR	erythrocyte sedimentation rate
ANCA	antineutrophil cytoplasmic antibody	EOX	oxaliplatin and capcytabine combination chemotherapy
APTT	activated partial thromboplastin time	FDA	Food and Drug Administration (USA)
ARDS	acute respiratory distress syndrome	FISH	fluorescent *in situ* hybridization
ASmAb	anti-smooth muscle antibody	FMF	familial Mediterranean fever
AST	aspartate transaminase	GABA	gamma-aminobutyric acid
BCG	Bacille Calmette-Guérin	GI	gastrointestinal
bpm	beats per minute	GGT	gamma glutamyl transpeptidase
BMI	body mass index		
BSG	British Society of Gastroenterology	GIST	gastrointestinal stromal tumour
C^{14}	carbon-14	HAART	highly active antiretroviral therapy
Ca	cancer antigen		
CBD	common bile duct	HAV	hepatitis A virus
CDAD	*Clostridium difficile*-associated diarrhoea	HBcAb	antibody to the hepatitis B core antigen
CDT	*Clostridium difficile* toxin	HBeAg	hepatitis B e antigen
CEA	carcinoembryonic antigen	HBsAb	antibody to the hepatitis B surface antigen
CFTR	cystic fibrosis transmembrane regulator		
		HBsAg	hepatitis B surface antigen
CMV	Cytomegalovirus	HBV	hepatitis B virus
CRP	C reactive protein	HCV	hepatitis C virus
CT	computerized tomography	HELLP	haemolysis, elevated liver enzymes, low platelet count syndrome
EBV	Epstein–Barr virus		

HFE	High iron FE (haemochromatomosis gene)	Na	sodium
HIV	human immunodeficiency virus	NAFLD	non-alcoholic fatty liver disease
HMB	hydroximethylbilane synthesase	NASH	non-alcoholic steatohepatitis
HHV 8	human herpesvirus 8	NAT2	N-acetyltransferase 2
IBD	inflammatory bowel disease	NSAIDs	non-steroidal anti-inflammatory drugs
IBS	irritable bowel syndrome	OLT	orthotopic liver transplantation
IFL	irinotecan with 5-fluorouracil combination chemotherapy	pANCA	antineutrophil cytoplasmic antibodies reacting with myeloperoxidase
IFN	interferon	PBC	primary biliary cirrhosis
IL	interleukin	PCR	polymerase chain reaction
INR	international normalized ratio	PET	positron emission tomography
IPMN	intraductal papillary mucinous neoplasm	PICC	peripherally inserted central catheter
IPSID	immunoproliferative small intestinal disease	PPARγ	peroxisome proliferator-activated receptor gamma
IVF	*in vitro* fertilization	PPI	proton pump inhibitor
K	potassium	PSC	primary sclerosing cholangitis
LOLA	ʟ-ornithine ʟ-aspartate	PUD	peptic ulcer disease
LFT	liver function test	PVC	polyvinyl chloride
LKM1	liver kidney microsomal antibody type 1	RUQ	right upper quadrant
LP	lumbar puncture	SCA	serous cystadenoma
MAC	*Mycobacterium avium* complex	SIRS	systemic inflammatory response syndrome
MALT	mucosa-associated lymphoid tissue	SLA	soluble liver antigen
MARS	molecular absorbent re-circulating system	SLE	systemic lupus erythematosus
MCN	mucinous cystic neoplasm	SMA	spinal muscular atrophy
MCV	mean cell volume	SSRI	Selective serotonin reuptake inhibitor
MDR	multi-drug resistant	TB	tuberculosis
MELD	Model for Endstage Liver Disease	TFR2	transferrin receptor 2
Mg	magnesium	TIPSS	transjugular intrahepatic portal systemic shunt
MMR	mismatch repair	TNF	tumour necrosis factor
MRCP	magnetic resonance cholangiopancreatography	TSH	thyroid stimulating hormone
MRI	magnetic resonance imaging	U&E	urea and electrolytes
MRSA	methicillin resistant *staphylococcus aureus*	WCC	white cell count
MSI	microsatellite instability	XDR	extensively drug resistant
		ZES	Zollinger–Ellison syndrome

Normal ranges

Normal ranges in the laboratories of the John Radcliffe Hospital, Oxford

Hb	13–17g1dL (men)	GGT	15–40 IU/L
	12–15g/dL (women)	Albumin	35–50 g/L
MCV	83–101fL (men)	Amylase	25–125 IU/L
	76–96fL (women)	AFP	0–7 IU/mL
WCC	4–11 x 10^9/L	CEA	0–3 µg/L
Platelets	150–400 x 10^9/L	Ca_{125}	0–30 IU/L
Prothrombin time	12–15 secs	Ca_{19-9}	0–31 U/mL
INR	0.7–1.1	Ferritin	20–300 µg/L (Men)
APTT	24–34 secs		10–200 µg/L (Women)
Haptoglobin	0.5–2.65 g/L		
Na	135–145 mmol/L	Folate	4–24 µg/L
K	3.5–5.0 mmol/L	Vitamin B_{12}	180–900 ng/L
Urea	2.5–6.7 mmol/L	Copper	11–20 µmol/L
Creatinine	54–145 umol/L (range usually corrected for age or weight)	Caeruloplasmin	16–60 mg/dL
		CD4 lymphocyte count	0.6–1.5 x10^9/L
Calcium	2.12–2.65 mmol/L	TSH	0.35–5.5 mU/L
Magnesium	0.75 – 1.05 mmol/L	Free T_4	10.5–20 pmol/L
Phosphate	0.80–1.45 mmol/L	Fecal elastase	>200 µg elastase/g of stool
CRP	0–8 mg/L		
ESR	need range	IgA	0.8–3.0 g/L
Glucose (fasting)	3.0–5.5 mmol/L	IgG	6–13 g/L
Bilirubin	3–17 µmol/L	Ascitic fluid WCC	none
AST	15–42 IU/L		
ALT	10–45 IU/L		
ALP	95–320 IU/L (notably different between laboratories, depending on the analytical technique)		

Case 1

A 22-year-old male porter from South Africa was admitted to hospital after being found by his landlord with confusion. On arrival at the hospital his Glasgow Coma Score was 13. He was apyrexial, with a blood glucose of 5.4mmol/L, pulse rate 60 beats/min and regular, and blood pressure 114/58mmHg. Heart sounds were normal and his chest was clear. He was noted to be jaundiced. Asterixis was present. There were no focal neurological signs. There were no spider naevi, muscle wasting, or gynaecomastia.

His only medical history was pulmonary tuberculosis 6 months earlier, diagnosed by pleural biopsy and pleural fluid analysis. He had last been followed up 2 months previously and was well at that time. He had completed 2 months of rifampicin, isoniazid, pyrazinamide and ethambutol, followed by rifampicin and isoniazid alone. There was no record of any other medications or over the counter preparations. There was no known alcohol or drug history. HIV testing had been negative.

Investigations showed:

- Hb 15.2g/dL, WCC 9.1 x 10^9/L, platelets 173 x 10^9/L
- Na 135mmol/L, K 3.7mmol/L, urea 2.8mmol/L, creatinine 78μmol/L
- Bilirubin 357μmol/L, ALT 1307 IU/L, ALP 436 IU/L, albumin 32g/L
- Prothrombin time 53.8 sec.

Questions

1a) What is the clinical syndrome illustrated by this case?

1b) Give a differential diagnosis for the cause of (a).

1c) What blood tests would you request?

1d) What radiological tests would you request?

1e) What is the management?

1f) What is the most likely cause in this patient and why? What is the mechanism of injury?

1g) How might this problem have been prevented?

Answers

1a) **What is the clinical syndrome illustrated by this case?**

This is acute liver failure (ALF), which is defined by three criteria:

- Rapid development of hepatocellular dysfunction (e.g. jaundice, coagulopathy)
- Encephalopathy
- Absence of a prior history of liver disease.

1b) **Give a differential diagnosis for the cause of (a)**

The differential diagnosis for ALF in this patient includes:

- Drugs (paracetamol, antituberculosis medications, propylthioracyl)
- Hepatotropic viruses (hepatitis B, hepatitis A, hepatitis E, with hepatitis B being the most common)
- Acute cryptogenic (non-A, non-B, non-C) hepatitis
- Autoimmune hepatitis
- Ischaemia
- Metabolic disorders such as Wilson's disease
- Malignant infiltration.

A careful history of past and present medications needs to be taken, together with a travel history and assessment of risk factors to determine the likelihood of acute viral hepatitis. Routine viral testing should be done for all patients (see below). In the presence of tense ascites **Budd Chiari syndrome** (hepatic venous outflow obstruction) should be considered, because ascites is unusual in early acute liver failure from other causes. **Wilson's disease** may present with acute liver failure and should always be considered in patients presenting at a young age, but usually there is accompanying haemolysis or renal failure, which were absent in the present case. Furthermore, the alkaline phosphatase is usually normal in Wilson's disease, whereas in this case it was elevated. Fulminant hepatic failure is an unusual presentation of hepatic neoplasms, whether primary or metastatic.

Although this patient had ALF, it may be difficult to distinguish this from **acute decompensation of chronic liver disease** in patients in whom the past medical history is unknown. For example, exacerbation of chronic viral hepatitis (B and C) may produce a similar picture to ALF. Patients with chronic liver disease, however, usually show stigmata, including spider naevi, muscle wasting, testicular strophy, or gynaecomastia, none of which were present in this patient. Furthermore, in chronic liver disease it would be rare for the prothrombin time to be over 40 sec (usually it would be about 25 sec). In this patient it was 53.8 sec. In alcoholic hepatitis, the alanine transaminase (ALT) rarely exceeds 300 IU/L, (see box 2) whereas in this case it was 1370 IU/L.

1c) **What blood tests would you request?**

A 'liver screen' should be performed to look for the cause of ALF including:

- Paracetamol concentration (although N-acetyl cysteine should be started before the result is known, to cover the possibility of toxicity). Note that paracetamol may be undetectable if the overdose was over 72 hours before blood testing
- Hepatitis A IgM
- Hepatitis B core IgM
- Autoimmune markers: antinuclear antigen (ANA), anti-smooth muscle antibody (ASmAb), liver kidney microsomal antibody type 1 (LKM1), and immunoglobulins
- Copper and caeruloplasmin to screen for Wilson's disease.

1d) **What radiological tests would you request?**

An ultrasound of the abdomen should be performed, since this will help distinguish between acute and chronic liver disease (splenomegaly is more common in chronic liver disease). This is particularly helpful in the context of a less severe coagulopathy, where it may be unclear whether this represents ALF or an acute exacerbation of chronic disease. Ultrasound will not help to differentiate between different causes of ALF.

1e) **What is the management?**

The management of ALF includes:

- **Intravenous rehydration**: most patients require liberal volume expansion, since such patients are often vasodilated, volume depleted and acidotic. The choice of fluid is not crucial and is usually a mixture of crystalloid and colloid. Fluid resuscitation can often reverse the acidosis.
- The **blood glucose** should be measured hourly and replaced: with intravenous glucose (10–50%) as necessary, since there is a high risk of hypoglycaemia. Glucose concentrations need to be maintained to prevent the cerebral and systemic effects of hypoglycaemia.

- **Arterial blood gas** to monitor acidosis: correction of lactic acidosis is important, because it can affect circulatory function and aggravate cerebral hyperaemia.
- **N-acetyl cysteine** should be given to cover the possibility of paracetamol overdose.
- **Antibiotics**: prophylaxis with an intravenous cephalosporin is recommended. Patients with ALF have a high risk of infection and sepsis from bacterial and/or fungal infection. The use of prophylactic antibiotics is associated with lower rates of infection complicating ALF. Without prophylaxis, infection develops in up to 80% of patients with ALF, and bacteraemia occurs in 20–25% (usually gram-negative organisms). If definite infection is proven, this should be treated aggressively (e.g. vancomycin and a third-generation cephalosporin).
- **Vitamin K** is not indicated: bleeding is unusual in ALF despite the increased prothrombin time. Fresh frozen plasma is not advocated, because the risks (fluid overload, normalization of the prothrombin time artificially) outweigh the benefits. Plasma product should be used only if the patient is bleeding or an invasive procedure is being performed. The prothrombin time is also a good prognostic indicator.
- Lactulose is of no proven benefit in ALF.
- **Intensive care management**: if the patient is not protecting their airway (grade 3 or 4 encephalopathy), intubation and ventilation is indicated. This applies especially during transfer to a transplant unit, because grade 4 encephalopathy can develop rapidly.
- **Liver transplant**: In patients with acute liver failure, liver transplantation should be considered at an early stage and the regional liver transplant unit contacted for advice. In paracetamol-induced ALF, referral to a transplant unit should be made if the prothrombin time is >60 sec. For non-paracetamol acute liver failure, the criteria are listed below.

The King's College Hospital criteria for liver transplantation in non-paracetamol ALF are:

- INR >6.5 or prothrombin time >100 sec

OR three of the following:

- patient age <11 years old or >40 years old
- serum bilirubin >300μmol/L
- time from onset of jaundice to development of coma >7 days

- INR >3.5 or prothrombin time >50 sec
- aetiology: non-A, non-B, or drug toxicity (not paracetamol).

It should be noted that patients should be transferred *well before* the development of these criteria. The patient in this case met the criteria on admission, since he had a prothrombin time of 53.8 sec, bilirubin of 357μmol/L, and drug toxicity as the aetiology (below).

1f) **What is the most likely cause of ALF in this patient and why? What is the mechanism of injury?**

The most likely cause of ALF in this patient is **isoniazid toxicity**. One to two percent of patients receiving isoniazid develop severe liver injury, defined as an ALT being at least 3 times the upper limit of normal. Fulminant hepatotoxicity is well described and has 10–20% mortality if the isoniazid is continued. The **mechanism** of injury is the production of toxic metabolites through isoniazid oxidation in the cytochrome p450 pathway. These metabolites accumulate in people who are slow acetylators and in those on concurrent enzyme-inducing medication such as rifampicin or alcohol. Although it remains controversial, certain polymorphisms of N-acetyltransferase 2 (NAT2) and glutathione-S-transferase genes are also thought to be risk factors. Other risk factors for hepatotoxicity include underlying liver disease (especially coexistent hepatitis B or hepatitis C), other hepatotoxic medications (such as protease inhibitors for treatment of HIV), excessive alcohol consumption, age >35 years, and female gender. It is unclear whether race or malnutrition contributes to the risk of toxicity.

1g) **How might this problem have been prevented?**

Before starting antituberculous treatment the patient requires education regarding the medication. Detection of risk factors for toxicity (1f, above) is important and every patient should have baseline LFTs. Individual patients need to be aware that they should see a doctor if non-specific symptoms occur. If the **ALT is >5 times** normal, or if symptoms arise, then antituberculous medications need to be stopped. If the **ALT is 2–4 times** normal, then liver function tests should be checked weekly for 2 weeks and then fortnightly until they have improved. If treatment needs to be continued, alternative agents such as ethambutol or fluoroquinolones should be considered, since these are the least hepatotoxic. Once the LFTs have normalized, antituberculous drugs should be reintroduced one by one. Rifampicin is usually introduced first and then isoniazid. Pyrazinamide should be omitted if possible. These drugs are often tolerated on reintroduction.

Further reading

Devlin J, O'Grady J (1999). Indications for referral and assessment in adult liver transplantation: a clinical guideline. *Gut*; **45**(Suppl. 6): V11–V121.

Jalan R (2005). Acute liver failure: current management and future prospects. *J Hepatol*; **42**: S115–S123.

Sass DA, Obaid Shakil A (2005). Fulminant hepatic failure. *Liv Trans*; **11**: 594–605.

Case 2

A 24-year-old female hairdresser presented with a 5-day history of jaundice, right upper quadrant discomfort, and general malaise. Her stool was of normal colour and not pale, nor did she have dark urine. She admitted to recent alcohol excess while on holiday in Ibiza, from where she had returned 10 days before. Her usual alcohol intake was 24 units/week, with binges during social events. She had no past medical history and used no prescription drugs, over-the-counter medications or NSAIDs, no nutritional supplements or herbal remedies, and no illicit drugs. She had not recently had a course of antibiotics. There was no history of previous blood transfusion, contact with hepatitis, or previous jaundice, and she had no tattoos. She had last had unprotected sex 8 months previously. There was no significant family history.

On examination she was clinically well, haemodynamically stable, and apyrexial. She was jaundiced, without lymphadenopathy, peripheral oedema, or finger clubbing. There were no signs of chronic liver disease or portal hypertension. She had a liver edge, palpable 3 cm below the costal margin, which was firm, smooth and non-tender. Cardiac and respiratory examination was unremarkable.

Investigations showed:

- Hb 13.4g/dL, WCC 4.22 x 10^9/L, platelets 182 x 10^9/L
- Prothrombin time 13.2 sec, APTT 36.1 sec
- Bilirubin 56µmol/L, ALT 2858 IU/L, ALP 626 IU/L, albumin 40g/L
- Ultrasound scan of the abdomen: mild splenomegaly with a span of 13.5cm. No gallstones, but there was slight thickening of the gallbladder wall. The liver was homogeneous and of normal size. The pancreas, bile duct, kidneys, and spleen appeared sonographically normal.

Questions

2a) What is the clinical problem and the differential diagnosis in this case?

2b) What is the significance of the ultrasound findings?

Further investigation revealed: hepatitis A IgM negative, hepatitis B surface Ag negative, cytomegalovirus IgM negative, EBV IgG positive, ANA positive 1/640, smooth muscle antibody negative, antimitochondrial antibody negative, IgG 35.6g/L, IgM 1.76g/L, IgA 2.81g/L.

2c) What is the most likely diagnosis given these investigation results?

2d) What would be your next investigation?

2e) How would you treat this patient?

Answers

2a) **What is the clinical problem and the differential diagnosis in this case?**

The clinical features of this case are consistent with **acute hepatitis**. Acute hepatitis is characterized by mild jaundice, lethargy, and markedly elevated transaminases. The sudden onset of symptoms in the presence of a normal albumin suggests acute liver injury. There is no evidence of acute liver failure, because the prothrombin time is normal (see Case 1, acute liver failure).

The differential diagnosis in this case includes:

- Viral hepatitis
- Toxins
- Autoimmune disease.

Viral, toxic (drug), and autoimmune causes may be responsible for markedly elevated transaminases. Recent travel to a coastal resort raises the possibility of shellfish consumption, which increases the risk of **hepatitis A** virus infection. The return from Ibiza 10 days prior to presentation is compatible with the incubation period for hepatitis A virus infection (see Case 16). There is no history of high-risk sexual behaviour within the past 90 days, and no contact with blood or blood products, so acute **hepatitis B** virus infection is unlikely. **Hepatitis A** (see Case 16), **hepatitis B** (see Case 44), **cytomegalovirus and Epstein–Barr** virus infections should, nevertheless, be excluded by appropriate serology. If other investigations are negative, **Hepatitis E** virus infection should be considered. Acute presentation of **hepatitis C** virus infection (see Case 43) is rare, but should be considered once other aetiologies have been excluded, especially if risk factors such as intravenous drug abuse are present. **Drug-induced hepatitis** in our patient is effectively excluded by the history, but checking a paracetamol concentration on admission would be a sensible precaution. Even though she has a history of binge drinking, the markedly elevated ALT is against an acute **alcoholic hepatitis**, in which transaminases rarely exceed 300 IU/L (see Case 1). In our patient, hepatomegaly was not marked and the leucocyte count was normal, which makes alcoholic hepatitis less likely, since it is associated with peripheral leucocytosis. Excess alcohol consumption may lead to fatty liver with hepatomegaly (see Case 45). **Autoimmune hepatitis** should be excluded, and investigation should include autoantibodies and immunoglobulin fractions.

2b) **What is the significance of the ultrasound findings?**

The ultrasound features of note are splenomegaly and gall bladder wall thickening.

Splenomegaly may occur in acute viral hepatitis. Alternatively, autoimmune hepatitis may present acutely, superimposed on chronic autoimmune liver disease, in which case splenomegaly could represent underlying portal hypertension. Thickening of the wall of the gall bladder has been well described in acute hepatitis and is thought to be proportional to the degree of liver cell necrosis, illustrated by the transaminitis.

2c) **What is the most likely diagnosis, given these investigation results?**

The most likely diagnosis is **autoimmune hepatitis**. A strongly positive ANA and serum IgG elevation more than twice the upper limit of normal, are highly suggestive of autoimmune hepatitis. This, together with the fact that viral serology was negative with no suggestion of biliary disease and no history of exposure to hepatotoxic drugs, makes autoimmune hepatitis the likely underlying cause. The fact that the patient is female also strengthens the likelihood.

2d) **What would be your next investigation?**

A **liver biopsy** should be performed. A needle biopsy of the liver is essential for confirming the diagnosis of autoimmune hepatitis, grading disease activity, and staging the fibrosis. Histopathological features of autoimmune hepatitis include portal inflammation with a mononuclear cellular infiltrate including plasma cells, extending beyond the limiting plate of hepatocytes into the lobule (interface hepatitis). If severe, confluent areas of necrosis may isolate groups of liver cells and form rosettes. Varying degrees of fibrosis may be present. Fatty change, iron excess, and biliary pathology are not features. Although a prominent plasma cell infiltrate is highly suggestive of autoimmune hepatitis, the biopsy features are not entirely specific.

In our patient interface hepatitis and plasma cells were seen in the mononuclear portal cellular infiltrate (see Figs 2.1 and 2.2 in the central colour section).

An international scoring system to aid in the diagnosis of autoimmune hepatitis has been developed as a research tool (Czaja 2006). This scoring system (Table 2.1) accommodates the diverse manifestations of the disease and produces an aggregate score, reflecting the probability of the diagnosis. It may be used when the diagnosis of autoimmune hepatitis is in doubt.

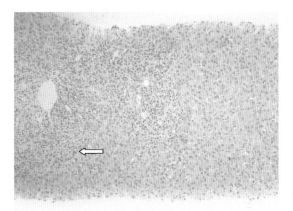

Fig. 2.1 (see colour plate 1) A low-power magnification image of a liver biopsy, showing a severe inflammatory infiltrate at the interface between the portal triad and lobule (arrow).

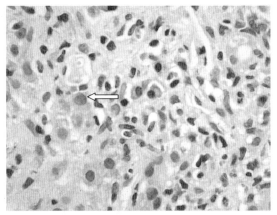

Fig. 2.2 (see colour plate 2) A higher magnification showing distinct plasma cells (arrow).

Using the scoring system, this patient's aggregate score was 17 prior to therapy (female gender, ALP:ALT ratio <1.5, IgG >twice upper limit, antinuclear antigen >1/80, negative viral serology, interface hepatitis, and plasma cell infiltrate on liver histology). A pre-treatment score of >15 gives a definite diagnosis.

2e) **How would you treat this patient?**

Treatment is with immunosuppression. The mainstay of treatment is **corticosteroids**. **Azathioprine** may be added once liver function tests have normalized, often allowing the prednisolone dose to be reduced to 5–7.5mg/day, or stopped completely. In our patient there was no

Table 2.1 International scoring system for autoimmune hepatitis

Criterion	Component	Score	Criterion	Component	Score
Sex	Female	+2	HLA	DR3 or DR4	+1
AP:AST (or ALT) ratio	> 3.0	−2	Immune disease	Thyroiditis, colitis, others	+2
	< 1.5	+2			
Gamma-globulin or IgG level above normal	> 2.0	+3	Other markers	Anti-SLA/LP, actin, LC1, pANCA	+2
	1.5–2.0	+2			
	1.0–1.5	+1			
	< 1.0	0			
ANA, SMA, or anti-LKM1 titres	> 1:80	+3	Histological features	Interface hepatitis	+3
	1:80	+2		Plasmacytic	+1
	1:40	+1		Rosettes	+1
	< 1:40	0		None of above	−5
				Biliary changes	−3
				Other features	−3
AMA	Positive	−4	Treatment response	Complete	+2
				Relapse	+3
Viral markers	Positive	−3			
	Negative	+3			
Drugs	Yes	−4	**Pre-treatment score**		
	No	+1	Definite diagnosis: > 15		
			Probable diagnosis: 10–15		
Alcohol	< 25g/day	+2	**Post-treatment score**		
	> 60g/day	−2	Definite diagnosis: > 17		
			Probable diagnosis: 12–17		

contraindication to azathioprine, so this was given in combination with prednisolone. Remission is defined as transaminases less than twice the upper limit of normal. Immunosuppression is usually required **long term**, but patients do not routinely require repeat liver biopsy. After withdrawal of therapy, only around 20% of patients have a sustained remission. Most relapses occur within 12 weeks of cessation of therapy and can be severe. However, relapse may occur months or years later, so there is a need for continued follow-up. Life expectancy of treated patients exceeds 85% at 10 years and 74% at 20 years. In around 10% of patients, therapy fails to prevent progression of liver disease, with eventual hepatic decompensation, leading to liver transplantation.

This patient responded well to treatment with corticosteroids and aza-thioprine, with normalization of liver biochemistry, so she was maintained on immunosuppression. Alternatives exist for those patients who do not tolerate first-line drugs. Mycophenolate mofetil and tacrolimus have both been used, although there are no controlled data.

Further reading

Czaja AJ (2007). Corticosteroids or not in severe acute or fulminant autoimmune hepatitis: therapeutic brinksmanship and the point beyond salvation. *Liver Transpl*; **13**: 953–5.

Czaja AJ (2006). Autoimmune hepatitis – approach to diagnosis. *Med Gen Med*; **8**: 55.

Juttner H-U, Ralls PW, Quin MF, Jenney JM (1982). Thickening of the gallbladder wall in acute hepatitis: Ultrasound presentation. *Radiology*; **142**: 465–6.

Montano Loza AJ, Czaja AJ (2007). Current therapy for autoimmune hepatitis. *Nat Clin Pract Gastroenterol Hepatol*; **4**: 202–14.

Heathcote J (2006). Treatment strategies for autoimmune hepatitis. *Am J Gastroenterol*; **101**(Suppl. 12): S630–2.

Case 3

A 35-year-old florist, 26 weeks pregnant, was referred to the outpatient department because of mild jaundice, a 1-month history of intense pruritus and fatigue.

Her first pregnancy, 3 years previously, was complicated by hypertension, but was otherwise uneventful and the child remained healthy. The current pregnancy followed three miscarriages. During this period, she was diagnosed with systemic lupus erythematosus (SLE) and antiphospholipid syndrome. There were no cerebral or renal manifestations of SLE. Current medications included azathioprine 200mg/day, prednisolone 5mg/day, low-dose aspirin, and low molecular weight heparin. She had been on azathioprine for 2 years.

On examination, she was fully orientated. Her pulse rate was 72bpm, and blood pressure 130/80mmHg. There was mild icterus, no spider naevi, no abdominal tenderness, and no hyper-reflexia.

Investigations showed:

- Hb 12.5g/L, WCC 10 x 10^9/L, platelets 312 x 10^9/L
- Na 135mmol/L, K 4.2mmol/L, urea 4.3mmol/L, creatinine 82μmol/L
- Bilirubin 102μmol/L, AST 475 IU/L, ALT 157 IU/L, ALP 350 IU/L, GGT 52 IU
- Serum bile acids 192μmol/L(normal 0–10)
- Urine dipstix – negative for protein.

Questions

3a) What is the differential diagnosis?

3b) Is a liver biopsy necessary?

3c) What treatment should be instituted?

3d) What are the maternal and fetal prognoses?

Answers

3a **What is the differential diagnosis?**

The differential diagnosis includes pregnancy-related liver disease and non-pregnancy related liver disease, including complications of SLE.

Pregnancy-related liver disease:

- Intrahepatic cholestasis of pregnancy
- Pre-eclampsia and eclampsia
- HELLP syndrome (Haemolysis (H), elevated liver enzymes (EL), low platelet count (LP)
- Acute fatty liver of pregnancy.

Non-pregnancy related liver disease:

- Autoimmune hepatitis (see Case 2)
- Viral hepatitis (see Cases 16, 43, 44)
- Drug-induced hepatitis (see Case 1)
- Biliary obstruction (see Case 9)
- Primary biliary cirrhosis (see Case 4)
- Primary sclerosing cholangitis (see Case 50).

The most likely pregnancy-related diagnosis is **intrahepatic cholestasis of pregnancy**. Pruritus is the primary clinical symptom of intrahepatic cholestasis of pregnancy. The pruritus can range from mild and tolerable to severe and disabling. Pruritus is typically worse in the evening, with a predilection for the palms or soles of the feet, and is not associated with any specific skin lesions. Mild jaundice occurs in 10–15% of cases, usually occurring 1–4 weeks after the onset of the pruritus. The main biochemical alterations are elevations of serum bile acids, and transaminase concentrations. The serum concentration of GGT may be modestly elevated. ALP is difficult to interpret during pregnancy, due to elevation of the placental isoenzyme.

Diagnosis of intrahepatic cholestasis of pregnancy is one of exclusion. It is important to exclude other causes of liver disease and cholestasis. This case does not fit with the rare **HELLP syndrome**, because there is no evidence of haemolysis or thrombocytopenia, and the patient is relatively well. Patients with SLE are, however, at increased risk of **pre-eclampsia**. Although there is hypertension, which raises the suspicion of pre-eclampsia, there is no proteinuria (making either pre-eclampsia or lupus nephritis most unlikely) or hyper-reflexia. **Acute fatty liver of pregnancy** is a sudden, catastrophic illness occurring almost exclusively in the third trimester, where microvesicular fatty infiltration results in encephalopathy and hepatic failure. The typical patient has 1–2 weeks of anorexia, nausea and vomiting, headache, and right upper quadrant pain; she looks ill, with jaundice, hypertension, oedema, ascites, a small liver, and hepatic encephalopathy.

Non-pregnancy related causes of liver disease must always be considered and **autoimmune hepatitis** in particular, not least because this is more common in SLE. Autoimmune hepatitis was sometimes (incorrectly) called lupus hepatitis in the past, although it is a condition quite separate from SLE.

Investigation should include screening for viral hepatitis, and radiological imaging of the biliary tract for biliary obstruction due to gallstones, which are more common during pregnancy. This can be done safely by abdominal ultrasound or magnetic resonance imaging. Drug-induced liver disease is also important to consider. Although **azathioprine** can cause hepatitis, this is usually an acute event that occurs within 3 weeks of starting the drug and very rarely in patients who have been established on the drug for more than a month. There are anecdotes of azathioprine-induced nodular-regenerative hyperplasia, but these are exceptional. Wide experience of azathioprine in pregnancy for the treatment of many conditions (including inflammatory bowel disease) indicates that it is not only safe, with no increase in miscarriage, still birth or congenital anomaly, but also that stopping the drug leads to a relapse of the underlying condition, which is more harmful to the fetus.

3b) **Is a liver biopsy necessary?**

Liver biopsy is not ordinarily necessary for the diagnosis of intrahepatic cholestasis of pregnancy. Nevertheless, in this case, a biopsy was performed to exclude autoimmune hepatitis and the remote possibility azathioprine-induced liver damage. The biopsy was consistent with intrahepatic cholestasis of pregnancy, showing centrilobular cholestasis without inflammation and cannalicular bile plugs among hepatocytes. Coexistent drug-induced hepatitis could not be excluded, but the considerations above (3a) made this unlikely. The important finding was that there were no features of autoimmune hepatitis, so she was treated as having intrahepatic cholestasis of pregnancy.

3c) **What treatment should be instituted?**

The primary objective of pharmacological treatment of intrahepatic cholestasis of pregnancy is to alleviate maternal symptoms and improve fetal outcome. Currently, **Ursodeoxycholic acid** is the most effective treatment for intrahepatic cholestasis of pregnancy, and appears to work as a choleuretic, to promote the flow of bile (see Case 4). It is effective at alleviating pruritus and restoring bile acids towards normal. Ursodeoxycholic acid is safer and more effective than cholestyramine, an anion-binding resin that is a bile acid sequestrant. Antihistamines are frequently used for treating pruritus, but it is their sedative effect that appears to relieve symptoms, rather than any effect on histamine production. **Vitamin K** should be administered regularly throughout pregnancy in patients with intrahepatic cholestasis of pregnancy, due to the increased risk of fetal haemorrhage and postpartum haemorrhage. Specialist advice is appropriate.

3d) **What are the maternal and fetal prognoses?**

The maternal prognosis is good and symptoms resolve rapidly after delivery, accompanied by normalization of the liver function tests. There is a predisposition to post-partum haemorrhage, probably because of vitamin K deficiency related to cholestasis. Persistent cholestasis after delivery should prompt reconsideration of other underlying liver disease, such as primary biliary cirrhosis, primary sclerosing cholangitis, or chronic hepatitis C, which may all cause pruritus during late pregnancy. Intrahepatic cholestasis of pregnancy **recurs** during subsequent pregnancies in 45–70%.

There are, however, significant **risks to the fetus**. Intrahepatic cholestasis of pregnancy increases the risk of preterm delivery, meconium staining of amniotic fluid, fetal bradycardia, fetal distress, and fetal loss. Most fetal death occurs after 37 weeks of gestation, so there is general agreement that all women with intrahepatic cholestasis of pregnancy should be **delivered no later than 37–38 weeks of gestation**. Delivery prior to 36 weeks should be considered for severe cases with jaundice, progressive elevation in serum bile acids, and suspected fetal distress. In terms of the SLE, there is an increased risk of spontaneous abortion (note that this patient had three miscarriages prior to this pregnancy), intrauterine fetal death, intrauterine growth retardation, and preterm birth.

This patient was delivered at 31 weeks because of increasing pruritus and slowing fetal growth. Her itching and liver function tests improved immediately post-partum, but did not completely normalize. The azathioprine was subsequently stopped with normalization of liver blood tests. Although the patient had been on azathioprine for over 2 years, the final diagnosis was felt to be a combination of intrahepatic cholestasis of pregnancy and azathioprine-induced hepatotoxicity.

Further reading

Saleh M, Abdo K (2007). Intrahepatic cholestasis of pregnancy: review of the literature and evaluation of current evidence. *J Womens Health*; **16**: 833–41.

Pusl T, Beuers U (2007). Intrahepatic cholestasis of pregnancy. *Orphanet J Rare Dis*; **2**: 26.

Hay E (2008). Liver disease in pregnancy. *Hepatology*; **47**: 1067–76.

Gisbert JP, González-Lama Y, Maté J (2007). Thiopurine-induced liver injury in patients with inflammatory bowel disease: a systematic review. *Am J Gastroenterol*; **102**: 1518–27.

Case 4

A 60-year-old woman, originally from Belgium was first seen in 1987 with asymptomatic abnormal liver blood tests.

Investigations at the time showed:

- Hb 12g/dL, WCC 4.0 x 10^9/L, platelets 233 x 10^9/L
- Bilirubin 7μmol/L, ALP 516 IU/L, GGT 217 IU/L, AST 42 IU/L, albumin 42g/L
- Ultrasound of the abdomen: normal.

The patient had a history of treated hypothyroidism. She had been well until 2005, when she had been admitted for a single episode of haematemesis and had undergone a gastroscopy. This showed her to have small oesophageal varices, with no signs of recent or imminent haemorrhage. They were too small for therapeutic intervention. She had recently suffered a fall and had fractured her right humerus. She was now complaining of general fatigue and itching, especially at night, localized to her forearms.

Further investigations showed:

- Platelets 117 x 10^9/L
- Bilirubin 28μmol/L, ALT 139 IU/L, ALP 1173 IU/L, albumin 37g/L.

Questions

4a) What is the likely diagnosis and how was it confirmed?

4b) What is the significance of the humeral fracture?

4c) What is the significance of the portal hypertension?

4d) How would you treat the disease?

4e) How would you manage the patient's symptoms?

Answers

4a) **What is the likely diagnosis and how was it confirmed?**

The clinical picture is of **progressive cholestatic liver disease** with the development of portal hypertension, fatigue and itching. The differential diagnosis of asymptomatic cholestatic liver function tests at presentation is **intrahepatic biliary disease** such as primary biliary cirrhosis and primary sclerosing cholangitis.

Other causes of a high alkaline phosphatase (ALP) include **hepatic infiltration** (e.g. sarcoidosis, granulomatous hepatitis, hepatic metastases, amyloid, see Case 42). It is important to remember that the ALP also rises with chronic heart failure and active systemic connective tissue disease. Primary biliary cirrhosis is (by far) the most likely diagnosis, because she is female, has no history of colitis (as might occur with primary sclerosing cholangitis due to association with colitis, see Case 50), and has a history of autoimmune disease (hypothyroidism). **Antimitochondrial antibodies** (AMA) are positive in 90% of patients with primary biliary cirrhosis, being highly sensitive and specific. Whether antimitochondrial antibodies are involved in the pathogenesis of primary biliary cirrhosis, or merely an epiphenomenon, is unclear. If they are involved in the pathogenesis, it is difficult to explain why bile ducts should be targeted, since mitochondria are present in most nucleated cells. Patients with primary biliary cirrhosis may also have a raised total IgM and may have elevated total cholesterol.

The role of liver biopsy in making the diagnosis of primary biliary cirrhosis is often debated, because the biliary disease is often patchy and the degree of fibrosis can be under-staged histologically. This woman was AMA positive and had liver fibrosis stage 3/4 on biopsy of the liver.

Primary biliary cirrhosis is a chronic autoimmune disease that leads to slowly progressive destruction and loss of small intralobular bile ducts, with resulting cholestasis, liver injury, inflammation, and necrosis. This leads to fibrosis and ultimately to cirrhosis. The designation as primary biliary cirrhosis is a misnomer, since patients only have cirrhosis near the end of the disease course. A more accurate description is chronic non-suppurative destructive cholangitis, but there is little chance that this catchy designation will replace PBC! Primary biliary cirrhosis is found predominantly in females, with a **female to male ratio** of 8:1. The peak **incidence** is in the fifth decade of life and the disease is uncommon in patients younger than 25 years. The **prevalence** in women in the UK is 940 cases per million. It is thought that environmental factors, including toxins, viruses, or bacteria may precipitate an autoimmune reaction in a genetically susceptible host.

A genetic predisposition is suggested, because primary biliary cirrhosis is more common in first-degree relatives. No single infectious agent has been reproducibly detected in the livers of patients with primary biliary cirrhosis, but candidates have included *Escherichia coli*, *Chlamydia pneumoniae*, *Helicobacter pylori*, *Mycobacterium gordonae*, *Novosphingobium aromaticivorans*, and human β-retrovirus. Appendectomy and tonsillectomy seem to have been performed more commonly in patients with primary biliary cirrhosis, but how this might predispose to the disease is unclear.

Patients may present clinically with **symptoms** of fatigue and pruritus, which often dominate the course of the disease. However, more than half of newly diagnosed patients will be asymptomatic. This probably represents the investigation of incidentally detected abnormal liver function tests, or elevated serum cholesterol. Primary biliary cirrhosis may also be found on further investigation of a substantial list of other associated conditions. The strongest **disease association** is with scleroderma, but others include Sjøgren's syndrome, Raynaud's phenomenon, systemic lupus erythematosus, rheumatoid arthritis, pernicious anaemia, type I diabetes, Addison's disease, autoimmune thyroid disease, coeliac disease, and inflammatory bowel disease, to name a few.

In early primary biliary cirrhosis with or without symptoms, physical **examination** may be normal. Xanthelasma are rarely seen. Patients may have scratch-marks of pruritus. Signs and symptoms of associated diseases may be present. As the disease progresses with the development of portal hypertension, splenomegaly may develop and collateral vessels found. Jaundice is a late finding in primary biliary cirrhosis and may not occur until the last 2–3 years of life. Referral for **liver transplantation** is considered when the bilirubin rises to >100μmol/L. Variceal bleeding or increasing jaundice are often the first signs of progressive liver disease. The 10-year survival in asymptomatic patients varies from about 60% to 90%. The most common cause of death is liver failure.

4b) **What is the significance of the humerus fracture?**

Primary biliary cirrhosis is associated with **osteoporosis** and a small, but significant increase in the risk of sustaining a fracture. Cirrhosis itself is also associated with an increased risk of fracture. About 20% of patients with primary biliary cirrhosis and endstage liver disease will have osteoporosis. Management includes the modification of general risk factors for osteoporosis, including the avoidance of alcohol excess, smoking cessation and steroid therapy. Our patient had already had one fragility fracture from minimal trauma and had a bone mineral density in the osteoporotic range (T-score <−2.5). Treatment is with bisphosphonates, which are well tolerated and appear to be safe in the presence of small varices. All patients with cirrhosis or a sustained bilirubin more than 3 times the upper limit of normal had best receive calcium 1000mg and Vitamin D_3 800 IU per day, regardless of bone mineral density, because a fracture can be associated with decompensation of liver disease as a consequence of analgesics or anaesthetics.

4c) **What is the significance of the portal hypertension?**

Portal hypertension in primary biliary cirrhosis develops in the pre-cirrhotic stage because of fibrosis around the portal tracts. The presence of **oesophageal varices** implies portal hypertension with collateral circulation. Patients with primary biliary cirrhosis who have blood platelets <200 x 10^9/L, albumin <40g/L and a bilirubin of >20μmol/L should be screened for oesophageal varices. Our patient has small varices, and annual follow-up endoscopy was arranged. Once varices enlarge to 50% of the lumen, primary therapy to reduce portal hypertension with non-selective beta-blockers or prophylactic endoscopic banding appears to reduce the risk of an index variceal bleed (see Case 5).

4d) **How would you treat the disease?**

The only therapy thought to have any effect on the progression of disease is **ursodeoxycholic acid**. Ursodeoxycholic acid is a bile acid that reduces cholestasis (see Cases 3 and 50). It occurs naturally in humans as a small proportion of the bile acid pool (2%). The optimal dose is thought to be 13–15mg/kg/day, so that it becomes the dominant bile acid in the bile acid pool. It enhances endogenous secretion (choleuretic effect), is less cyto-toxic than other bile acids, and is associated with less cytokine expression as well as a reduction in aberrant HLA expression by biliary endothelium. It is clinically associated with improvement in liver enzyme tests, with an initial response evident at 6 weeks. The rapid initial response slows to a steady subsequent improvement. Within 2 years 20% will have normal liver enzymes, which increases to 35% at 5 years. Early histological stages (I and II) may have slower progression on ursodeoxycholic acid, but a significant survival benefit has not yet been shown.

The indication for treatment with ursodeoxycholic acid is a positive antimitochondrial antibody with abnormal liver enzymes. Ursodeoxycholic acid may interact with clofibrate and colestyramine, so should be taken 4 hours apart from these medications. Clinical trials of other drugs have found no benefit in primary biliary cirrhosis, including colchicine, methotrexate, penicillamine, azathioprine or cyclosporin, either alone or in combination with ursodeoxycholic acid. Despite the use of ursodeoxycholic acid, progression to liver transplantation still occurs in a minority. Primary biliary cirrhosis recurs in the graft organ in 20%, but progression is slow, seldom leading to retransplantation. Associated conditions need treatment independently of the primary biliary cirrhosis.

4e) **How would you manage the patient's symptoms?**

Pruritus and fatigue are common and often debilitating symptoms. Both are poorly understood and benefit of therapy is often difficult to measure objectively. Eighty percent of patients with primary biliary cirrhosis have pruritus at some stage.

Pruritus occurs in cholestasis of any cause and may be the first manifestation of primary biliary cirrhosis before diagnosis. It is alleviated by sunlight and ultraviolet light and may yet improve as liver disease progresses. Bile acids are thought to be directly pruritogenic although opinions differ. For this reason, the bile acid sequestrant, **colestyramine**, is used as first-line therapy. Note the potential interaction with ursodeoxycholic acid (above). It is safe at a dose of 4–12g/day, but is unpalatable, poorly tolerated due to gastrointestinal symptoms, and the evidence for efficacy in pruritus is scant. It should be taken at the time that the gallbladder empties at meal times and the dose can be divided, half before and half after breakfast. For those who cannot tolerate colestyramine, the bile acid sequestrant **colesevalam** is available in capsule form, but is still undergoing clinical trials in pruritus. In addition to the pruritogenic effect of bile acids, cholestasis is thought to be associated with an increase in endogenous opioids. **Opioid antagonists** may reduce the central neurotransmission of pruritic signals. Opioid withdrawal, acute pain, the development of a pain syndrome, and hepatotoxicity may occur with opioid antagonists. **Naltrexone** has been shown to have a clear benefit in relieving pruritus. **Rifampicin**, which appears to act by reducing transfer of bile acids across the hepatocytes, has also been shown to relieve pruritus. **Sertraline** has been tried and exposure to **ultraviolet** light may help, keeping in mind the risks of overexposure. Ultimately intractable pruritus may only be successfully treated with **liver transplantation**.

Fatigue is a troublesome symptom to treat and a well-recognized feature of cholestatic liver disease. Fatigue in primary biliary cirrhosis does not correlate with severity or duration of disease, pruritus, liver function impairment, age, thyroid status, or mental acuity, but does correlate with autonomic dysfunction, sleep disorders, and depression. Fatigue is thought to be centrally mediated. Postulated mechanisms include the reaction to the diagnosis of primary biliary cirrhosis (although fatigue often precedes the diagnosis), a cytokine effect, excessive manganese, and altered function of the hypothalamic-pituitary-adrenal axis. It is of fundamental importance to exclude other, treatable causes of fatigue that may be associated with primary biliary cirrhosis, including Addison's disease, coeliac disease, or hypothyroidism. Trials with the 5-hydroxitryptamine 3 (5 HT_3) receptor antagonist, ondansetron to alter serotonergic neurotransmission, have shown no benefit. Daytime somnolence may be helped by modafenil, a stimulant used in narcolepsy.

Further reading

Kumagi T, Heathcote EJ (2008). Primary biliary cirrhosis. *Orphanet J Rare Dis*; **3**: 1.

Mayo MJ (2008). Natural history of primary biliary cirrhosis. *Clin Liver Dis*; **12**: 277–88.

Lindor K (2007). Ursodeoxycholic acid for the treatment of primary biliary cirrhosis. *N Engl J Med*; **357**: 1524–9.

Tandon P, Rowe BH, Vandermeer B, Bain VG (2007). The efficacy and safety of bile-acid binding agents, opioid antagonists, or rifampin in the treatment of cholestasis-associated pruritis. *Am J Gastroenterol*; **102**: 1528–36.

Case 5

A 52-year-old retired army major presented with recurrent haematemesis and melaena. The patient had been previously diagnosed with liver cirrhosis, secondary to alcohol abuse. He had had two episodes of variceal haemorrhage 2 years previously, which had been controlled by oesophageal variceal banding. He continued to drink up to six standard alcoholic drinks per day. He had type 2 diabetes, for which he was taking metformin 500mg twice daily. He was also taking spironolactone 50mg/day.

On examination, he was very unwell with a pulse rate of 110bpm, blood pressure 95/55mmHg, oxygen saturation 95%, and temperature 35.8°C. There were multiple spider naevi, but no jaundice or ascites. The patient was not confused and there was no asterixis.

Investigations showed:

- Hb 11.4g/dL, WCC 7.1 x 10^9/L, platelets 83 x 10^9/L
- Prothrombin time: 15.3 sec
- Na 134mmol/L, K 4.8mmol/L, urea 11.0mmol/L, creatinine 104μmol/L
- Glucose 24.2mmol/L
- Bilirubin 35μmol/L, ALT 75 IU/L, ALP 100 IU/L, GGT 320 IU/L, albumin 32g/L
- Gastroscopy showed four oesophageal varices protruding half way across the lumen. Seven variceal bands were applied with a good result.

Questions

5a) How would you manage this patient prior to endoscopy and what initial therapy would you introduce following endoscopy?

5b) What are the predictors of failure to control variceal bleeding?

Unfortunately, the patient did re-bleed and required another endoscopy, but the endoscopist was unable to control the bleeding. By this stage the patient had had 10 units of red packed cells and remained tachycardic and hypotensive.

5c) What management should be considered at this stage?

5d) Why did the patient became confused and disorientated several days later?

5e) What is the subsequent management plan for patients in whom acute variceal bleeding is controlled endoscopically?

Answers

5a) **How would you manage this patient prior to endoscopy and what initial therapy would you introduce following endoscopy?**

The immediate management includes:

- Correct hypovolaemia
- Prophylactic antibiotics
- Vasoactive drugs
- Endoscopic therapy
- Treat and prevent encephalopathy.

Correct hypovolaemia

'Cautious and conservative' blood volume restitution is currently recommended, using packed red blood cells to maintain the haemoglobin at approximately 7–9g/dL, and intravenous colloid to maintain haemodynamic stability. Crystalloid, including saline, can be given in an emergency but continuous saline infusion should be avoided, because this will precipitate ascites and peripheral oedema. Monitoring central venous pressure helps avoid hypovolaemia, which is a common cause of renal failure in such patients. On the other hand, over transfusion should also be avoided, because volume overload increases portal pressure, which can precipitate further bleeding. Although cirrhotic patients with gastrointestinal bleeding often have a coagulopathy, there is no evidence that fresh frozen plasma or platelet administration is helpful, and there is some evidence that it is harmful due to volume expansion.

Prophylactic antibiotics

The use of prophylactic antibiotics (oral quinolone or intravenous ceftriaxone) should be standard therapy for patients with cirrhosis who have variceal bleeding. and should be instituted from admission and continued for approximately 5 days. An association with bacterial infection and variceal bleeding has been shown in randomized trials. Antibiotics decrease the rate of bacterial infections including spontaneous bacterial peritonitis, decrease the incidence of early re-bleeding, and significantly improve survival.

Vasoactive drugs

In suspected variceal bleeding, vasoactive drugs (such as **terlipressin**) should be started as soon as possible, before diagnostic endoscopy.

Vasopressin and its analogues, such as terlipressin, cause **splanchnic vasoconstriction**, leading to a reduction in portal pressure. Randomized controlled trials have shown that early administration of vasoactive drugs reduces the rate of active bleeding, facilitates diagnostic and therapeutic endoscopy, improves the control of bleeding and may decrease bleeding-related mortality. Vasoactive drug therapy should be administered for about 5 days, because this is the period in which early re-bleeding is most frequent.

Several drugs are available to treat acute variceal haemorrhage; the choice depends on local availability, bearing in mind that the only drug shown to improve survival is terlipressin. Somatostatin and octreotide have a similar effect on bleeding, but have not been shown to improve survival. Randomized controlled trials have shown that the efficacy of vasoactive therapy is significantly improved when **combined with endoscopic therapy**. If vasoactive drugs are started as soon as possible *before* endoscopy, the incidence of active variceal bleeding during the endoscopy decreases from 50% (when drugs are not used), to 20–25%. Terlipressin and octreotride have fewer systemic side effects, such as angina or gut ischaemia, than vasopressin, but should still be used with caution in people with a history of coronary artery disease.

Endoscopic therapy

Endoscopy should be performed as soon as possible after resuscitation, especially in patients with active bleeding and features suggesting cirrhosis. The aim is to stop bleeding by **banding** (ligation) or sclerotherapy, and subsequently to obliterate the **oesophageal varices**. Variceal wall tension is the key factor that determines variceal rupture. Endoscopic therapy reduces variceal wall tension by reducing variceal size until obliteration, and by increasing the thickness of the vascular wall. Variceal banding has proved more effective and safer than **sclerotherapy** (with ethanolamine) and is currently the endoscopic treatment of choice for oesophageal varices. Nevertheless, the choice is also influenced by the availability of equipment and expertise. Variceal obturation with tissue adhesives such as cyanoacrylate or with thrombin are generally limited to the treatment of **gastric varices**.

The current recommended therapy for variceal bleeding (combining vasoactive drugs, emergency endoscopic variceal banding and antibiotic prophylaxis), has reduced 5-day re-bleeding rates from 30% to 10–15%. Endotracheal intubation may be required for airway protection during endoscopy, particularly in patients with encephalopathy.

Treat and prevent encephalopathy

Hepatic encephalopathy can be precipitated by bleeding in patients with cirrhosis. Patients who present or develop encephalopathy should be treated with lactulose. Although there are no studies to evaluate the value of lactulose for preventing hepatic encephalopathy, either lactulose or phosphate enemas are usually given to prevent encephalopathy following a variceal bleed.

Following endoscopy a proton pump inhibitor should be given, because acid suppression has been shown to reduce the risk of bleeding from oesophageal ulcers following variceal banding. Proton pump inhibitors should be continued until varices have been eradicated. A non-selective beta-blocker should also be started (below).

5b) **What are the predictors of failure to control variceal bleeding?**

Clinical factors associated with failure to control bleeding and mortality are:

- Active bleeding at endoscopy
- Shock at admission
- Early re-bleeding (<5 days)
- Severity of liver disease (Child–Pugh grade: mortality in patients with Class C = 70–80%)
- Raised bilirubin
- Prothrombin time (reflecting severity of liver disease)
- Thrombocytopenia (indirect measure of portal hypertension)
- Encephalopathy
- Recent use of corticosteroids for alcoholic hepatitis within 7 days of bleeding
- Age >60 years
- Complicating hepatocellular carcinoma.

Portal hypertension increases with increasing severity of cirrhosis. The best predictor of re-bleeding is, however, an increased hepatic venous pressure gradient. The hepatic venous pressure gradient is a measure of the severity of portal hypertension. A hepatic venous pressure gradient >20mmHg has been shown to be independently associated with mortality and early re-bleeding. Measurement of hepatic venous pressure gradient is performed by transjugular venous cannulation, and requires access to skilled interventional radiology. Although accurate and reproducible, with a low coefficient of variation in measurement and few complications, it is rarely used outside the research setting except in one or two centres.

Unfortunately, the patient did re-bleed and required another endoscopy, but the endoscopist was unable to control the bleeding. By this stage the patient had had 10 units of packed red cells and remained tachycardic and hypotensive.

5c) **What management should be considered at this stage?**

This patient has uncontrolled variceal bleeding despite medical and endoscopic therapy. Such patients are best managed with a transjugular intrahepatic portal systemic shunt (TIPSS) (Figs 5.1a and 5.1b). TIPSS is an interventional treatment to decompress the portal system by creation of an intrahepatic shunt between the portal and hepatic veins. TIPSS is only indicated for 'salvage therapy' when first-line methods (medical and endoscopic) have failed. Studies report immediate control of bleeding in 91–100% of cases, 30-day re-bleeding in 7–30% and a 1-month mortality of 28–55%, reflecting the severity of the underlying liver disease .

If access to TIPSS is not immediately available, mechanical balloon tamponade is accepted as a temporary measure until definitive therapy can be instituted. Most commonly used is the three-lumen, double balloon Sengstaken-Blakemore tube. Only the gastric balloon need be used (filled with about 250ml of water mixed with 50ml radiological contrast) in most cases. Insertion is best achieved using a well lubricated stiffening guidewire, and should be carried out by an experienced physician, because of the risk of oesophageal perforation. The oesophageal balloon is rarely necessary and should not be insufflated for more than 8 hours.

Surgical shunting, (portocaval or splenorenal) does not appear to improve survival, and is associated with a substantial incidence of encephalopathy. Surgery should only ever be considered in patients with non-severe (Child–Pugh A) liver disease. Liver transplantation is not indicated for an acute bleeding episode, but all such people should be considered as transplant candidates, if only to exclude this as an option if (for instance) the person continues to drink or has substantial comorbidity.

5d) **Why did the patient became confused and disorientated several days later?**

The most likely explanation for the confusion in this patient is post-TIPSS hepatic encephalopathy. Hepatic encephalopathy is the main complication that has limited the application of TIPSS. Clinically evident hepatic encephalopathy develops in approximately 35% of patients after TIPSS, most often within the first 7 days. It is often short lived when managed

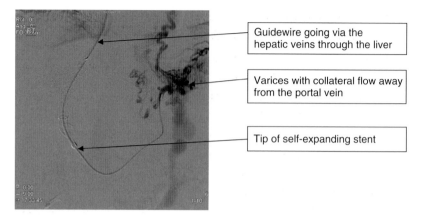

Guidewire going via the hepatic veins through the liver

Varices with collateral flow away from the portal vein

Tip of self-expanding stent

Fig. 5.1a This picture shows the wire through the hepatic vein into the portal vein, with metal TIPSS stent visible. There are varices visible on the right.

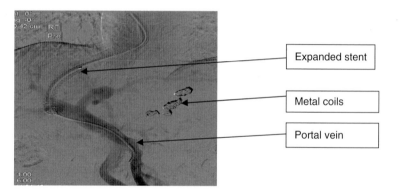

Expanded stent

Metal coils

Portal vein

Fig. 5.1b This picture shows the metal TIPSS stent, which is just proximal to the opacified portal vein. The varices seen on the right have been coiled.

with regular lactulose, but in severe cases the shunt has to be reduced in diameter or occluded, with all the implications for increasing the hepatic venous pressure gradient and re-bleeding. Our patient responded well to treatment with lactulose. Interestingly, the development of post-TIPSS encephalopathy is not associated with a poor prognosis, and minor degrees of hepatic encephalopathy are no more prevalent after TIPSS than expected in a general cirrhotic population.

5e) **What is the subsequent management plan for those patients in whom acute variceal bleeding is controlled endoscopically?**

The current regimen to prevent re-bleeding in those patients who have controlled acute oesophageal variceal bleeding is:

- Endoscopic **eradication of varices** (repeat banding every 1–2 weeks until varices eradicated)

- Combined with oral, **non-selective beta-blockers**

The combination is more effective than beta-blockers alone in preventing late re-bleeding. Haemodynamic responders (i.e. those with a decrease in hepatic venous pressure gradient to <12mmHg, or by >20% of baseline) have a marked reduction in the risk of haemorrhage, but this is not measured routinely, and there is unfortunately no surrogate marker at present.

Further reading

Bendtsen F, Krag A, Møller S (2008). Treatment of acute variceal bleeding. *Dig Liver Dis*; **40**: 328–36.

Dell' A, deFranchis R, Iannuzzi F (2008). Acute variceal bleeding: pharmacological treatment and primary/secondary prophylaxis. *Best Pract Res Clin Gastroenterol*; **22**: 279–94.

Triantos CK, Burroughs AK (2008). Predicting failure to control bleeding in acute variceal bleeding. *J Hepatology*; **48**: 185–88.

Villanueva C, Colomo A, Aracil C, Guarner (2008). Current endoscopic therapy of variceal bleeding. *Best Pract Res Clin Gastroenterol*; **22**: 261–78.

Case 6

A 70-year-old Irish man presented to his doctor with a skin rash on his right lower leg. Routine blood tests were performed and mildly disordered liver function tests were found, with a markedly raised serum ferritin. He was referred to the hepatology clinic for assessment. There was no history of liver disease and he was not taking any medication. He had stopped smoking 30 years earlier and drank heavily until 10 years before, but now only drank two units of alcohol per day. He had no other risk factors for chronic liver disease and had undergone a hip replacement for arthritis 7 years previously.

Examination revealed a pulse rate of 80 beats/minute and blood pressure 115/65mmHg. His skin appeared pigmented. Examination of cardiac and respiratory systems was normal. He had no clinical evidence of chronic liver disease or portal hypertension, although the liver was palpable 4cm below the costal margin.

Investigations showed:

- Hb 13.5g/dL, WCC 5.6 x 10^9/L, platelets 155 x 10^9/L
- Bilirubin 15μmol/L, ALT 56 IU/L, ALP 536 IU/L, albumin 41g/L
- Fasting glucose 8.2mmol/L
- Ferritin 4838μg/L
- Prothrombin time 12.4 sec
- Autoimmune and viral markers were negative
- Ultrasound of the abdomen: normal liver echogenicity and no lesions, no ascites, normal spleen.

Questions

6a) Discuss the most likely diagnosis and how you would confirm it.

6b) What are the disease manifestations?

6c) Discuss the types of genetic iron overload.

6d) Discuss the pathophysiology of haemochromatosis.

6e) Discuss the management and aspects of screening for this disease.

Answers

6a) **Discuss the most likely diagnosis and how you would confirm it.**

The most likely diagnosis is **hereditary haemochromatosis**. The combination of hepatomegaly, skin pigmentation, arthritis, abnormal liver function tests, and a markedly raised serum ferritin is highly suggestive of hereditary haemochromatosis. The arthritis in this case, however, is of the hip joint, which is atypical and may simply represent degenerative joint disease in a 70-year-old man, unrelated to iron overload. The raised ferritin is a measure of body iron stores and is consistent with (but not diagnostic of) iron overload. Other causes of a raised ferritin include inflammatory conditions, obesity, and excess alcohol intake, although it would be exceptional for any of these to cause a ferritin >1500μg/L.

Confirmation of the diagnosis involves a **liver biopsy** when the ferritin is >1000μg/L. Staining with Prussian blue (Perl's) confirms iron overload in the hepatocytes and is used for staging of the degree of fibrosis, since cirrhosis may be present in asymptomatic individuals. Cirrhosis can be predicted, however, in 80% of people homozygous for C282Y with a ferritin >1000μg/L, AST >40 and a platelet count of <200 x 10^9/L, without liver biopsy. **Genotyping** for the common HFE gene mutations (C282Y and H63D, below) is suggestive, but not necessarily diagnostic. Liver fibrosis is unusual in patients who are homozygous for the C282Y mutation with a ferritin <1000μg/L, so a liver biopsy is not indicated unless there is diagnostic doubt.

Our patient was found to be homozygous for C282Y, and a liver biopsy was performed. The biopsy showed a severely fibrotic liver, bordering on cirrhosis with grade 4 haemosiderosis (Fig. 6.1 in central coloured section). This was compatible with the diagnosis of haemochromatosis. Liver synthetic function was still normal, and on ultrasound of the abdomen there was no evidence of focal liver lesions (hepatocellular carcinoma) or portal hypertension (normal spleen and portal vein).

6b) **What are the disease manifestations?**

Manifestations include liver disease, arthropathy, hyperpigmentation, diabetes, cardiac disease and hypogonadism. Pituitary failure is a feature of the rare juvenile form of haemochromatosis. **Liver disease** is the most prominent manifestation, being found in 95% of patients who have clinical disease. It ranges from abnormal liver function tests to hepatomegaly, liver fibrosis, and overt cirrhosis. Patients with cirrhosis are at increased risk of developing hepatocellular carcinoma. The **arthropathy** of haemochromatosis typically affects the **second and third metacarpophalangeal** joints.

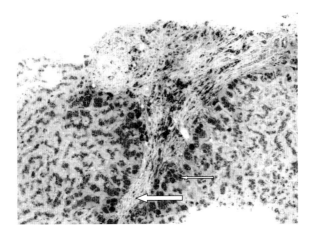

Fig. 6.1 (see colour plate 3) Photomicrograph of a liver biopsy stained with Prussian blue (Perl's stain) showing features of parenchymal iron deposition (small arrow) and advanced fibrosis (large arrow).

Diabetes is typically associated with haemochromatosis, along with **skin pigmentation** ('bronze diabetes'). Diabetes may be due to hypoinsulinaemia, but insulin resistance is also a feature. Interestingly, the prevalence of diabetes in patients with haemochromatosis is no different from the general population. A useful clinical tip is to consider haemochromatosis should a patient have liver disease and disease in one other organ (diabetes, cardiac failure etc). **Cardiac involvement** is much less common and usually manifests as congestive cardiac failure, although arrhythmias may occur. Like pituitary failure, it is more common in the juvenile forms of the disease.

6c) **Discuss the types of genetic iron overload.**

Genetic forms of iron overload may be divided into **haemochromatosis** and **other forms**. Haemochromatosis refers to a particular phenotype of hereditary iron overload, characterized by normal erythropoiesis, increased transferrin saturation, and parenchymal iron deposition because of reduced activity of **hepcidin**. Haemochromatosis consists of five different genetic disorders, of which by far the most common form (90%) is type 1 haemochromatosis or 'HFE' haemochromatosis. The genetic defect in the HFE gene is a mutation on chromosome 6p21.3, resulting in substitution of tyrosine for cysteine at position 282 (C282Y). The condition is **autosomal recessive** and homozygotes with the C282Y mutation are at risk of developing iron overload. In the European population homozygocity is found in around 1:250 people, but only a tiny proportion of homozygotes (perhaps 1%) develop clinical haemochromatosis, for reasons unknown.

A second mutation (H63D) has also been identified, but homozygocity for this mutation or compound heterozygosity with C282Y, rarely leads to iron overload. It was initially thought that C282Y homozygotes would invariably lead to progressive iron overload and resulting disease manifestations. High penetrance was assumed based on studies performed in patients with symptomatic disease.

It is now known that **penetrance** is variable and that environmental or genetic factors influence the development of manifestations. The incomplete penetrance of haemochromatosis in patients who are homozygous for C282Y is illustrated by a 50–75% prevalence of biochemical expression (increased ferritin and transferrin saturation), a 25% prevalence of non-specific asthenia or arthropathy, and <10% prevalence of severe organ damage with cirrhosis, hepatocellular carcinoma, diabetes, or cardiomyopathy. From another perspective, approximately 20% of men and 40% of women who are homozygous for C282Y have a normal serum ferritin. One clear influence on clinical expression of the disease is that of female gender. Lower disease penetrance in woman may be due to physiological blood loss, but this may not be the only factor. Coinheritance of other gene mutations (for hepcidin or haemojuvelin for example, see below) are associated with earlier clinical disease and a greater iron burden.

An important **environmental factor** influencing clinical expression of haemochromatosis is alcohol consumption, since alcohol increases the iron burden and has independent toxic effects on end-organs affected by haemochromatosis.

Other mutations associated with clinical expression of iron overload are much less common. **Type 2 haemochromatosis** (juvenile haemochromatosis) is caused by mutations in the gene for haemojuvelin or hepcidin. It is autosomal recessive and results in early onset severe disease presenting with cardiac or endocrine manifestations (hypopituitarism). A mutation in the transferrin receptor 2 (TFR2) gene causes **type 3 haemochromatosis**, which is similar to HFE haemochromatosis and autosomal recessive. The only dominant mutation (SLC40A1) causing typical haemochromatosis is **ferroportin** disease type B and is rare.

Other genetic causes of iron overload include ferroportin disease type A, which is autosomal dominant and causes mesenchymal iron overload. It is rare. Two recessive conditions are hereditary acaeruloplasminaemia, which causes neurological, haematological, or endocrine disease, and hereditary hypotransferrinaemia, which causes microcytic anaemia with parenchymal iron overload. Both are the stuff of case reports, because of insights they give into physiological iron transport.

6d) **Discuss the pathophysiology of haemochromatosis.**

Iron balance is regulated solely by variation in intestinal absorption. **Hepcidin** is the central player, promoting iron export from enterocytes, macrophages, or placental cells. Hepcidin deficiency is to haemochromatosis what insulin is to diabetes. It works by modulating the delivery of iron to the plasma and consequently controls intestinal iron absorption. Hepcidin is a 25 amino acid polypeptide hormone that induces the degradation of the cellular iron exporter, ferroportin. Hepcidin concentrations are influenced by serum iron concentrations, hypoxia, anaemia, and inflammation, but the precise interaction of HFE gene expression with hepcidin remains unclear.

6e) **Discuss the management and aspects of screening for this disease.**

The mainstay of therapy is the depletion of iron stores by **phlebotomy**. Phlebotomy, with the removal of 500mL of whole blood each week until the serum ferritin is <50μg/L, is standard practice. The aim is to deplete iron stores to an extent that iron leaches from the tissues. This is subject to tolerance and patients who become anaemic naturally have a less intense regimen of bloodletting. Once the **target ferritin** has been reached, the frequency of maintenance phlebotomy is judged by ferritin measurements every 4–6 months. The rate of **reaccumulation** of iron is highly variable, since maintenance phlebotomy increases the rate of intestinal iron absorption. Effective phlebotomy has been shown to reverse fibrosis in the liver and reduce the risk of hepatocellular carcinoma in the presence of cirrhosis by reversing parenchymal iron deposition.

Hepatocellular carcinoma remains a leading cause of death and is more common than liver failure in patients with haemochromatosis and cirrhosis (see Case 14). Screening cirrhotic patients for a carcinoma every 6 months, with ultrasound of the liver and α-fetoprotein determination, is recommended. Orthotopic liver transplantation is uncommonly carried out for uncontrolled haemochromatosis, since the mortality from sepsis or cardiac decompensation is high.

Population screening for a condition that is common, may have serious and preventable consequences, is easily treatable, and readily diagnosed by a blood test, may seem appropriate. However, biochemical measures of iron overload (such as serum transferrin saturation) have a low positive predictive value for C282Y homozygocity. Since the genetic defect also has variable penetrance, this decreases the population benefit of screening, so it is not currently indicated.

Further reading

Adams PC, Barton JC (2007). Haemochromatosis. *Lancet*; **370**: 1855–60.

Deugnier Y, Brissot P, Loreal O (2008). Iron and the liver. *J Hepatol*; **48** (Suppl.): S113–S123.

Bacon BR, Britton RS (2008). Clinical penetrance of hereditary hemochromatosis. (Editorial). *N Engl J Med*; **358**: 291–2.

Case 7

A 40-year-old HIV-positive male theatre critic presented to the outpatient department with a 10-week history of watery diarrhoea associated with a 7kg loss of weight. He had been diagnosed with HIV 2 years earlier after he developed two AIDS-defining illnesses (*Pneumocystis jiroveci* pneumonia and cytomegalovirus retinitis). His current medications were zidovudine, lamivudine, and saquinavir. There had been no changes to the prescribed regimen for over 6 months.

On examination he was cachetic, afebrile, had a pulse rate of 96 beats per minute and blood pressure 125/78mmHg. There was no abdominal tenderness or distension.

Investigations showed:

- Hb 11.2g/dL, WCC 3.4 x 10^9/L, platelets 215 x10^9/L
- Na 130mmol/L, K 3.1mmol/L, creatinine 85μmol/L
- CRP 25mg/L
- CD4 lymphocyte count 100 cells/μL.

Questions

7a) What is the differential diagnosis?

7b) What should be the sequence of evaluation?

7c) What is the role of endoscopy?

7d) What does 'HIV enteropathy' mean?

Answers

7a) **What is the differential diagnosis?**

The differential diagnosis includes:

- Infection: protozoal, bacterial, mycobacterial, viral, and fungal
- Drug-induced diarrhoea: protease inhibitors, other medications
- Gut neoplasms: lymphoma, Kaposi's sarcoma
- Idiopathic: HIV enteropathy
- Pancreatic insufficiency
- Unrelated to HIV (microscopic colitis, coincidental coeliac disease).

The CD4+ count of 100 cells/mm³ means that infection is highly likely. Poor compliance with medication is probable. The most common cause of **infectious diarrhoea** in the HIV population is **protozoal** infection (*Ciclospora* spp., *Isospora belli*, *Microsporidium* sp. or *Cryptosporidium* sp.). Diarrhoea is generally self limited if the CD4+ count is normal. A CD4+ count <100 cells/mm³ means that severe disease is likely. **Bacterial** diarrhoea also occurs more frequently in patients with low CD4 counts, with more virulence. *Shigella* sp. and *Campylobacter* sp. generally present with severe abdominal pain and bloody diarrhoea. *Clostridium difficile* diarrhoea is common, because antibiotic use is commonplace and hospitalization is frequent.

Intestinal tuberculosis caused by *Mycobacterium avium* complex (MAC) or drug-resistant *Mycobacterium tuberculosis* needs to be considered, especially if the CD4+ count is <50 cells/mm³. **Viral** colitis may also cause diarrhoea in HIV-positive patients. Cytomegalovirus (CMV) is the most common cause of diarrhoea in patients with multiple negative stool tests, especially if the CD4+ count is <100 cells/mm³. Other viruses (herpes simplex, adenovirus, norovirus, or rotavirus) are occasional causes. HIV itself has also been implicated (see below). **Fungal** infections of the gut include *Histoplasma capsulatum*, coccidioidomycosis, and cryptococcosis, but generally occur in the context of systemic infection.

Diarrhoea in the era of highly active antiretroviral therapy (HAART) is very often drug induced (**antiretroviral therapy**), but in this case is unlikely in view of the very low CD4+ count, profound weight loss, and stable medication. Diarrhoea due to HAART is generally not associated with weight loss and the mechanism is not understood. The incidence of diarrhoea associated with protease inhibitors (most commonly with saquinavir and nelfinavir when therapy is initiated) ranges between 5% and 50%, and usually resolves even if the medication is continued. The temporal relationship of the diarrhoea to any medication change is relevant.

Intestinal lymphoma associated with HIV is usually rapidly progressive and associated with 'B' symptoms. Kaposi's sarcoma is possible, but tends to cause bleeding. Irritable bowel syndrome can be excluded given the marked weight loss, but **microscopic colitis** or **coeliac disease** is possible.

7b) **What should be the sequence of evaluation?**

Evaluation of this patient should include:

- **History**: drug history, symptoms such as weight loss, nocturnal or bloody diarrhoea, abdominal pain, and symptoms of systemic infection. Chronic diarrhoea with profound weight loss is strongly suggestive of an underlying opportunistic infection.

- **Examination**: fever, cachexia, abdominal tenderness or mass, and signs of opportunistic infection (oral candidiasis) or malabsorption (glossitis).

- **Stool tests**: three stool samples will identify about 80% of identifiable bacterial pathogens and should be sent for:
  - microscopy, culture, and sensitivity
  - ova, cysts, and parasites
  - *Clostridium difficile* toxin assay

- If the CD4+ count is <200 cells/µL, specific stool tests for cryptosporidia and microsporidia should be carried out.

- If the CD4+ count is <100 cells/µL, mycobacterial culture of stool and colonic mucosal biopsy should be carried out.

7c) **What is the role of endoscopy?**

Upper gastrointestinal endoscopy and colonoscopy increase the diagnostic yield if the stool tests are negative. The endoscopist should be alerted to the need for biopsies for microscopy and culture. If the CD4+ count is <100/mm³, the patient is at risk of CMV, for which mucosal biopsy is needed for diagnosis. Although there is some controversy about whether to do a sigmoidoscopy (involving a simple phosphate enema preparation, usually available the same day, without sedation) or a full colonoscopy (needing full bowel preparation and less readily available), the most appropriate test is usually indicated by the clinical features. If the patient is unwell with metabolic disturbance (as in this case), colonoscopy is best avoided unless the diagnosis is not detected by flexible sigmoidoscopy.

Some studies report that CMV is missed in 40% of cases if right-sided colonic biopsies are not taken, but this seems an over estimate.

Upper gastrointestinal endoscopy with duodenal biopsy for microscopy and, very importantly, for culture is required to diagnose MAC (consider if CD4+ <100/mm^3), *Microsporidium* spp., or *Cryptosporidium* sp. infection. Endoscopic procedures are less helpful if there is no weight loss.

7d) **What does 'HIV enteropathy' mean?**

The role of HIV as a diarrhoeal pathogen remains controversial. HIV enteropathy is a term used to account for diarrhoea in AIDS patients who lack an identifiable cause. Although the precise features are not agreed, the term implies a chronic diarrhoeal illness in patients with AIDS where no cause can be found despite extensive evaluation. With improvement in diagnostic techniques, greater awareness of the spectrum of diarrhoeal pathogens, and endoscopy with small intestinal biopsies in patients with negative stool tests, a diminishing proportion have 'idiopathic diarrhoea'.

In this case, the patient had cryptosporidiosis, diagnosed by an acid-fast stain of the stool, (organisms appear as bright red spherules). He was encouraged to comply with HAART, which cleared the infection. This is the most effective therapy for treatment of cryptosporidiosis.

Further reading

Abubakar I, Aliyu SH, Arumugam C, Hunter PR, Usman NK (2007). Prevention and treatment of cryptosporidiosis in immunocompromised patients. *Cochrane Database Syst Rev*; **1**: CD004932.

Cello JP, Day LW (2009). Idiopathic AIDS enteropathy and treatment of gastrointestinal opportunistic pathogens. *Gastroenterology*; **136**: 1952–65.

Nemechek PM, Polsky B, Gottlieb MS (2000). Treatment guidelines for HIV-associated wasting. *Mayo Clin Proc*; **75**: 386–94.

Wilcox CM, Saag MS (2008). Gastrointestinal complications of HIV infection: changing priorities in the HAART era. *Gut*; **57**: 861–70.

Case 8

A 39-year-old restaurant owner was seen in the hepatology clinic with abdominal distension. Wilson's disease had been diagnosed 25 years before. One of his siblings also had Wilson's disease. He had been prescribed penicillamine, but had taken it erratically over the years: generally for just 3 weeks before each clinic appointment.

His weight had increased by 6kg and he had ankle oedema in addition to abdominal distension, which had improved on spironolactone 100mg/day. He had restarted penicillamine 1g/day. He had travelled to Africa 5 months before. He drank eight units of alcohol per week. He had never had a blood transfusion and had no tattoos.

On examination his pulse was 72bpm and blood pressure 140/80mmHg. He was apyrexial, with normal cardiorespiratory examination. He had spider naevi, but was not jaundiced. He had 4cm hepatomegaly, shifting dullness and a brownish discoloration around the periphery of the iris, in keeping with Kayser–Fleischer rings. Neurological examination was normal.

Investigations in clinic showed:

- Hb 13.3g/dL, WCC 5.8 x10^9/L, platelets 96 x10^9/L
- Prothrombin time 20.5 sec, INR 1.5
- Na 137mmol/L, K 3.8mmol/L, creatinine 83 μmol/L
- Bilirubin 46μmol/L, ALT 126 IU/L, ALP 275 IU/L, albumin 28g/L
- IgG 21.9g/L
- Caeruloplasmin <9.7mg/dL
- Copper 11.4 μmol/L.

He was strongly advised to take regular penicillamine, and was then seen again 5 weeks later in clinic. He was now jaundiced and had tense ascites. There was no evidence of encephalopathy. He was admitted to hospital from clinic and on admission he had a temperature of 38°C.

Investigations on admission showed:

- Hb 12.5g/dL, WCC 16.6 x10^9/L, platelets 76 x10^9/L
- Prothrombin time 28.1 sec
- Na 126mmol/L, K 3.6mmol/L, creatinine 80μmol/L
- Bilirubin 125μmol/L, ALT 114 IU/L, ALP 318 IU/L, albumin 22g/L

- Ascitic fluid: macroscopically clear, yellow fluid, protein <10g/L, albumin<5g/L
- WCC 460/mm^3, polymorphonuclear leucocytes 254/mm^3, Gram stain negative, culture negative.

Questions

8a) Define the clinical problem at presentation to the clinic. How would you assess the severity and what would be your initial management?

8b) What precipitated the deterioration that lead to the hospital admission?

8c) What treatment would you give?

8d) Describe whether and how you would perform a therapeutic paracentesis?

8e) How should this patient be managed in the future?

Answers

8a) **Describe the clinical problem at presentation to the clinic. How would you assess the severity and what would be your initial management?**

This patient presents with decompensated chronic liver disease. There is likely to be cirrhosis, owing to stigmata of chronic liver disease, a low platelet count, and a long history of inadequately treated Wilson`s disease. Ascites indicates portal hypertension complicating chronic liver disease, but does not always indicate cirrhosis. The absence of a clear precipitant (e.g. gastrointestinal bleed, infection, or acute toxic liver insult), suggests that the decompensation results from progression of the underlying liver disease alone.

Assessment of severity

The degree of liver dysfunction in cirrhosis is graded using the **Child–Pugh classification**. This classification scores the serum levels of bilirubin, albumin, and prothrombin time, and the presence/severity of ascites and encephalopathy. The total score ranges from 5 to 15 and places a patient in one of three groups that reflect increasing severity of disease (Table 8.1).

The groups (and corresponding scores) are: **Child–Pugh A (5–6), B (7–9) and C (10–15)**. There are several limitations to the score. The five variables were selected empirically and not based on statistical regression; cut-off values are arbitrary; and each variable is given the same weight. Renal function, which is an important prognostic variable, is not taken into account. However, it is user friendly and has stood the test of time, because it relates to outcome. Survival at 5 years and 10 years in cirrhotic patients are 95% and 90%, respectively in Child A, 75% and 60% in Child B, and 55% and 30% in Child C.

Another score, the **Model for Endstage Liver Disease (MELD)**, was initially devised to predict prognosis in patients being considered for

Table 8.1 Child–Pugh Score

Measure	1 point	2 points	3 points	units
Bilirubin	<34 (<2)	34–50(2–3)	>50 (>3)	μmol/L (mg/dL)
Albumin	>35	28–35	<28	g/L
INR	<1.7	1.71–2.20	>2.20	N/A
Ascites	None	Diuretic responsive	Refractory	N/A
Encephalopathy	None	Gr I-II	Gr III-IV	N/A

transjugular intrahepatic portal systemic shunts (TIPSS). It is derived from statistical regression analysis, with each variable given the appropriate weight, and it includes renal function. It requires a calculator, is not user friendly at the bedside, but is used in the USA for patients being considered for transplantation.

Model for Endstage Liver Disease:

$9.6 \log_e$(creatinine in mg/dL) $+ 3.8 \log_e$ (bilirubin in mg/dL) $+ 11.2 \log_e$ (INR) $+ 6.4$

Calculator: www.unos.org/resources/meldpeldcalculator.asp

Interpretation of score (predicted 3-month mortality):

- 40 or more: 100% mortality
- 30–39: 83% mortality
- 20–29: 76% mortality
- 10–19: 27% mortality
- <10: 4% mortality.

This patient was Child–Pugh B (score 9) at presentation, with a MELD score of 15.

Management

Management at this stage would be aimed at **control of fluid retention**, which is the main reason that the patient was referred. His ascites had already improved on spironolactone, which had been prescribed by the family practitioner. Therapeutic drainage of the ascites was not indicated at this stage. **Spironolactone** has a long half-life and should be given at a once daily dose of 100–400mg/day. It is an aldosterone antagonist, which promotes renal sodium loss and conserves potassium. Dose adjustments should consider the serum potassium, because hyperkalaemia is a major adverse effect. It is antiandrogenic and may lead to gynaecomastia. Fluid restriction is not required at this stage, but salt (NaCl) restriction is advisable. Sodium intake should be restricted to 90mmol/day (5.2g of salt/day), which can be achieved by a '**no-added-salt**' dictum and avoiding pre-prepared or canned food.

The patient does not yet have neurological signs of Wilson`s disease, so penicillamine should initially be continued at a dose of 500mg twice a day, in the hope that liver function will improve. Adherence to therapy is a complex topic and should be addressed empathetically, with appropriate support to ensure that medication is taken.

Complete abstinence from alcohol is also advisable, even though his previous intake was low. Percutaneous liver biopsy is too risky at this stage, in view of the pressure of ascites and the prothrombin time which is already prolonged and would not alter management. It is important, nevertheless, to exclude concomitant liver disease, and a full liver screen should be performed (see Case 1), to exclude viral hepatitis in view of the travel history. An ultrasound scan of the abdomen should be requested to document liver size, exclude hepatocellular carcinoma (which is rare in Wilson's disease) or portal vein thrombosis, and to document spleen size. An endoscopy would be appropriate to look for varices.

8b) **What precipitated the deterioration that led to the hospital admission?**

The acute deterioration resulted from **spontaneous bacterial peritonitis**. Five weeks after his initial clinic appointment the patient presented with marked deterioration of his condition, with tense ascites, rising bilirubin, further prolongation of prothrombin time and a decline in serum albumin. He had a systemic inflammatory response (tachycardia, fever, and elevated WCC), but no encephalopathy or evidence of gastrointestinal haemorrhage. Bacterial infection is by far the most likely cause. The following should be carried out:

- blood cultures
- diagnostic paracentesis, with ascitic fluid analysis for albumin, cell count, and culture.

Spontaneous bacterial peritonitis is diagnosed when the ascitic fluid polymorphonuclear leucocyte count exceeds $250/mm^3$ of fluid. In this patient the cell count was marginal ($254/mm^3$ of fluid), but diagnostic in the circumstances. The Gram stain was negative, which is typical in spontaneous bacterial peritonitis, because there is a low bacterial load. Fluid culture was also negative, which is also typical, because it depends on the method used. Cultures are positive in 40% (fluid sent in a sterile container for inoculation onto culture medium) to 80% (inoculation into blood culture medium at the bedside). An obsolete term 'culture-negative neutrocytic ascites' is now thought to represent the 20–60% of patients who have spontaneous bacterial peritonitis and a false-negative ascitic fluid culture. The very low ascitic fluid albumin concentration, resulting in a high **serum-ascites albumin gradient** (>11g/L), indicates portal hypertension as the cause of the ascites. Low protein concentration in the ascitic fluid is a risk factor for spontaneous bacterial peritonitis. Secondary bacterial peritonitis should be suspected if a polymicrobial infection is detected on culture.

8c) **What treatment would you give?**

Intravenous **third generation cephalosporin antibiotics or oral quinolones** are the mainstay of therapy. The most common bacterial isolates are *Escherichia coli*, *Klebsiella* sp., enterococci, and streptococci. Antibiotics given for 5 days seem to be as effective as 10 days, so the shorter course should be given. Oral fluoroquinolones are an alternative to intravenous cefotaxime in patients who are not encephalopathic or vomiting. Aminoglycoside antibiotics are best avoided in patients with decompensated liver disease, because of an unpredictable volume of distribution (ascites) and the risk of precipitating renal failure. Antibiotic therapy should be started as soon as the ascitic polymorphonuclear leucocyte count confirms the diagnosis, so an urgent request for analysis is appropriate.

Patients with spontaneous bacterial peritonitis are at risk of hepatorenal syndrome (see Case 11), due to bacterial translocation triggering inflammatory pathways in patients with intravascular hypovolaemia. To reduce the risk, volume expansion with albumin is appropriate. A 19% absolute risk reduction in mortality (from 29% to 10%) has been reported when albumin is given. When albumin infusion is compared with another colloid, albumin appears to be superior in maintaining circulatory function, although studies have been underpowered to show a reduction in renal failure or mortality. Albumin should be given at a dose of 1.5g/kg on day 1, followed by 1g/kg on day 3 to patients with an increased or rising serum creatinine.

8d) **Describe whether and how you would perform a therapeutic paracentesis**

In view of the tense ascites, 'total' paracentesis (until no further fluid can be drained) is best performed. This removes a large volume of ascitic fluid (>5L), which can potentially cause circulatory dysfunction, renal impairment, and hyponatraemia. Ascites can, however, be removed rapidly as long as it is combined with the administration of 6–8g albumin for every litre of fluid removed. The drainage catheter should be removed as soon as possible, ideally within 6 hours, in order to minimize secondary infection.

8e) **How should this patient be managed in the future?**

Management of ascites and hyponatraemia

Management includes fluid restriction to less than 1.5L/day and 'no-added salt' dictum. Spironolactone is continued unless hyponatraemia gets worse or the urea rises, in which case it should be reduced or stopped. A loop diuretic (e.g. frusemide (at a starting dose of 20mg/day)) may be added once spironolactone has been given at a maximum dose (400mg/day) for 5 days, if ascites reaccumulates, but particular caution is necessary to avoid exacerbating hyponatraemia and renal impairment. Further paracentesis may be needed.

Prevention of further spontaneous bacterial peritonitis

Patients who develop spontaneous bacterial peritonitis have a mortality in the following 12 months of 20–40% after their first episode and 40–70% after a second episode. Secondary antibiotic prophylaxis with cipro-floxacin 500mg/day or norfloxacin 400mg/day reduces infection and mortality. In one study prophylactic antibiotics reduced recurrent spontaneous bacterial peritonitis from 68% to 20%, and Gram-negative infection to 3%, although it may increase in Gram-positive infections including MRSA.

Orthotropic liver transplantation

Referral for orthotropic liver transplantation (OLT) should be considered (see Case 1 and Case 47).

Further reading

Moore KP, Aithal GP (2006). Guidelines on the management of ascites in cirrhosis. *Gut*; **55**(Suppl. VI): VI1–VI12.

Durand F, Valla D (2005). Assessment of the prognosis of cirrhosis: Child–Pugh versus MELD. *J Hepatol*; **42**: S100–S107.

Koulaouzides A, Bhat S, Karagiannidis A, Tan WC, Linaker BD (2007). Spontaneous bacterial peritonitis. *Postgrad Med J*; **83**: 379–83.

Sort P, Navasa M, Arroyo V et al. (1999). Effect of intravenous albumin on renal impairment and mortality in patients with cirrhosis and spontaneous bacterial peritonitis. *N Eng J Med*; **341**: 403–9.

Neuberger J, Gimson A, Davies M et al. (2008). Selection of patients for liver transplantation and allocation of donated livers in the UK. *Gut*; **57**: 252–7.

Case 9

A 59-year-old man presented with a 4-week history of jaundice, 6kg weight loss, pale stools, and dark urine. He had not experienced any abdominal pain. There was no previous medical history and he was not taking any regular medication. Alcohol intake was 25 standard drinks per week and the patient smoked 40 cigarettes/day.

On examination, he was afebrile, jaundiced, and the liver edge was palpable 2cm below the costal margin. There were no stigmata of chronic liver disease.

Investigations showed:

- Hb 13.5g/dL, WCC 4.5 x 10^9/L, platelets 124 x 10^9/L
- Na 134mmol/L, K 3.7mmol/L, urea 4.1mmol/L, creatinine 100μmol/L
- Bilirubin 240μmol/L, ALT 120 IU/L, ALP 1506 IU/L, albumin 36g/L
- Prothrombin time 19 sec
- Abdominal ultrasound: dilated common bile duct (12mm), with mildly dilated intrahepatic ducts, no stones in the gallbladder. Pancreas not seen
- ERCP is shown in Figs 9.1a and 9.1b
- CT scan of the abdomen is shown in Fig. 9.2.

Questions

9a) What investigations need to be done prior to ERCP? What does the ERCP show (Figs 9.1a and 9.1b)?

9b) What does the CT show (Fig. 9.2)?

9c) Give a differential diagnosis.

9d) How would you treat this patient and what is the prognosis?

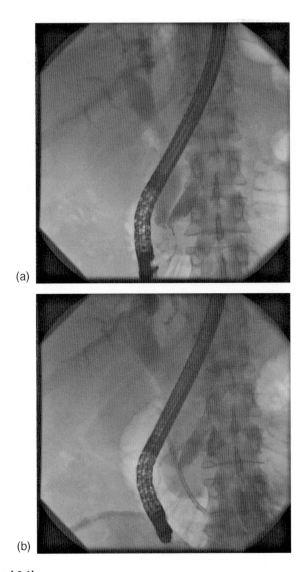

(a)

(b)

Fig. 9.1a and 9.1b

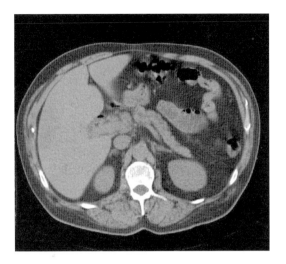

Fig. 9.2

Answers

9a) What investigations need to be done prior to ERCP? What does the ERCP show (Figs 9.1a and 9.1b)?

Correct INR

If a sphincterotomy or pre-cut is being considered, then the prothrombin time should be corrected prior to the procedure. In biliary obstruction the prothrombin time corrects rapidly with vitamin K (unlike in chronic liver disease), which is best given the day before the procedure. If a biliary stent is being inserted without sphincterotomy, then an INR of ≤2 is acceptable.

Magnetic resonance cholangiography

This is a non-invasive approach to imaging an obstructed biliary system. Current protocols consider this a necessary investigation before ERCP; the investigation is debatable in a jaundiced patient such as this, with objective evidence on ultrasound of biliary obstruction, but much depends on local availability of MR scanning and access to ERCP.

Prophylactic antibiotics

Ascending cholangitis results from bacterial infection of an obstructed biliary system, usually from enteric Gram-negative microorganisms, resulting in bacteraemia. There is incomplete drainage of the biliary system after ERCP in up to 10% of patients after stenting. Antibiotics started in these patients may reduce the frequency of cholangitis by 80%. If antibiotics are restricted to this group, ≈90% of all patients having an ERCP will avoid antibiotics, but 80% of cholangitic episodes will be prevented.

The British Society of Gastroenterology Guidelines suggest the following prophylaxis:

- Oral ciprofloxacin 750mg 60–90 min before procedure

- **OR** gentamicin 120mg intravenously just before the procedure

- **OR** a parenteral quinolone, cephalosporin or ureidopenicillin, given intravenously, just before the procedure.

Explain risks of ERCP to the patient

Complications of ERCP occur in 5–10% of patients. The precise risk depends on the particular patient, disease, and type of procedure. Pancreatitis is the most common complication of ERCP; it occurs in 3–5%. Pancreatitis usually resolves in 1–3 days, but severe pancreatitis occurs in about 1% of ERCP procedures. Severe pancreatic damage can result in the formation of a pseudocyst or abscess, which may require a prolonged stay in hospital. Rare fatal cases of pancreatitis related to ERCP have been reported. Other complications are less common and occur mainly after intervention such as sphincterotomy. This includes bleeding, which may necessitate a blood transfusion or surgery. Sphincterotomy can also result in perforation when the cut extends into the tissues behind the duodenum and pancreas. Some perforations can be treated medically (with intravenous fluids, antibiotics and a nasogastric tube); other cases may require surgery and prolonged hospital treatment. Very rarely, the endoscope itself can perforate the oesophagus, stomach, or duodenum. This type of perforation usually requires surgery.

Images

The ERCP (Fig. 9.1a) shows a dilated common bile duct and pancreatic duct (double duct sign, highly suggestive of an obstructing carcinoma), and a dilated intrahepatic biliary tree. Fig. 9.1b shows the biliary stent *in situ* and a dilated pancreatic duct.

9b) **What does the CT show?**

It is important that the CT scan is performed prior to the ERCP, because stent insertion or post-ERCP pancreatitis makes interpretation of the

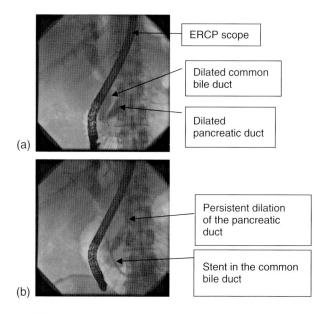

(a)

ERCP scope

Dilated common bile duct

Dilated pancreatic duct

(b)

Persistent dilation of the pancreatic duct

Stent in the common bile duct

Fig. 9.1a and 9.1b

CT scan very difficult. It is for this reason that current protocols also recommend magnetic resonance cholangiopancreatography prior to ERCP. The CT (Fig. 9.2) shows a dilated pancreatic duct. This determines that the level of biliary obstruction is low. There is no visible lesion in the head of the pancreas, no evidence of lymphadenopathy, or metastatic disease.

9c) **Give a differential diagnosis:**

- Ampullary tumour
- Carcinoma of the head of the pancreas
- Bile duct stones
- Cholangiocarcinoma
- Benign bile duct stenosis.

See Fig. 9.3 for an investigation algorithm.

The two most common causes of the **'double duct sign'** (simultaneous dilatation of both the pancreatic and bile ducts) are carcinoma of the head of the pancreas and **carcinoma of the ampulla of Vater**. Both conditions present with obstructive jaundice and weight loss. The endoscopic photograph of the ampulla (Fig. 9.4 in central colour section) makes it very likely that this is an ampullary carcinoma. Cholelithiasis with impaction of a gallstone in the ampullary area could cause simultaneous dilatation of the pancreatic and bile duct; however, this would generally be accompanied by biliary colic and not associated with weight loss. It is uncommon for a cholangiocarcinoma to cause a double duct sign, and benign bile

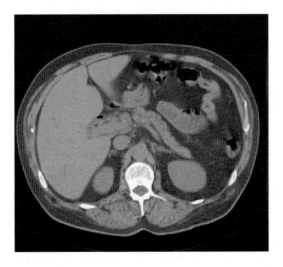

Fig. 9.2

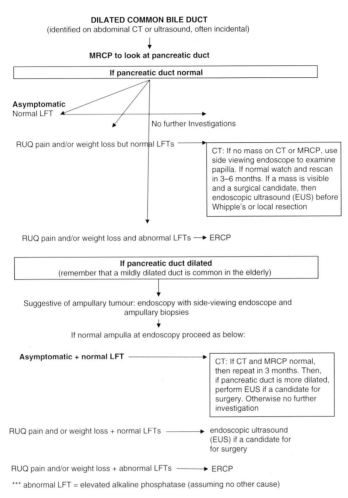

DILATED COMMON BILE DUCT
(identified on abdominal CT or ultrasound, often incidental)

↓

MRCP to look at pancreatic duct

| If pancreatic duct normal |

Asymptomatic
Normal LFT

No further Investigations

RUQ pain and/or weight loss but normal LFTs

CT: If no mass on CT or MRCP, use side viewing endoscope to examine papilla. If normal watch and rescan in 3–6 months. If a mass is visible and a surgical candidate, then endoscopic ultrasound (EUS) before Whipple's or local resection

RUQ pain and/or weight loss and abnormal LFTs → ERCP

| If pancreatic duct dilated |
(remember that a mildly dilated duct is common in the elderly)

Suggestive of ampullary tumour: endoscopy with side-viewing endoscope and ampullary biopsies

↓

If normal ampulla at endoscopy proceed as below:

Asymptomatic + normal LFT

CT: If CT and MRCP normal, then repeat in 3 months. Then, if pancreatic duct is more dilated, perform EUS if a candidate for surgery. Otherwise no further investigation

RUQ pain and or weight loss + normal LFTs → endoscopic ultrasound (EUS) if a candidate for for surgery

RUQ pain and/or weight loss + abnormal LFTs → ERCP

*** abnormal LFT = elevated alkaline phosphatase (assuming no other cause)

Fig. 9.3 Algorithm for managing patients with biliary obstruction

duct stenosis generally follows iatrogenic injury; there was no previous surgery in this case.

9d) **How would you treat this patient and what is the prognosis?**

Pancreatoduodenectomy (Whipple's procedure) is the treatment of choice for patients with an ampullary carcinoma. Resectability rates approach 90%, compared with 25% in pancreatic adenocarcinoma. The explanation for the greater resectability rate for ampullary adenocarcinoma is multifactorial. It can partly be explained by earlier presentation (because the anatomic location of the tumour provokes jaundice at an early stage), but may also reflect a different biological behaviour compared with pancreatic cancer.

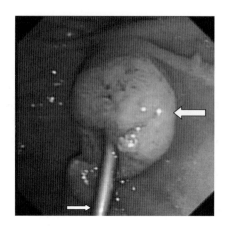

Fig. 9.4 (see colour plate 4) Endoscopic photograph of the tumour (large arrow) after stent (small arrow) insertion

Nodal metastases are present at diagnosis of ampullary carcinoma in 35% (usually adjacent periampullary nodes). Overall 5-year survival after resection is 40–50%, but this increases to 80% if there are no nodal metastases. This is much better than pancreatic or cholangiocarcinoma, which have 5-year survival rates of 10–20%, so it is important to make the distinction. Poor prognostic factors include advanced stage, tumour size >2.5cm, perineural invasion, angiolymphatic invasion, nodal metastases, signet-ring or poorly differentiated histopathology, and positive (R1) resection margins.

Patients with ampullary adenocarcinoma can benefit from 5-fluorouracil (5FU)-based chemoradiotherapy after resection, especially node positive (N1) patients. If metastatic or unresectable local disease is found at the time of surgery, palliation with a Roux-en-Y hepaticojejunostomy bypass is appropriate.

In this patient, the tumour was resected and histology showed a moderately differentiated ampullary adenocarcinoma, with 11/25 nodes positive. Neo-adjuvant chemotherapy with weekly 5FU was given after surgery. The patient remains well 3 years later.

Further reading

Clarke DL, Pillay Y, Anderson F, Thomson SR (2006). The current standard of care in the periprocedural management of the patient with obstructive jaundice. *Ann R Coll Surg Engl*; **88**: 610–16.

Coss A, Enns R (2009). The investigation of unexplained biliary dilatation. *Curr Gastroenterol Rep*; **11**: 155–9.

Dittrick GW, Mallat DB, Lamont JP (2006). Management of ampullary lesions. *Curr Treat Options Gastroenterol*; **9**: 371–6.

Tran TC, Vitale GC (2004). Ampullary tumors: endoscopic versus operative management. *Surg Innov*; **11**: 255–63.

Case 10

A 78-year-old woman from Yorkshire was referred with a 5-year history of diarrhoea that was predominantly nocturnal. Symptoms had worsened over the preceding 12 months. She would have to get up three or four times to open her bowels, on 3 or 4 nights a week. Daytime frequency was only twice, but stools were often explosive, pale and sometimes left a residue after flushing. She had lost 10kg in 2 years, but her appetite was normal. She had been referred 2 years previously and been investigated. A barium enema had shown sigmoid diverticular disease, but no other abnormality. A macrocytic anaemia (Hb 10.8g/dL, MCV of 132fL) had been found, attributable to vitamin B12 deficiency. Her folate was normal, towards the upper limit of the range. Vitamin B12 replacement every 3 months had been started. On examination, she was cachectic and weighed 51kg.

Investigations showed:

- Hb 12.7g/dL, WCC 8.0 x 10^9/L, platelets 224 x 10^9/L, MCV 98fL
- CRP 9mg/L
- U&E normal
- Albumin 31g/L
- Faecal elastase 248μg/g (normal >200μg/g)
- Endomysial antibody serology negative.

A small bowel enema was requested and the patient was started on empirical treatment.

Questions

10a) What is the differential diagnosis?
10b) Name three conditions that predispose to the most likely diagnosis.
10c) How is the diagnosis made?
10d) How would you manage this patient?
10e) Discuss the underlying condition.

Answers

10a) **What is the differential diagnosis?**

Small intestinal bacterial overgrowth results from an excess of bacteria in the small bowel, often associated with abnormal small bowel anatomy and/or motility. It characteristically causes painless, explosive and malodorous diarrhoea, weight loss, and B12 deficiency. Bacteria deconjugate bile acids and prevent effective emulsification of dietary fat, with subsequent steatorrhoea. Anaerobic organisms metabolize dietary vitamin B12 into inactive cobamides. These cobamides then compete with ileal binding sites for vitamin B12 absorption, limit absorptive capacity, and eventually lead to deficiency. In contrast, folic acid absorption is unaffected and bacterial production of folate may lead to high folic acid concentrations. Reduced disaccharidase activity in the brush border, secondary to small intestinal bacterial overgrowth, causes lactose intolerance, which contributes to the diarrhoea.

Exocrine pancreatic insufficiency is also characterized by steatorrhoea (see Case 12) and may cause vitamin B12 deficiency, because pancreatic enzymes are needed to release vitamin B12 from R-binding protein. R-binder combines with vitamin B12 in the stomach to protect it from degradation when exposed to gastric acid. In our patient, however, the faecal elastase concentration was normal (>200µg/g), which makes pancreatic insufficiency unlikely. In younger people, a faecal elastase of 200–500µg/g still raises the possibility of exocrine pancreatic insufficiency.

Small bowel mucosal pathology (such as coeliac or Whipple's disease) may cause steatorrhoea and occasionally vitamin B12 deficiency. Coeliac disease with negative endomysial antibody serology is very unusual (<5% in most published series, although may be slightly more common in practice).

Nocturnal diarrhoea should always be considered to have an organic cause and not attributed to a functional bowel disorder (such as irritable bowel syndrome) until proven otherwise. Other conditions that cause chronic nocturnal diarrhoea (such as microscopic colitis) do not cause B12 deficiency. Any condition resulting in B12 deficiency needs to have been present for years, because the physiological daily requirement for vitamin B12 is about one thousandth of total body stores. In this woman, the most likely cause was small intestinal bacterial overgrowth.

A small bowel enema was requested to define small bowel anatomy and **extensive jejunal diverticulosis** was identified (Fig. 10.1).

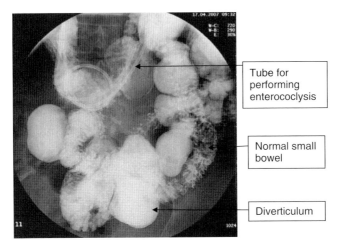

Fig. 10.1 A small bowel enema showing multiple jejunal diverticula.

10b) **Name three conditions that predispose to the most likely diagnosis**

Small intestinal bacterial overgrowth is typically associated with anatomical abnormalities of the small bowel, either spontaneous or acquired after surgery, and from conditions that affect small bowel motility. Stasis of luminal fluid promotes bacterial growth. Small intestinal resection and anastomosis may create a **blind loop**, while resection of the ileocaecal valve promotes retrograde flow of colonic contents and bacteria into the small bowel. The most common postoperative association with small intestinal bacterial overgrowth is **ileocolic resection** for Crohn's disease, but in the past partial gastrectomy with a Bilroth II or Roux-en-Y anastomosis were often complicated by a 'blind loop syndrome' that include diarrhoea due to bacterial overgrowth.

Acquired conditions include **small bowel strictures** and **small bowel diverticulosis**. Strictures are commonly caused by Crohn's disease, but radiation enteropathy and non-steroidal drugs may also cause strictures and upstream stasis. Small bowel dysmotility in **systemic sclerosis** and **autonomic neuropathy** (most commonly complicating diabetes) may cause small intestinal bacterial overgrowth. Nevertheless, small intestinal bacterial overgrowth may occur with normal intestinal anatomy, including achlorhydria and old age. It is conceivable that proton-pump inhibitors in the elderly may predispose to small intestinal bacterial overgrowth. Old age may be associated with small intestinal bacterial overgrowth due to multiple factors including reduced intestinal motility, reduced IgA secretion, small bowel diverticulosis, which is more common in old age, previous intestinal surgery, and achlorhydria. Small intestinal bacterial overgrowth should be considered in patients with coeliac disease whose symptoms persist despite avoiding dietary gluten, and in patients with rheumatoid arthritis, who may have small intestinal bacterial overgrowth associated with disease activity.

10c) **How is the diagnosis made?**

Small intestinal bacterial overgrowth is an epiphenomenon associated with other gastrointestinal conditions. The diagnosis is often **clinical**, since the explosive, malodorous, painless diarrhoea with or without weight loss is characteristic in a patient with a predisposing condition. A low B12 and high folate are characteristic, but relatively uncommon in practice.

Bacterial concentration and composition changes from the proximal to the distal small intestine: the number of colony forming units (cfu)/mL increase and the composition changes from predominantly Gram-positive bacteria to Gram-negative and anaerobic bacteria. Colonization of the proximal small bowel with coliforms and anaerobes is abnormal and may cause symptoms at lower concentrations than Gram-positive bacteria.

Culture of small bowel aspirate is the **gold standard** for diagnosis of small intestinal bacterial overgrowth (generally defined as more than 10^5 cfu/mL), but rarely employed. The threshold of 10^5 cfu/mL is based on early studies of patients with surgically constructed blind loops. Nevertheless, small bowel culture is difficult and invasive, because it requires an aspirate that may itself become contaminated.

Non-invasive tests are far more attractive. A variety of breath-tests exist, based on the ability of bacteria to produce hydrogen (H_2) or carbon dioxide (CO_2), through the metabolism of specific carbohydrate substrates that may be radio-labelled. These include glucose, lactulose and D-xylose. If glucose or lactulose are used, H_2 is measured in the breath. Bacteria are the only producers of hydrogen in the intestine and detection of >20ppm within 2 hours of ingestion implies bacterial production from the small intestine. However, 15–20% of patients produce methane or hydrogen sulphide, which are undetectable by conventional hydrogen analysers and may give rise to false-negative results. Glucose is almost entirely absorbed in the first metre of small intestine, so a positive test implies proximal small intestinal bacterial overgrowth. Lactulose, however, is not absorbed at all, but is subsequently fermented in the colon, giving a late peak (>2 hours) in breath hydrogen, which is normal. An early peak (<2 hours) is considered positive, but the test is difficult or impossible to interpret in patients with rapid intestinal transit or after small bowel resection. The **glucose hydrogen breath** test, when compared with culture of small bowel aspirate, has a sensitivity of 27–58% and specificity of 30–83%. The **lactulose hydrogen breath** test has a sensitivity of 17–89% and a specificity of 44–100%, so the latter is generally preferred. In contrast to hydrogen, ^{13}C-D-xylose or ^{14}C-D-xylose administration enables the measurement of $^{13}CO_2$ or $^{14}CO_2$ in the breath. The **^{14}C-D-xylose breath** test has a sensitivity of 40–100% and a specificity of 40–100%, but the use of a radioisotope is a drawback.

Formal assessment of small intestinal bacterial overgrowth is therefore fraught with difficulty, because there is not only heterogeneity in studies comparing non-invasive tests to bacterial culture, but the gold standard is itself also of questionable validity. A systematic review has questioned the validity of current non-invasive breath tests based on an inadequate gold standard. Correlation in studies is recommended between a compatible clinical syndrome, non-invasive tests, and an appropriate response to therapy. In **clinical practice** it is reasonable to give empirical antibiotic therapy to a patient with compatible symptoms and a predisposing cause. This is simple and usually sufficient.

In our patient the diagnosis of small intestinal bacterial overgrowth was based on the clinical syndrome of steatorrhoea, weight loss, and vitamin B12 deficiency, with small intestinal diverticulosis and a rapid response to antibiotics.

10d) **How would you manage this patient?**

Any predisposing factors should be corrected, but this is rarely possible, especially for anatomical abnormalities. Nutritional deficiencies should be corrected. In addition to vitamin B12 deficiency, fat-soluble vitamins A, D, and E may be deficient. Vitamin K is produced by bacteria and not deficient in these patients. Thiamine and nicotinamide may rarely be deficient. **Antibiotic therapy** is highly effective in the treatment of small intestinal bacterial overgrowth. Metronidazole 400mg three times daily, or ciprofloxacin 500mg twice daily for a week, is usually effective. Cyclical (occasionally continuous) antibiotics, for 1 week every month, alternating between these antibiotics is an appropriate way of managing patients with abnormal anatomy.

We managed our patient on 1 week of antibiotics per month, alternating between ciprofloxacin and metronidazole. She had an excellent response with resolution of symptoms and stabilization of her weight. After 14 months we decided to stop the antibiotics because she was well.

Seven months later she remained well off antibiotics, but relapse at some stage can be expected.

10e) **Discuss the underlying condition**

Small intestinal diverticulosis is uncommon and although autopsy series report a prevalence of 0.06–1.3%, the true prevalence is unknown. It occurs more frequently with advancing age and the peak clinical prevalence is in the 6th and 7th decades of life. Most diverticula (80%) are jejunal. In general diverticula become fewer and smaller more distally. An association between small bowel and colonic diverticula has been postulated, but the latter are almost universal with advancing age. Small bowel diverticula are thought to represent herniation of mucosa and sub-mucosa through the muscle layers of the intestine, on the mesenteric border. Unlike colonic diverticula, acute emergencies from diverticulitis, perforation, or haemorrhage are exceptionally uncommon.

Further reading

Rana SV, Bhardwaj SB (2008). Small intestinal bacterial overgrowth. *Scand J Gastroenterol*; **43**: 1030–37.

Khoshini R, Dai SC, Lezcano S, Pimentel M (2008). A systematic review of diagnostic tests for small intestinal bacterial overgrowth. *Dig Dis Sci*; **53**: 1443–54.

Kassahun W, Fangmann J, Harms J, Bartels M *et al.* (2007). Complicated small-bowel diverticulosis: A case report and review of the literature. *World J Gastroenterol*; **13**: 2240–42.

Case 11

A 53-year-old unemployed man with known alcoholic liver cirrhosis presented to the emergency department with jaundice, ascites, and oedema to the thighs. He reported drinking 6 pints of beer/day for over 30 years. He was not on any medication.

On examination, the pulse rate was 88bpm and blood pressure 120/60mmHg. There was firm hepatomegaly, with the liver edge palpable 6cm below the costal margin, and definite ascites. There was no asterixis, but multiple spider naevi were present.

Investigations showed:

- Na 123mmol/L, K 3.7mmol/L, urea 2.0mmol/L, creatinine 93μmol/L
- Bilirubin 235μmol/L, ALT 133 IU/L, ALP 708 IU/L, albumin 22g/L
- CRP 26mg/dL
- Prothrombin time 17.0 sec
- Abdominal ultrasound: course liver texture, splenomegaly, and ascites.

He was started on chlordiazepoxide and intravenous thiamine. A diagnostic (20ml) ascitic tap was carried out, which showed no evidence of spontaneous bacterial peritonitis. He had high gradient ascites (Serum-ascites albumin gradient >11g/L).

Two days after admission, he developed severe cellulitis in his right leg. He was started on intravenous ceftriaxone. The next day his creatinine had risen to 266μmol/L, with the bilirubin increasing to 300μmol/L. Moderate confusion developed and the blood pressure decreased to 100/50mmHg.

Questions

11a) What are the possible causes of the decline in renal function?

11b) What is the pathophysiology of renal dysfunction in chronic liver disease?

11c) What management should be instituted?

11d) His ascites became very uncomfortable. What would you recommend?

Answers

11a) **What are the possible causes of the decline in renal function?**

As in any case of acute renal failure, pre-renal, renal, and post-renal causes need to be considered. Specific to patients with liver disease, hepatorenal syndrome (in the pre-renal category) should always be considered.

The two most likely causes in this particular case are both pre-renal in origin. Sepsis from cellulitis causing **hypovolaemia** and therefore decreased renal perfusion may be the sole cause or there may be underlying **hepatorenal syndrome**. A normal creatinine at presentation does not exclude underlying renal dysfunction. Patients with liver cirrhosis often have apparently normal renal function, because the creatinine is not a good marker of glomerular filtration rate in such patients. The creatinine is 'falsely' low because of decreased hepatic creatinine synthesis and decreased skeletal muscle mass.

Other pre-renal and renal causes in the presence of cirrhosis should be considered. These include spontaneous bacterial peritonitis, excessive diuretic use, hypovolaemia from gastrointestinal bleeding, dehydration, and renal tubular damage from nephrotoxic drugs, or contrast agents. None of these causes were present in this case. There are multiple causes of intrinsic renal failure.

In order to differentiate any cause of pre-renal failure or hepatorenal syndrome from intrinsic renal failure, a **urinary sodium** should be performed. It should be <10mmol/L in the former two conditions (due to avid sodium retention by functioning renal tubules) and >30mmol/L in intrinsic renal failure (attributable to renal tubular dysfunction). **Urine microscopy** is likely to show urinary casts or cellular debris in intrinsic renal disease. IgA nephropathy can occur in alcoholics, and glomerulonephritis is associated with hepatitis C infection. Although obstructive or **post-renal dysfunction** is not specifically associated with liver disease, it is wise to request a renal ultrasound to exclude a hydronephrosis.

11b) **What is the pathophysiology of renal dysfunction in chronic liver disease?**

The pathophysiological hallmark of advanced cirrhosis is systemic, particularly splanchnic, vasodilatation which is caused by endogenous vasodilators (especially nitric oxide) entering the circulation, due to porto-systemic shunting of blood. Systemic vasodilatation is associated with decreased systemic vascular resistance, which in turn leads to peripheral and splanchnic blood pooling resulting in a reduction of the effective arterial blood volume. This activates the renin-angiotensin-aldosterone system and other vasoconstrictive neurohumoral systems, including catecholamines, in order to replenish the intravascular blood volume. On the one hand, this leads to sodium and water retention, while on the other, it induces renal vasoconstriction. Any event that further decreases renal perfusion (e.g. sepsis, gastrointestinal bleed), will cause deterioration in renal function and precipitate acute renal failure.

11c) **What management should be instituted?**

Management should follow the general principles for the management of renal failure of any aetiology, as well as specific measures for the liver disease. In patients with chronic liver disease, the management of acute renal failure must focus on pre-renal causes and hepatorenal syndrome.

Initial management comprises correction of life-threatening abnormalities such as hyperkalaemia and hypoglycaemia. Sepsis should be treated (as in our case). The patient should have appropriate fluid replacement (crystalloid/colloid) to ensure that any reversible pre-renal component has been treated. 5% dextrose is best avoided in patients who are hyponatraemic, but it is important to **avoid sodium loading** with repeated normal saline infusions, since this will increase total body sodium and lead to worsening of ascites. Initial resuscitation with normal saline is acceptable. The balance is difficult and volume expansion with albumin or other colloid and central venous pressure monitoring is appropriate. The importance of reversing the decline of renal failure by correcting hypovolaemia cannot be over-emphasized, because once renal failure is established it is difficult to reverse in patients with liver disease. Any gastrointestinal bleeding should be treated promptly, including volume replacement. All diuretic therapy and nephrotoxic medication should be discontinued. If there is no improvement in the renal function after volume replacement, the diagnosis is most probably hepatorenal syndrome.

There are two types of hepatorenal syndrome. **Type 1 hepatorenal syndrome** is rapidly progressive, with the creatinine increasing to >250μmol/L within 2 weeks. Precipitating factors include spontaneous bacterial peritonitis, major surgical procedures, and acute alcoholic hepatitis. It follows a fulminant course, with the development of oliguria, encephalopathy, and marked hyperbilirubinaemia The prognosis is poor. **Type 2 hepatorenal syndrome** is characterized by a more benign course, with a stable reduction in glomerular filtration rate over weeks to months, accompanied by diuretic-resistant ascites and avid sodium retention. Our patient had developed Type 1 hepatorenal syndrome.

The following treatment options are potentially effective for hepatorenal syndrome:

- First-line therapy: vasoconstrictor drugs (e.g. bolus doses of terlipressin) in combination with albumin to expand the circulating blood volume. This improves renal function in more than 50% of patients. **Terlipressin** predominately causes splanchnic vasoconstriction, but should be used with care in patients with angina, because it can provoke coronary vasoconstriction.

- Liver transplantation remains the definitive treatment, but many patients die awaiting transplantation. Transplantation has a greater role in Type 2 hepatorenal syndrome.

- Artificial liver support (such as the molecular absorbent re-circulating system [MARS]), is being explored, but convincing evidence of benefit in hepatorenal syndrome is lacking.

11d) **His ascites became very uncomfortable. What would you recommend?**

Sodium and water retention, caused by hypovolaemia and activation of the renin-angiotensin-aldosterone system in patients with cirrhosis, often leads to tense ascites, requiring large volume paracentesis. **Paracentesis** itself, however, can provoke hypovolaemia. Albumin is therefore given during paracentesis, either as 20% or a 4.5% solution, a dose of 6–8g of albumin per litre of ascitic fluid removed (see Case 8). The choice depends in part on availability, but also on the estimated degree of hypovolaemia (with more concentrated albumin, there is a danger of exacerbating fluid overload). This prevents deterioration of renal function and helps avoid exacerbating hepatorenal syndrome. Once a patient has established hepatorenal syndrome and tense ascites, there is no evidence that draining the ascites improves renal blood flow, so paracentesis can be left until there is an improvement in renal function unless it is causing discomfort.

This patient's renal function did not improve following fluid resuscitation and he was treated with intravenous terlipressin 0.5mg twice daily, and 4.5% albumin infusions for 7 days. Within 3 days his creatinine had decreased to 150μmol/L and the bilirubin to 36mmol/L. He remains off alcohol 2 years later, with a creatinine of 78μmol/L on spironolactone 100mg/day.

Further reading

Betrosian AP, Agarwal B, Douzinas EE (2007). Acute renal dysfunction in liver disease. *World J Gastroenterol*; **13**: 5552–9.

Colle I, Durand F, Pessione F *et al.* (2002). Clinical course, predictive factors and prognosis in patients with cirrhosis and type 1 hepatorenal syndrome treated with terlipressin. A retrospective analysis. *J Gastroenterol Hepatol*; **17**: 882–8.

Fabrizi F, Dixit V, Messa P, Martin P (2009). Terlipressin for hepatorenal syndrome: A meta-analysis of randomized trials. *Int J Artif Organs*; **32**: 133–40.

Ortega R, Gines P, Uriz J *et al.* (2002). Terlipressin therapy with and without albumin for patients with hepatorenal syndrome: Results of a prospective nonrandomised study. *Hepatology*; **36**: 941–8.

Schepke M (2007). Hepatorenal syndrome: current diagnostic and therapeutic concepts. *Nephrol Dial Transplant*; **22**(Suppl. 8): viii2–viii4.

Case 12

A 76-year-old man from London presented with a 2-year history of diarrhoea. He reported passing 4–7 loose, oily stools per day. He described the stool as looking like 'axle grease'. Over the 2-year period he had lost 4kg, but his weight had recently been stable. He had a history of cerebrovascular disease with dementia, ischaemic heart disease, and gout, and had had a gastroenterostomy and vagotomy in 1961 for duodenal ulceration. He neither smoked nor drank alcohol.

Vital signs were normal. He was not pale and not jaundiced. Abdominal examination was unremarkable, apart from a scar in the midline.

He had been investigated a year before for the same problem. A flexible sigmoidoscopy at the time had shown him to have diverticulosis, but biopsies of the colonic mucosa were normal. Antiendomysial antibodies were negative.

Investigations showed:

- Hb 11.1g/dL, WCC 5.3 x 10^9/L, platelets 100 x 10^9/L, MCV 89fL
- Bilirubin 12µmol/L, ALT 9 IU/L, ALP 169 IU/L, albumin 42g/L
- CRP 4mg/L.

Questions

12a) What is the clinical problem?

12b) What is the differential diagnosis?

12c) How would you investigate?

12d) What is the diagnosis in this case?

12e) How would you treat this patient?

Answers

12a) **What is the clinical problem?**

The description of greasy stools suggests **steatorrhoea due to malabsorption.**

12b) **What is the differential diagnosis?**

The differential diagnosis includes:

- Intraluminal maldigestion (pancreatic insufficiency, bacterial over-growth, biliary obstruction)
- Mucosal malabsorption. (Coeliac disease, Whipple's desease)

Intraluminal maldigestion resulting from either **exocrine pancreatic insufficiency** or **bacterial overgrowth** are the likely causes. Weight loss is often not prominent in these disorders and the serum albumin is usually normal. Pancreatic insufficiency presenting in an elderly patient is usually *not* due to alcohol-related chronic pancreatitis, which presents in the fourth and fifth decade. Pancreatic atrophy is common in the elderly and does not itself imply exocrine pancreatic insufficiency, but some do have insufficiency without another discernible cause. Bacterial overgrowth is common in the elderly even in the absence of anatomical abnormalities of the small bowel (see Case 10). Biliary obstruction may also cause steatorrhoea, but this patient was not jaundiced. Mucosal malabsorption resulting from coeliac disease is unlikely (but not totally excluded) from the negative endomysial antibody serology. Coeliac disease only rarely causes steatorrhoea and then only in severe cases with other features, including anaemia with iron and folate deficiency. Small bowel biopsies have not been performed in this case, so rare causes of mucosal malabsorption (such as Whipple's disease) have not been excluded, but are unlikely. A low albumin in a patient with steatorrhoea is usually associated with mucosal malabsorption.

12c) **How would you investigate?**

The **faecal elastase** is usually diagnostic of exocrine pancreatic insufficiency, but mild cases may be missed. It is a simple, indirect measure of pancreatic exocrine function and can be requested on the first outpatient appointment. A concentration <200µg/g of stool is consistent with exocrine pancreatic insufficiency, but in younger people the concentration should be >500µg/g. Stool water affects the measurement, so the test cannot be done on liquid stool. Faecal elastase is stable, so the test can be performed on a sample that is days old, and pancreatic enzyme supplementation does *not* affect the assay. In a population-based study to quantify the prevalence of exocrine pancreatic insufficiency in people aged 50–75, 12% had a faecal elastase <200µg/L and 5% had a concentration <100µg/L, so this should be considered as a cause of unexplained weight loss.

A normal faecal elastase with steatorrhoea is suggestive of bacterial overgrowth. Measuring stool fat content, however, rarely contributes to the diagnosis, and 3-day or 5-day stool fat collections are obsolete. Direct testing of exocrine pancreatic function is inconvenient and rarely used (e.g. pancreolauryl test), because of poor sensitivity. Pancreatic imaging is appropriate, if exocrine pancreatic insufficiency is confirmed.

Further investigations showed:

- Faecal elastase < 15µg/g
- IgG normal
- CT scan of the pancreas showed an atrophic pancreas, no pancreatic mass and no ductal dilatation (Fig. 12.1).

12d) **What is the diagnosis?**

The patient has **severe exocrine pancreatic insufficiency**. Although alcohol is the most common cause for chronic pancreatitis, it is unlikely in an elderly patient presenting for the first time with exocrine pancreatic insufficiency. Our patient had no pain and did not drink. Obstruction of the pancreatic duct by a tumour at the ampulla is an important potential cause of exocrine pancreatic insufficiency in elderly patients. Pancreatic insufficiency may be of unknown aetiology and our patient falls into this group. Pancreatic atrophy is *not* a measure of

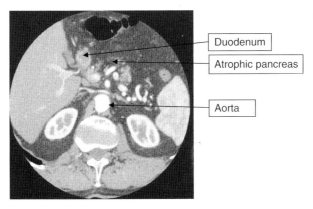

Fig. 12.1 A CT scan showing an atrophic pancreas.

function and may be seen in advanced age without exocrine pancreatic insufficiency.

12e) **How would you treat this patient?**

Pancreatic enzyme replacement is appropriate. The vital constituent is lipase and the dose is determined by the lipase content. Enteric coated mini-microspheres of pancreatic enzymes (e.g. Creon™) are designed to release enzymes at a pH >5. Lipase is then not inactivated by gastric acid. Some patients, however, have markedly reduced pancreatic bicarbonate secretion and benefit from the addition of a proton pump inhibitor to ensure that the pH is high enough for the microspheres to release the lipase in the proximal small bowel. Acid suppression would be inappropriate in our patient, because of the previous vagotomy. Patients are usually started on the equivalent of 25,000 units of lipase during (*not* after or before!) each meal, and 10,000 during snacks. The dose is adjusted according to response.

Further reading

Gloor B, Ahmed Z, Uhl W, Buchler MW (2002). Pancreatic disease in the elderly. *Best Prac Res Clin Gastroenterol*; **16**: 159–70.

Rothenbacher D, Low M, Hardt PD *et al.* (2005) Prevalence and determinants of exocrine pancreatic insufficiency among older adults: Results of a population-based study. *Scand J Gastroenterol*; **40**: 697–704.

Domingues-Munoz JE, Iglesias-Garcia J, Iglesias-Rey M, Vilarino-Insua M (2006). Optimising the therapy of exocrine pancreatic insufficiency by the association of a proton pump inhibitor with enteric-coated pancreatic extracts. *Gut*; **55**: 1056–7.

Case 13

A 70-year-old retired Korean mechanic presented with a 12-month history of epigastric discomfort and 5kg weight loss. A laparoscopic cholecystectomy had been carried out for multiple gallstones. The discomfort continued post-cholecystectomy. His past medical history included a seronegative arthritis and a salivary gland biopsy consistent with Sjøgren's syndrome. The patient denied drinking alcohol and was a non-smoker. He had become jaundiced over the preceding 3 weeks.

On examination, the patient was jaundiced and wasted. There were no ascites or spider naevi.

Investigations showed:

- Na 135mmol/L, K 5.0mmol/L, urea 13mmol/L, creatinine 112μmol/L, glucose 9.5mmol/L
- Bilirubin 260μmol/L, ALT 67 IU/L, ALP 1028 IU/L
- Prothrombin time: 13.0 sec
- Amylase 15 IU/L (normal 25–125 IU/L)
- Abdominal ultrasound showed a dilated bile duct and an abnormality in the pancreatic head
- CT scan (Fig. 13.1)
- ERCP: two distal common bile duct strictures and mild irregular narrowing of the pancreatic duct. Brushings were negative for malignancy.

Questions

13a) What are the two most likely possible diagnoses and what are the clinical and laboratory features of each?

13b) What is the main abnormality on the CT scan and how does this assist with the diagnosis?

13c) What two additional tests would help in confirming the diagnosis?

13d) What is the prognosis for the two most likely diagnoses and describe the treatment for each.

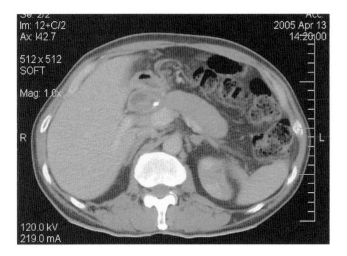

Fig. 13.1 CT scan of the abdomen in a 70-year-old man with jaundice.

Answers

13a) **What are the two most likely possible diagnoses and what are the clinical and laboratory features of each?**

The two principal differential diagnoses to consider are

- pancreatic carcinoma
- autoimmune pancreatitis (rare).

Pancreatic carcinoma is the second most frequent gastrointestinal cancer after colorectal cancer. Care is needed to ensure that pancreatic cancer is not assumed just because it is common. Misdiagnosis is relatively common if only one imaging modality (such as CT scanning) is used, and biopsy is often appropriate, especially since therapeutic use of chemotherapy depends on biopsy-proven cases. About 2% of pancreatic masses resected for suspected malignancy are found to be due to autoimmune pancreatitis and these are over-represented in long-term survivors of Whipple's procedure for 'pancreatic cancer'.

Autoimmune pancreatitis is a benign systemic fibro-inflammatory disorder, in which the pancreas is one of several potentially affected organs. Other affected organ systems include the bile ducts, salivary glands (note the previous diagnosis of Sjøgrens syndrome in this man), and retroperitoneal lymph nodes. Autoimmune pancreatitis can be difficult to differentiate from malignancy. Conversely, it is important not to miss the diagnosis of pancreatic carcinoma.

The difficulty in diagnosis in our case is because both conditions can present with obstructive jaundice, a mass, and obstruction or stricturing of the bile duct. Pancreatic cancer (affecting the head of the pancreas) generally presents with painless jaundice, with pain as a late feature. It commonly needs to be distinguished from an ampullary cancer (see Case 9). The principal symptom of **autoimmune pancreatitis** is also obstructive jaundice. Severe abdominal pain is rare in autoimmune pancreatitis, but most patients complain of abdominal discomfort. Recent onset diabetes is present in about half of patients with autoimmune pancreatitis, but can also occur in pancreatic cancer. Both conditions can be associated with decreased appetite and weight loss.

The concentrations of serum pancreatic enzymes are inconsistently elevated in both pancreatic cancer and autoimmune pancreatitis, and are therefore not of any use in distinguishing between the two. CA19-9 is elevated in the presence of jaundice and so is not helpful in differentiating autoimmune pancreatitis and pancreatic carcinoma. Various patterns of elevated concentrations of serum autoantibodies have been described in patients with autoimmune pancreatitis. These include antinuclear factor, rheumatoid factor, antimitochondrial antibody, anti-smooth muscle antibody, antibodies against carbonic anhydrate II, and lactoferrin.

Cholangiocarcinoma and primary sclerosing cholangitis may also cause distal common bile duct strictures, but not pancreatic duct strictures. Chronic pancreatitis may also cause a distal common bile duct stricture and is associated with a dilated pancreatic duct, with or without duct strictures. Nevertheless, a 'double duct sign' strongly suggests malignancy (see Case 9). Pancreatic calcification is common in chronic pancreatitis, identified by CT scanning (about 60%) or plain abdominal radiograph (about 20%). There was no pancreatic calcification on the CT scan, which makes chronic pancreatitis unlikely in this case.

13b) **What is the main abnormality on the CT scan and how does this assist with the diagnosis?**

The characteristic appearance of autoimmune pancreatitis on CT scan is a diffusely enlarged **'sausage-shaped' pancreas**. In autoimmune pancreatitis there is generally a sharp outline, homogenous appearance to the pancreas, and minimal or absent peripancreatic stranding. These appearances are consistent whether on CT, MRI or transabdominal ultrasonography. Contrast-enhancement sometimes shows a low-contrast margin, described as a rim or capsule on CT. Nevertheless, an appreciable number of patients with autoimmune pancreatitis do not have diffuse pancreatic involvement, but have a focal swelling or mass that mimics pancreatic carcinoma. Dilatation, stricture, or irregularity of the main pancreatic duct, as well as the common bile duct, can occur in autoimmune pancreatitis with or without focal swelling of the pancreatic head. Enlarged peripancreatic lymph nodes are commonly seen and can reach a diameter of up to 30mm. A suspicion of autoimmune pancreatitis should occur if the patient is unduly young, has coexistent autoimmune conditions, or if there are multiple strictures on the CT scan. Fortunately, the diagnosis is readily confirmed if considered (below).

The method of choice for diagnosing and staging pancreatic cancer is also CT scanning. The pancreatic protocol for CT consists of a **dual-phase scan** with intravenous and oral contrast agents. The first (pancreatic) phase is obtained 40 sec after administration of the intravenous contrast. At this time, maximum enhancement of the normal pancreas is obtained, allowing identification of non-enhancing (potentially neoplastic) lesions. The second (portal venous) phase is obtained 70 sec after

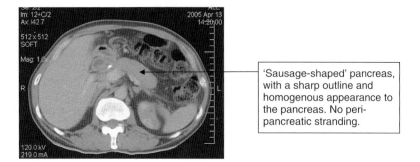

'Sausage-shaped' pancreas, with a sharp outline and homogenous appearance to the pancreas. No peri-pancreatic stranding.

Fig. 13.1 CT scan of the abdomen in a 70-year-old man with jaundice.

injection of the intravenous contrast, which allows accurate detection of liver metastases and assessment of tumour invasion of portal or superior mesenteric veins.

13c) **What two additional tests would help in confirming the diagnosis?**

The two tests that distinguish between pancreatic cancer and autoimmune pancreatitis are:

- **Serum IgG4 concentration**
- Pancreatic biopsy.

Once considered, the diagnosis of autoimmune pancreatitis is fortunately relatively straightforward. An **elevated IgG4** concentration (normal range 0.1–1.3g/L) has a sensitivity of 90%, a specificity of 98% and a positive predictive value of 95% for the diagnosis of autoimmune pancreatitis. Why the inflammatory process (unlike other conditions) is so specific for the IgG4 is unclear. Nevertheless, pancreatic biopsy may still be required to differentiate autoimmune pancreatitis from pancreatic carcinoma. Endoscopic ultrasound examines the pancreas in detail and allows fine-needle aspiration of lesions in the head. Although fine-needle aspiration is generally inadequate for diagnosing autoimmune pancreatitis, it has a high positive predictive value if malignant cells are found. Percutaneous pancreatic biopsy is the alternative, although it carries a 5% risk of provoking acute pancreatitis. A periductal lympho-plasmacytic infiltrate associated with fibrosis and containing >10 IgG4-positive cells per high-power field (on immunostaining) is pathognomonic for autoimmune pancreatitis (Fig. 13.2).

13d) **What is the prognosis for the two most likely diagnoses and describe the treatment for each.**

Pancreatic cancer carries an extremely poor prognosis with less than 20% of affected patients surviving the first year, and only 4% alive 5 years after diagnosis. Some of these may have autoimmune pancreatitis in historical series. Surgical resection is the only curative treatment, but only 15% are candidates for curative resection, because of local invasion at the time of presentation. Metastases are an absolute contraindication for resection. The standard operation is pancreaticoduodenectomy (**Whipple's procedure**), which has a mortality rate of <3% in experienced hands. Positive lymph nodes in the resection specimen carry a poor prognosis. For those patients who do not have a resectable lesion, palliation is appropriate by biliary stenting to relieve jaundice, coeliac plexus block for pain relief, surgical bypass for gastric outflow tract obstruction, or palliative chemotherapy.

In contrast, autoimmune pancreatitis carries a good prognosis, which is why it is an important diagnosis. Until recently, diagnosis and treatment generally involved surgical excision to exclude malignancy, or because of a preoperative presumption of carcinoma. After simple, serological diagnosis (an elevated IgG4), **corticosteroids** are now indicated to induce complete clinical and radiological remission that is generally sustained with a return to normal serology, improvement or disappearance of duct stenoses, often with restoration of endocrine and exocrine function. The initial dose of prednisolone is usually 30–40mg/day and tapered by 5mg every 2 weeks. Relapse may occur, requiring reintroduction of corticosteroids with immunomodulators. To avoid delay in treating malignancy, any corticosteroid-treated pancreatic mass should show near-complete resolution when reimaged 2–4 weeks after starting therapy. Any residual mass should be explored surgically. Diabetes and pancreatic insufficiency requiring enzyme supplements may still need treatment despite corticosteroids.

This patient had autoimmune pancreatitis. He had an IgG4 of 4.0g/L (reference range 0.1–1.3g/L), and was treated with prednisolone. His jaundice resolved and CT scan returned to normal. Five years later he remains well with no recurrence of jaundice or weight loss.

Further reading

Kawa S, Hamano H (2007). Clinical features of autoimmune pancreatitis. *J Gastroenterol*; **42** (Suppl. XVIII): 9–14.

Pickartz T, Mayerle J, Lerch MM (2007). Autoimmune pancreatitis. *Nature Clin Practice Gastroenterol*; **4**: 314–23.

Sugumar A, Chari S (2009). Autoimmune pancreatitis: an update. *Expert Rev Gastroenterol Hepatol*; **3**: 197–204.

Toomey DP, Swan N, Torreggiani W, Conlon KC (2007). Autoimmune pancreatitis. *Brit J Surg*; **94**: 1067–74.

Case 14

A 68-year-old retired book keeper with alcoholic liver disease was seen in the gastroenterology clinic with symptoms of gastro-oesophageal reflux. Thirteen years previously, she had been found to have liver cirrhosis with portal hypertension and oesophageal varices, which had bled. She had then remained abstinent of alcohol, with improvement in her liver function. She had also had a mastectomy for breast cancer 3 years before.

Investigations showed:

- Hb 12.9g/dL, WCC 4.6 x 10^9/L, platelets 148 x 10^9/L
- Prothrombin time 12.7 sec
- Na 139mmol/L, K 4.3mmol/L, creatinine 95μmol/L
- Bilirubin 23μmol/L, ALT 19 IU/L, ALP 126 IU/L, albumin 40g/L
- Ultrasound scan of the abdomen revealed a 25mm hypoechoic lesion in the right lobe of the liver. The remainder of the liver was heterogeneous and had an irregular margin. The spleen was mildly enlarged, with a bipolar length of 13cm.
- CT scan of the abdomen confirmed the presence of a 33mm exophytic nodule arising from the tip of the right lobe of the liver. This enhanced avidly in the arterial phase and was isodense with the rest of the liver in the portal phase. There was no other focal liver lesion. The liver had a grossly irregular surface, in keeping with cirrhosis. There was splenomegaly (16cm), but no significant collaterals. The portal vein was patent and there were no ascites. (Figs 14.1 and 14.2).

Questions

14a) What is the likely diagnosis?

14b) What are the risk factors for the development of this condition?

14c) How is this condition staged?

14d) Discuss the therapeutic options.

14e) Discuss therapy for this patient.

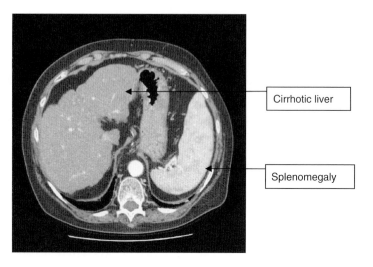

Fig. 14.1 CT scan showing the cirrhotic liver. Note the shrunken liver with irregular outline and enlarged spleen, due to portal hypertension.

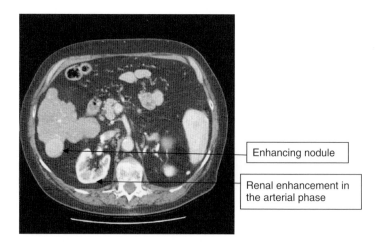

Fig. 14.2 A CT scan showing a round lesion at the tip of the right lobe of the liver, with intense contrast enhancement seen during the arterial phase.

Answers

14a) **What is the likely diagnosis?**

An isolated space-occupying lesion in a cirrhotic liver is highly suspicious of **hepatocellular carcinoma**. In this case, the lesion was >2cm in diameter and hypervascular, shown by contrast enhancement in the arterial phase of the CT scan, which is characteristic of hepatocellular carcinoma.

The diagnosis of hepatocellular carcinoma is probable in a cirrhotic liver when two radiological modalities show a focal lesion, with contrast enhancement in at least one imaging technique. A lesion seen on a single imaging modality with contrast enhancement plus serum α-fetoprotein >400ng/ml is also considered diagnostic. A false-positive elevation in α-fetoprotein may occur in chronic viral hepatitis with active replication and no focal liver lesion, or acute hepatic necrosis from any cause. Furthermore, the serum α-fetoprotein may be within the normal range if the hepatocellular carcinoma is <2cm in diameter. Preoperative sequential radiological imaging is 98% sensitive and 100% specific for predicting hepatocellular carcinoma by these criteria. Needle biopsy of a liver lesion suspected of being a hepatocellular carcinoma is best avoided, because there is a 1.5–5% risk of tumour seeding in the needle tract. Biopsy, however, is reasonable in lesions of >2cm if radiological findings are indeterminate, or if the tumour is unresectable, and a decision on systemic therapy depends on the histopathology.

The characterization of **liver lesions <2cm** in diameter, remains difficult. Lesions <1cm still carry a 50% chance of being malignant. Consequently interval ultrasound scanning (about 3-monthly) is recommended to identify enlargement. For lesions 1–2cm in diameter, biopsy may well be appropriate, but should be discussed with the hepatobiliary surgeon who will potentially resect the lesion. Small tumours may be well differentiated and difficult to distinguish histologically from normal liver. Fluorescent *in situ* hybridization (FISH) analysis, which is already used in the diagnosis of cholangiocarcinoma from cytological sampling of biliary strictures, may help by demonstrating aneuploidy in suspicious liver lesions. Aneuploidy is diagnostic of neoplastic transformation.

14b) **What are the risk factors for the development of this condition?**

Liver cirrhosis of any cause is the main risk factor for the development of hepatocellular carcinoma, since 80% develop in cirrhotic livers. Hepatitis C virus infection accounts for most cases in the developed world and up to a third will develop hepatocellular carcinoma in their lifetime. The annual incidence is 3–5% in this group. In Asia and Africa, chronic hepatitis B virus infection is the major cause, with an annual incidence of 2–6% in those with cirrhosis. Consequently, screening for hepatocellular carcinoma is recommended for patients with cirrhosis, usually by ultrasound of the liver at 6-monthly intervals. Even though the sensitivity of ultrasound is low (20–50%), specificity is 92–96% in cirrhotic patients and it is readily available, relatively low cost, and carries no risk. Sensitivity is least for small lesions.

Magnetic resonance imaging with angiography has a high sensitivity for lesions 1–2cm in diameter, but is expensive, insensitive for lesions <1cm, and not uniformly available. It is (with CT) used mainly to confirm a diagnosis of hepatocellular carcinoma when ultrasound has detected a liver lesion. Positron emission tomography has low sensitivity for lesions <2cm in diameter. Nevertheless, there are no data that show a survival benefit from screening in cirrhosis, although patients who have a hepatocellular carcinoma detected in the context of a screening programme have smaller tumours with a higher application of potentially curative therapies.

14c) **How is this condition staged?**

Staging of hepatocellular carcinoma is complicated, because the severity of the underlying liver disease affects survival, as well as the tumour-related stage. The **Barcelona-Clinic Liver Cancer stage** takes into account tumour characteristics (size, vascular invasion, and extra-hepatic spread), stage of liver disease (Child–Pugh score, portal hypertension, bilirubin), and the patient's performance status. This is currently the standard for management of hepatocellular carcinoma. Patients with hepatocellular carcinoma are divided into three groups, Stage 0, Stages A–C, and stage D:

- Stage 0 (very early stage): Child–Pugh A, performance status 0 with carcinoma *in situ* or a single mass <2cm

- Stages A–C (early stage [A], intermediate stage [B], and advanced stage [C]): all Child–Pugh A or B

  - Stage A: single to 3 nodules <3cm and performance status 0

  - Stage B: multiple nodules and performance status 0

  - Stage C: portal invasion, lymph node or distant metastases, and performance status 1–2

- Stage D (Terminal stage): Child–Pugh C, performance status 3–4 with extensive liver involvement (accounts for >50% of patients).

14d) **Discuss the therapeutic options**

Therapeutic options depend on the stage and can be divided into **resectable** or **unresectable disease**. Only stage 0 and stage A tumours are potentially resectable and only these are potentially curable. Stage A hepatocellular carcinoma has a 5-year survival of 50–70% if treated by orthotopic liver transplantation, resection, or complete local ablation. Even in this group, outcomes vary. Three subgroups (defined as a single tumour of <2cm, a single tumour 2–5cm and, up to three lesions with none larger than 3cm in diameter) each have different treatment outcomes. Orthotopic liver transplantation can be considered if there is a single tumour <5cm, or up to three lesions with none larger than 3cm (the so-called **Milan criteria**). **Transplantation** has the potential advantage of curing the underlying liver disease and removing the risk of subsequent tumours, and a 5-year survival of 70% has been reported.

For patients who have resectable disease but are not considered suitable for transplant, **hepatic resection** depends on the stage of liver disease. The best candidates for resection are patients with cirrhosis who are Child–Pugh A, have a normal bilirubin, and no clinical evidence of portal hypertension. Only 10% of patients fall into this category. Hepatocellular carcinoma without cirrhosis is uncommon in the west (5%), but much more common in Asia (40%). Resection is the therapy of choice. Within this group, outcomes are worse for larger tumours, since size is a surrogate marker for vascular invasion.

Local ablation is potentially appropriate for patients with Stage A hepatocellular carcinoma who are unsuitable for resection or transplantation. Eighty percent of tumours <3cm can be completely ablated, but only 50% of tumours 3–5cm in diameter. Five-year survival is 40–70%. Patients who are Child–Pugh A, with single, small tumours (<3cm) fare best. Techniques include percutaneous ethanol injection and radiofrequency ablation. Radiofrequency ablation is more effective than ethanol, but there are no data comparing outcomes between ablation and resection. Patients who have unresectable disease have a median survival <1 year, although heterogeneity is illustrated by the fact that 2-year survival ranges from 8% to 50%.

Intermediate (stage B) hepatocellular carcinoma is defined as an unresectable tumour in an asymptomatic patient and carries a median survival of 16 months. This can be extended to 20 months by **hepatic artery chemoembolization** in those patients with a patent portal vein.

Advanced (stage C) hepatocellular carcinoma (symptomatic patients with extrahepatic spread or vascular invasion) have a median survival of 6 months. **Sorafenib**, a multi-kinase inhibitor, has been shown to improve survival in these patients by a median of 3 months, becoming the first systemic therapy for hepatocellular carcinoma to show a clinically significant benefit. It stabilizes disease, as opposed to inducing tumour shrinkage, which is the traditional measure of response to cytotoxic chemotherapy.

End-stage hepatocellular carcinoma (Stage 0, performance status 3–4, severe tumour related symptoms), or patients with Child–Pugh C cirrhosis have a dismal prognosis, with a median survival of 3 months. Palliative care is appropriate.

14e) **Discuss therapy for this patient**

Our patient was asymptomatic, had stable cirrhosis, Child–Pugh A (see Case 8), but significant portal hypertension, with a 3.3cm lesion in her liver. The size made it unsuitable for hepatic resection, and the age of 68 years, with a history of breast cancer, excluded her from liver transplantation. She underwent local tumour ablation with radiofrequency ablation. A CT scan performed 11 months after ablation showed no local recurrence and no new liver lesions (Fig. 14.3).

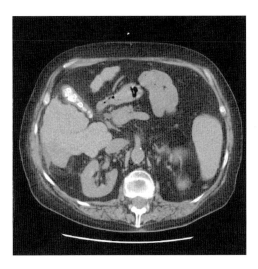

Fig. 14.3 A CT scan 11 months after ablation of the lesion at the tip of the right liver lobe (compare with Fig. 14.1).

Further reading

Talwalker JA, Gores GJ (2004). Diagnosis and staging of hepatocellular carcinoma. *Gastroenterology*; **127**: S126–32.

Llovet JM, Bruix J (2008). Novel advancements in the management of hepatocellular carcinoma in 2008. *J Hepatol*; **8**: S20–S37.

Llovet JM, Ricci S, Mazzaferro V *et al.* (2008). Sorafenib in advanced hepatocellular carcinoma. *N Engl J Med*; **359**: 378–90.

Lin SM, Lin CJ, Lin CC *et al.* (2004). Radiofrequency ablation improves prognosis compared with ethanol injection for hepatocellular carcinoma ≤4cm. *Gastroenterology*; **127**: 1714–23.

Case 15

A 50-year-old female schoolteacher presented to the outpatient department with a 12-year history of abdominal pain, straining at stool, a feeling of incomplete evacuation, and needing to return to the toilet several times after defecation. She often used per-vaginal digitation to assist the passage of stool and would spend up to 30 minutes on the toilet at any one time. She had seen a dietitian in the past and was on a high-fibre diet and using cracked linseed supplements, and occasional laxatives. Her bowels were currently opening about once daily, although 'always with difficulty'. She described daily flatus incontinence, but denied any faecal incontinence. Prior to the onset of these symptoms, her bowels had opened every 1–2 days with no difficulty. She had a 13-year-old son (weighing 3700g [8lb 8oz] at birth), born by vaginal delivery with the aid of forceps. She remembered having a vaginal tear at this time, requiring sutures.

Otherwise, her medical history included an epigastric hernia repair 4 years ago, and mild urinary stress incontinence. She had no urinary frequency.

On examination, she had a soft abdomen with no palpable masses. Her pulse was 76bpm and she was clinically euthyroid. Perineal examination revealed some perineal descent when the patient was asked to strain. Perineal and sacral sensation was normal. Rectal examination revealed small pellets of firm stool, but was otherwise normal. Sigmoidoscopy showed normal rectal mucosa. Proctoscopy showed moderate mucosal prolapse but no haemorrhoids.

Questions

15a) What is the most likely cause for the patient's constipation?

15b) What is the differential diagnosis?

15c) How would you further investigate this patient?

15d) What types of laxatives are used for different causes of constipation?

Answers

15a) **What is the most likely cause for the patient's constipation?**

The most likely cause of this patient's constipation is **functional outlet obstruction**, due to excessive perineal descent (descending perineum syndrome). The history of straining at stool for prolonged periods, feeling of incomplete evacuation, and need for digitation, are the symptomatic hallmarks. A history of a vaginal delivery of a large baby, requiring forceps, and symptoms of urinary stress incontinence are also consistent with this diagnosis. Such a history needs to be elicited empathetically and carefully, primarily by thinking of the possibility rather than dismissing any history of constipation as due to inadequate dietary fibre.

15b) **What is the differential diagnosis?**

Every patient with constipation needs a thorough **history** and careful examination of the perineum as well as a rectal examination. Systemic symptoms that might suggest hypothyroidism or hypercalcaemia should be considered. The duration of symptoms, maximum interval between defecation, sensitive questioning on the process of defecation, and an appropriate obstetric history are all important, although not specific for the diagnosis. **Examination** should include inspection of the perineum for any local tear or lesion, a request to strain as if the bowels were going to open so that perineal descent can be assessed (usually <2cm), assessment of sacral sensation (in case of a neurological cause), and rectal examination. Sigmoidoscopy is not essential unless there are symptoms such as bleeding. The **differential diagnoses** shown in Table 15.1 should be considered.

15c) **How would you further investigate this patient?**

Although the history does not suggest a non-gastroenterological cause of constipation, **blood tests** should be carried out for calcium, thyroid function tests, potassium, glucose, and renal function. Blood tests in this lady were normal and symptoms suggested a gastroenterological cause. **CT colonography** (also known as CT pneumocolon, or virtual colonoscopy) is appropriate at this age (our patient was 50) rather than colonoscopy to exclude a structural cause, because it is non-invasive, generally readily available, and does not need sedation. Colonoscopy is better reserved for those aged <45 years old, but it is exceptional to find anything other than pseudomelanosis coli from the use of stimulant laxatives when the history of constipation is so long. The CT colonography in this patient was normal.

Table 15.1 Differential diagnosis of constipation

Cause	Comment
Non-gastroenterological causes	
Drugs	Specifically ask about analgesics
	Also consider calcium antagonists, tricyclics, iron supplements, and many others
Environment and diet	Ask about soluble dietary fibre (linseed is more effective than bran), access to the toilet (delay can reduce the urge to defecate), and consider poor mobility as a contributing factor
	Occupational exposure to lead still occurs
Endocrine and metabolic	Hypothyroidism, hypercalcaemia, hypopituitarism, diabetes, hypokalaemia, rarely uraemia
	Always check thyroid function, calcium, and electrolytes
Neuromuscular	Parkinson's disease, autonomic neuropathy (usually diabetic), or spinal cord damage are occasional causes, but it is important to consider a lesion in the conus if constipation is progressive or associated with nocturnal back pain
	Many rare myopathies are associated with constipation
Psychiatric conditions	Constipation can be a feature of the psychomotor retardation of depression.
Gastroenterological causes	
Structural	Pain from an anal fissure or obstruction due to a neoplasm (may be pelvic rather than colorectal), stenosis from diverticular or Crohn's disease, volvulus, or intussusception (may be rectal-rectal intussusception)
Functional • normal transit • slow transit • functional outlet obstruction	Normal transit means constipation-predominant irritable bowel syndrome
	Slow transit is life-long and associated with extreme intervals between defaecation (often >1 week). Transit studies using radio-opaque markers are appropriate if the interval between defaecation is >5 days
	Functional outlet obstruction is suspected from the history and is an indication for defecation proctography to image the dynamics of defaecation

A functional cause seemed likely. A **transit study** is always indicated, as history alone does not discriminate between slow transit constipation and functional outlet obstruction. A **defaecating proctogram** (Fig. 15.1) showed 4cm descent of the perineal body during evacuation, a large anterior rectocele, and a recto-rectal intussusception. Thirty percent of the instilled barium paste was retained after evacuation.

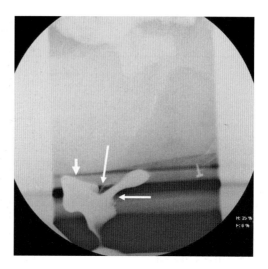

Fig. 15.1 Single lateral image from a defecating proctogram showing intra-rectal intussuscption (long arrows) and a moderate anterior rectocele (short arrows).

The radiological appearance was consistent with functional outlet obstruction due to the descending perineum syndrome. **Anorectal manometry** showed a low anal sphincter resting pressure and **endoscopic ultrasound** (Fig. 15.2) identified a defect in the external anal sphincter. The internal sphincter was normal.

The history and investigations were consistent with a defaecation disorder, although it may be debated whether a dynamic anatomical change causing obstruction is best classified as 'structural' or 'functional'.

Treatment includes biofeedback therapy, appropriate use of laxatives (15d), and surgery. **Biofeedback therapy** is only available at specialist centres. When a cause can be anatomically defined, patients are best referred to a colorectal surgeon with an interest in pelvic floor disorders for discussion about surgical intervention, although surgery is not appropriate for all patients. The decision about when *not* to operate for dynamic obstruction is as important as a decision to operate.

Our patient underwent a laparoscopic anterior mesh rectopexy to correct her recto-rectal intussusception and had a good result. Three months after surgery bowels were opening once daily, with no sensation of incomplete evacuation and no need to digitate.

15d) **What types of laxatives are used for different causes of constipation?**

There are four groups of laxatives and over 60 different preparations (Table 15.2), but adjusting dietary fibre intake and an osmotic laxative, with only an occasional stimulant, work for most. The diagnosis should be reassessed if two sorts of laxative are ineffective. Any laxative is dangerous in mechanical obstruction.

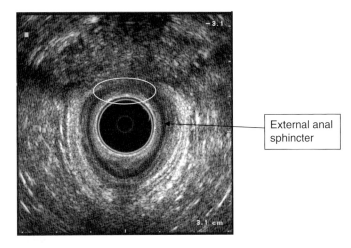

Fig. 15.2 Defect in the external anal sphincter (circled).

Table 15.2 Different types of laxatives

Type	Comment
Bulk-forming laxatives	For constipation-predominant irritable bowel syndrome or painful anorectal conditions, with extra fluid, isphagula husk (Fybogel®) can be prescribed, but is relatively expensive.
	Golden or cracked linseed, available in the cereal section of any supermarket, are good sources of soluble fibre that take up water readily.
	Fibre usually makes symptoms from neuropathic, structural, slow-transit constipation, or defaecation disorders worse
Osmotic laxatives	Indicated when bulk-forming laxatives are ineffective
	Lactulose (30–100mL/day, often too little given), polyethylene glycol 3350 (Movicol® 1–3 sachets/day), or sodium picosulphate (Laxoberal®, 5–20mL/day available over the counter in the UK)
	Generally take several days to work and need to be taken on a regular basis and the dose adjusted according to effect
Stimulant laxatives	For opioid-induced constipation, bowel clearance, neurological disorders or temporary use in stubborn constipation
	Long-term use should be avoided
	Anthraquinones (e.g. Senna – 2–4 tablets at night), bisacodyl (e.g. Dulcolax 5–10mg at bedtime), or codanthrusate (1–3 capsules, or 5–15mL at night) are appropriate for patients on long-term morphine, but the latter carries a small carcinogenic risk

(continued)

Table 15.2 (continued) Different types of laxatives

Type	Comment
Faecal softeners	For stubborn constipation
	Glycerine suppositories or an enema (e.g. Micralax®, or Fleet Enema) can be given 2–3 times a week to prevent recurrent faecal impaction
	Docusate sodium (100mg capsule once or twice daily, or as a liquid) is modestly effective

Further reading

D' Hoore A, Penninckx F (2003). Obstructed defaecation. *Colorectal Dis*; **5**: 280–7.

Andromanakos N, Skandalakis P, Troupis T, Filippou (2006). Constipation of anorectal outlet obstruction: Pathophysiology, evaluation and management. *J Gastroenterol Hepatol*; **21**: 639–46.

Muller-Lissner S (2007). The difficult patient with constipation. *Best Practice Research Clin Gastro*; **21**: 473–84.

Case 16

A 53-year-old South African woman was being followed up in cardiology clinic for ischaemic heart disease. She had been feeling unwell in the preceding week, with nausea and vomiting accompanied by general malaise. She had not recently travelled. She smoked 15 cigarettes per day. Her son, with whom she lived, had had a flu-like illness in the preceding weeks.

On examination, she was jaundiced. She had a tender liver, but no signs of chronic liver disease.

Investigations showed:

- Hb 18.4g/dL, WCC 7.0 x 10^9/L, platelets 143 x 10^9/L
- Na 137mmol/L, K 4.1mmol/L, creatinine 79μmol/L
- Bilirubin 95μmol/L , AST 1160 IU/L, ALT 3422 IU/L, albumin 39g/L
- Prothrombin time 15 sec
- INR 1.3
- Blood film: plasma cells noted.

Questions

16a) What is the differential diagnosis and what investigations are indicated?

16b) Considering the results given in Answer 16a), discuss the clinical course of this disease.

16c) Discuss the transmission and prevention of this disease.

16d) What is the significance of the plasma cells seen on the blood film?

Answers

16a) **What is the differential diagnosis?**

The differential diagnosis is that of an **acute hepatitis**. This includes acute viral hepatitis, autoimmune liver disease, drug toxicity (see Case 1) and in view of her ischaemic heart disease, it is important to consider ischaemic hepatitis. Ischaemic hepatitis is usually seen in patients with congestive heart failure who become hypotensive. It is a result of hepatic venous outflow obstruction combined with reduced hepatic arterial blood flow. In the absence of risk factors for acute hepatitis B infection, such as intravenous drug use, unscreened blood products or sexual exposure, the most common viral causes are hepatitis A and hepatitis E. Epstein–Barr virus and cytomegalovirus are uncommon causes in this age group. Alcoholic hepatitis does not cause a pronounced transaminitis (ALT is almost always <300 IU/L).

The pronounced transaminitis is most consistent with a viral cause. An ultrasound scan of the abdomen was unremarkable.

- HAV IgM positive, HBsAb negative, HBsAg negative

- Antinuclear antibody negative, anti-smooth muscle antibody negative, IgG 10.9g/L.

16b) **Discuss the clinical course of this disease.**

The patient has **acute hepatitis A**. The incubation period after ingestion of the virus is 15–50 days (mean 28 days). Patients typically have a flu-like prodrome that starts suddenly, lasts 5–7 days, and may be accompanied by nausea and vomiting. This is followed by jaundice. **Faecal shedding** of viral particles is greatest in the prodrome, with marked reduction in viral excretion after the onset of jaundice. Viraemia occurs. The onset of jaundice is preceded by darkening of urine. Clinically there may be mild enlargement of the liver, which is often tender. Serum transaminases may be elevated up to 100 times the upper limit of normal. The bilirubin is usually <170μmol/L. Symptomatic disease occurs more frequently and is more severe in adults: 70% develop symptoms with jaundice, whereas 70% of children under the age of 6 years will be asymptomatic. Even if young children have viral symptoms, they rarely become jaundiced. Most illnesses resolve completely within 3–6 months.

Occasionally hepatitis A may be complicated by acute liver failure, prolonged cholestasis or relapse. **Acute liver failure** occurs in <1% of patients and typically presents with progressive jaundice and subsequent encephalopathy. Risk factors include the elderly and those with pre-existing liver disease. Mortality is up to 95% without liver transplantation. Indicators of a poor prognosis once acute liver failure has developed include age >40 years or <10 years, jaundice for more than 7 days prior to encephalopathy, serum bilirubin >291µmol/L, and prothrombin time >25 sec. **Prolonged cholestasis** is uncommon, but is associated with worsening jaundice (bilirubin >340µmol/L), increasing ALP, reduction in ALT, and predominant pruritus. It may persist for months, but complete resolution usually occurs. **Relapse** of hepatitis rarely occurs weeks or months after initial resolution of hepatitis. Symptoms and transaminitis may be similar to the initial episode. The prognosis is good.

Treatment of hepatitis A is supportive. Admission is indicated for severe cases with hepatic decompensation, or if there is dehydration and electrolyte imbalances secondary to vomiting. Avoidance of hepatic toxins (alcohol, paracetamol) is advisable.

16c) **Discuss the transmission and prevention of this disease.**

Transmission is enteric (**faecal–oral**) and the usual source of contact is within a household in endemic areas. Up to 50% of household members of an index case may acquire infection without prompt and meticulous preventive measures. Daycare centres for babies and small children are an important source of infection. **Epidemics** are associated with poor sanitation, overcrowding, and low socioeconomic status. **Sporadic** outbreaks may be associated with a single source, shared by large numbers of people (such as drinking water or contaminated food). Contact with sewage (occupational or incidental), ingestion of uncooked shellfish, and travel by non-immune individuals to endemic areas are well-recognized risk factors and should be identified by a careful history. In **low-prevalence areas**, outbreaks are mainly food borne. Intravenous drug use is a risk factor through poor living conditions, although parenteral transmission by contaminated blood products has been documented.

Prevention is through adequate sanitation, primary vaccination, and post-exposure prophylaxis. An important component of secondary prevention is notification of local authorities of an index case. Hepatitis A is a **notifiable disease**.

Even before HAV serology was available, passive immunization with human immunoglobulin containing anti-HAV IgG was the mainstay of prophylaxis. Since 1992, inactivated HAV vaccine has been available in Europe (Havrix®). A second vaccine (Vaqta®) became available in 1996. Vaccine is given in two separate doses. After a single dose, 100% of people will have protective antibodies at 6 months. This persists for at least 1 year. A second dose provides effective immunity for up to 20 years. Antibody concentration in the serum after two doses of vaccine may be as high as those seen following natural infection.

Vaccination has markedly reduced the incidence of hepatitis A. Annual cases reported to the Centers for Disease Control in the USA have dropped from 30,000 before the introduction of vaccination to <4000 in 2006. Hepatitis A vaccination is part of the routine childhood vaccination schedule in the USA, given by the time the child is 2 years old. This is not the practice in all countries. Specific indications for immunization include travel from areas of low prevalence to areas of high prevalence, underlying chronic liver disease, clotting factor deficiencies requiring frequent administration of blood products, and intravenous drug use. Epidemic outbreaks in a community can be rapidly terminated by blanket immunization.

Intramuscular injection of pooled human immunoglobulin is effective **post-exposure prophylaxis** when given within 2 weeks of contact with an index case. Even if infection is not prevented, it is attenuated. The passive immunity lasts about 3 months. In people with IgA deficiency, immunoglobulin is contraindicated, due to the risk of anaphylaxis. It may be given during pregnancy or lactation and no viral transmission has been documented. A trial of vaccination versus immunoglobulin for post-exposure prophylaxis showed no difference between the two. The advantage of vaccination is the cost, availability, and long-lasting immunity.

Our patient had acquired the infection from her son. Since he had subclinical disease, his source could not be identified. Had his condition been diagnosed, post-exposure prophylaxis would have been desirable due to the increased risk of complicated disease at her age, but fortunately she made an uneventful recovery.

16d) **What is the significance of the plasma cells seen on the blood film?**

Peripheral plasmacytosis is usually a manifestation of a plasma cell dyscrasia (myeloma). This should be excluded in any patient with plasma cells on peripheral blood film. A reactive peripheral plasmacytosis has been described in association with other malignancies, autoimmune disease, and infections including septicaemia, EBV infection, parvovirus B19 infection, and dengue fever. It has also been described in association with acute hepatitis A.

Our patient had normal protein electrophoresis, no Bence–Jones proteinuria, and a normal bone marrow examination. The plasmacytosis was transient and resolved spontaneously.

Further reading

Baker CJ (2007). Another success for hepatitis A vaccine. *N Engl J Med*; **357**(17): 1757–9.

Gupta A, Chawla Y (2008). Changing epidemiology of hepatitis A infection. *Indian J Med Res*; **128**: 7–9.

Koff RS (1998). Hepatitis A. *Lancet*; **351**: 1643–9.

Victor JC, Monto AS, Surdina TY *et al.* (2007). Hepatitis A vaccine versus immune globulin for post-exposure prophylaxis. *N Engl J Med*; **357**: 1685–94.

Wada T, Maeba H, Ikawa Y *et al.* (2007). Reactive peripheral blood plasmacytosis in a patient with acute hepatitis A. *Int J Hematol*; **85**: 191–4.

Case 17

A 30-year-old woman came to seek advice about her risk of cancer. Her maternal aunt had just been diagnosed with bowel cancer at 43 years of age, and her mother had been treated for endometrial cancer over 15 years ago. Her father, 35-year-old brother, and 25-year-old sister were both well. Her maternal grandparents died at a young age in a motor vehicle accident. Her paternal grandparents were alive and well, with no history of malignancy. She went on to have a colonoscopy which discovered a poorly differentiated adenocarcinoma in the ascending colon.

Questions

17a) What is the name of the most likely syndrome?

17b) What clinical criteria should raise suspicion of this syndrome?

17c) How is the syndrome best diagnosed?

17d) What surveillance should the patient be offered?

17e) Who in this patient's family should be screened and by what method?

Answers

17a) **What is the name of the most likely syndrome?**

The most likely syndrome is **Lynch Syndrome** (hereditary non-polyposis colorectal cancer, also known as HNPCC). Approximately 10–15% of patients with colorectal cancer have a family history of colorectal cancer, while only 5% have a family history of early onset (<45 years) colorectal cancer. In this situation, a combination of environmental and genetic factors plays a role, but in a small fraction of cases, genetic factors play a dominant role. Lynch syndrome is the most common inherited form of colorectal cancer. The syndrome is due to a mutation in one of the **mismatch repair genes**: MSH2, MLH1, MSH6, PMS2, which leads to multiple errors in repetitive DNA sequences (microsatellites) throughout the genome of tumours. This instability is called **microsatellite instability (MSI)**.

The cardinal features of Lynch syndrome are:

- Autosomal dominant inheritance: *de novo* mutation is very rare, unlike in familial adenomatous polyposis
- Associated cancers: endometrium, stomach, ovary, ureter/renal pelvis, brain, small bowel, hepatobiliary tract, pancreas, or skin cancers
- Development of colorectal cancer at an early age
- Development of multiple cancers (synchronous colorectal cancers – occurring in more than one site at the same time, or metachronous – occurring after an interval)
- Features of colorectal cancer: located in the proximal colon; may be multiple (synchronous) tumours; have an improved survival compared with sporadic cancers at a young age, although more often poorly differentiated
- Features of adenomas: the number may vary from one to a few; a higher proportion have villous growth pattern or mucinous histology; tendency to have a high degree of dysplasia with rapid progression from adenoma to carcinoma
- High frequency of MSI identified by MSI analysis
- Immunohistochemistry: characterized by loss of MLH1, MSH2, MSH6, or PMS2 protein expression

17b) **What clinical criteria should raise suspicion of this syndrome?**

The **Revised Bethesda Criteria** are used to identify individuals suspected of having Lynch syndrome. If a patient meets just one of these criteria (Table 17.1), it is an indication for molecular genetic studies either by analysis of MSI in the tumour DNA, or immunohistochemical analysis of mismatch repair proteins. See also the Amsterdam II Criteria (Table 17.2).

The lifetime risk for carriers of a mismatch repair (MMR) gene varies from 30% to 80%. Risk depends on gender and type of MMR gene involved. For females, the risk of endometrial cancer is 30–60%. Risk of other cancers is 10–15%.

17c) **How is the syndrome best diagnosed?**

The mainstay of diagnosis of Lynch syndrome remains an accurate family history. Clinicians should suspect the condition in patients with early onset malignancy or multiple malignancies. Such patients are best referred to specialist family cancer clinics. If the Bethesda criteria are met by the index case, immunohistochemical analysis for MMR protein expression is appropriate, as well as examination of tumour DNA for MSI.

When grading **MSI** in colorectal tumours, the tumour is referred to as MSI-high when two of the five markers show instability. If only one of the markers shows instability, the tumour is referred to as MSI-low. If none of the markers show instability, the tumour is referred to as MSI-stable. **Immunohistochemistry** demonstrates loss of function of the MMR proteins by comparing normal host tissue to that of the tumour.

17d) **What surveillance should the patient be offered?**

Surveillance for this patient would include annual or biennial **colonoscopy**, because the risk of a metachronous colorectal cancer is high. The risk for developing an invasive colorectal cancer within a 2-year period is, however, very small. It remains uncertain whether subtotal colectomy should be performed instead of segmental resection in Lynch

Table 17.1 Revised Bethesda criteria for suspected Lynch syndrome

- Colorectal cancer diagnosed in a patient <50 years of age
- Presence of synchronous or metachronous colorectal cancer, or other Lynch-related tumour in the same patient, regardless of age
- Colorectal cancer with microsatellite instability ('MSI-high',) diagnosed in a patient <60 years of age
- Patient with colorectal cancer and a first-degree relative with a Lynch syndrome-related tumour, when one of the cancers was diagnosed <50 years of age
- Patient with colorectal cancer with two or more first-degree or second-degree relatives with a Lynch syndrome-related tumour, regardless of age

Table 17.2 Amsterdam II Criteria

- There should be at least three relatives with colorectal cancer or Lynch syndrome-associated cancer: one relative should be a first-degree relative of the other two
- At least two successive generations should be affected
- At least one tumour should be diagnosed <50 years of age
- Familial adenomatous polyposis should be excluded
- All tumours should be verified by histopathological examination and not by history alone

syndrome patients with a primary colorectal cancer, especially for patients <60 years of age.

Endometrial cancer is the second most common malignancy in Lynch syndrome and female carriers of mutations are best offered **endometrial cancer surveillance**. This may include biennial gynaecological examination and transvaginal ultrasound starting at 30–35 years of age. Nevertheless, the impact of endometrial cancer surveillance on mortality remains unclear. There is a higher risk of endometrial cancer in MSH6-mutation carriers, so hysterectomy might be considered for these women after the menopause.

Ovarian cancer is more likely if there are MSH2, MLH1, or MSH6 mutations. There is no established surveillance regimen for **ovarian** cancer. Bilateral salpingo-oöphorectomy should be considered after the completion of child bearing, especially if there is ovarian cancer in the family. The risk of **gastric** cancer in Lynch syndrome in the West is low. The yield from gastric cancer surveillance by endoscopy is very low, and surveillance is recommended only if there is a strong family history of gastric cancer. **Urothelial tract** screening is also debatable and only recommended if there is a family history of urothelial cancer. There are no formal surveillance programmes for brain, small bowel, pancreas, biliary tract, or skin cancers.

17e) **Who in this patient's family should be screened and by what method?**

After identification of a mutation in an affected individual, **genetic counselling** and presymptomatic mutation analysis should be offered to first-degree relatives. Detailed information from an experienced clinical geneticist and good psychological guidance are prerequisites for sensitive presymptomatic diagnosis based on DNA testing. Identification of subjects carrying a MMR mutation is important, because surveillance can be restricted to these individuals, while those without a gene defect can be reassured and spared from surveillance. Knowledge of a mutation may influence decisions about conception, but may also affect life assurance or other aspects of an individual's life.

Once a mutation is identified, surveillance is continued for life. Screening colonoscopy is probably best performed every 1–2 years, starting at 25 years of age. Endometrial, ovarian, gastric, and urothelial tract screening should be discussed with the individual, as above.

This family was diagnosed with an MSH6 mutation. This was initially identified in the colorectal cancer by MSI analysis. Her mother and her 35-year-old brother were found to carry the mutation, although her younger sister and her father did not.

Further reading

Vasen HFA (2007). Review article: the Lynch syndrome (hereditary non-polyposis colorectal cancer). *Aliment Pharmacol Ther*; **26** (Suppl. 2): 113–26.

Ramsoekh D, Van Leerdam ME, Wagner A, Kuipers EJ (2007). Review article: detection and management of hereditary non-polyposis colorectal cancer (Lynch syndrome). *Aliment Pharmacol Ther*; **26**(Suppl. 2): 101–11.

Case 18

A 22-year-old woman from Northampton, UK was seen in the gastroenterology clinic with a 2-year history of diarrhoea, iron deficiency anaemia, and a raised C-reactive protein (RP). She constantly felt below par. She passed liquid stool without visible blood up to 8 times a day and more recently up to 3 times at night. She had intermittent abdominal pain and had lost weight, but ascribed this to being on a diet, since she otherwise felt well. She had no other medical history and was taking the oral contraceptive pill. She smoked 10 cigarettes per day, but drank no alcohol. Travel history included a trip to Ireland a month previously, without any history of travel to developing countries.

Physical examination was unremarkable, apart from a slight tachycardia of 92 bpm. She was not particularly pale. A rectal examination and rigid sigmoidoscopy were not carried out.

Investigations showed:

- Hb 10.3g/dL, WCC 8.1 x 10^9/L, platelets 632 x 10^9/L, MCV 74 fL
- Ferritin 10µg/L
- CRP 20mg/L
- Na 139mmol/L, K 3.9mmol/L, creatinine 78µmol/L
- Albumin 46g/L, ALT 13 IU/L, ALP 253 IU/L, bilirubin 4µmol/L
- Thyroid-stimulating hormone 0.38 mU/L
- Endomysial antibody negative, IgA normal
- Gastroscopy: multiple small ulcers starting in the second part of the duodenum, extending beyond the limit of insertion of the endoscope. Biopsies from the second part of the duodenum reported chronic ulceration.
- Colonoscopy and ileoscopy: severe ulceration and stricturing in the terminal ileum (Fig. 18.1 in central colour section). Multiple small ulcers were present in the caecum, distal ascending colon, proximal transverse colon, and splenic flexure, with normal mucosa in interceding areas and between ulcers.
- Histopathology: biopsies from the terminal ileum showed severe acute or chronic inflammation with ulceration and granulomas (Fig. 18.2 in central colour section).

Questions

18a) What is the diagnosis and how is it best classified?

18b) What extraintestinal manifestations may occur?

18c) Describe the management.

18d) How does smoking and potential pregnancy affect the condition?

18e) What is the prognosis?

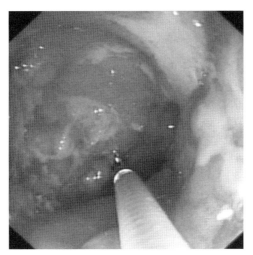

Fig. 18.1 (see colour plate 5) An endoscopic view of the terminal ileum showing inflammation and ulceration.

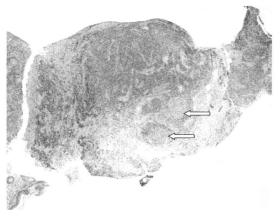

Fig. 18.2 (see colour plate 6) A photomicrograph showing non-caseating granulomas (arrows) in a biopsy from the terminal ileum.

Answers

18a) **What is the diagnosis and how is it best classified?**

The diagnosis is **Crohn's disease**. The diagnosis of Crohn's disease depends on four factors – the history, endoscopy, histopathology, and radiology. The history, endoscopic findings and histopathology are all consistent with Crohn's disease, although only a minority of biopsy specimens show submucosal granulomas.

Crohn's disease most commonly involves the terminal ileum and/or colon. Isolated terminal ileal disease occurs in about 30% at presentation and a further 30% have ileocolitis, with 30% having isolated colitis. Even though it can involve any part of the gut, it commonly stops where it starts: the pattern of involvement is usually stable over time in a single patient, particularly in adults. This is a common cause of misconception, because information about Crohn's disease usually starts by stating that it can affect any part of the gut. This gives the erroneous impression of creeping inflammation. Disease behaviour can change, however, and Crohn's disease may be progressive, with the development of complications. This includes stricturing and fistulization, requiring surgical intervention.

The Montréal classification classifies the disease according to:

- **Age at presentation** (i.e. 16 years or younger [A1], 17–40 years [A2], and >40 years [A3])

- **Maximal location of disease prior to first surgery** (i.e. terminal ileal [L1], colonic [L2], ileocolonic [L3], upper GI only [L4])

- **Disease behaviour** (i.e. inflammatory, non-stricturing, non-penetrating [B1], stricturing [B2], or penetrating [B3], and perianal disease modifier [p])

- With disease modifiers:

  - **Concomitant upper GI** involvement is indicated by adding L4 as a modifier to L1–3

  - **Perianal disease** is designated p and added to B1–3 where appropriate (see Case 19).

The Montréal classification recommends that disease behaviour is assessed >5 years after diagnosis, acknowledging that the pattern of disease can change. The cause of Crohn's disease is unknown, but it probably involves an abnormal immune response to luminal bacteria, in a genetically susceptible host. Multiple genes (32 in 2009, but rising) have been associated with Crohn's disease. These include genes involved in regulating the innate immune system (such as *NOD 2*), genes related to autophagy (such as *ATG16L1*), and genes involved in the adaptive immune system (such as *IL23R*). First-degree relatives of people with Crohn's disease have a slightly increased risk of developing the disease. There may be a primary defect in mucosal defence, as well as a dysregulated immune response.

18b) **What extraintestinal manifestations may occur?**

Extraintestinal manifestations affect about 15–20% of patients, most commonly women with colonic disease. Extraintestinal manifestations may involve the eyes, skin, musculoskeletal system, or hepatobiliary system. Involvement of the lungs, kidneys, pancreas, heart, or central nervous system has also been reported, suggesting systemic inflammation in some individuals. Arthropathies may be divided into **peripheral and axial arthropathies**. Peripheral arthritis may be pauciarticular (type 1), involving the large joints of the lower limbs and related to the activity of the underlying bowel disease. In contrast, a symmetrical polyarthropathy of the small joints (type 2), may run a more chronic course, unrelated to the activity of the bowel disease. Peripheral arthritis occurs in about 10% of patients with Crohn's disease, and is more prevalent in patients with colonic involvement, compared with isolated small bowel disease. Axial arthropathies, which include ankylosing spondylitis and sacroiliitis, are not associated with disease activity. Ankylosing spondylitis in patients with IBD is associated with HLA B27 in 50–80% of cases, which is a weaker association than ankylosing spondylitis without inflammatory bowel disease (94%).

Cutaneous manifestations include **erythema nodosum**, occurring in up to 10% of patients. It is a panniculitis, causing erythematous, tender nodules typically over the shins. It is usually associated with disease activity and commonly occurs with other extraintestinal manifestations, such as uveitis or arthritis. **Pyoderma gangrenosum** is a severe skin manifestation, often independent of disease activity. It is painful and may persist for years. Pyoderma gangrenosum occurs in <2% of patients with Crohn's disease and characteristically affects areas exposed to minor trauma. It appears particularly susceptible to treatment with anti-TNF therapy. **Sweet's syndrome** is another neutrophilic dermatosis causing a florid erythematous papular rash, associated with fever and arthropathy, on the face or trunk that is rarely associated with colonic Crohn's disease. **Ocular manifestations** include conjunctivitis, iritis, episcleritis, anterior uveitis, and very rarely ocular myositis. Precise, ophthalmological diagnosis should be considered essential. 'Eye Casualty' exists for this, because inaccurate diagnosis impairs vision. Episcleritis may reflect the activity of bowel disease, but uveitis can progress independently.

Primary sclerosing cholangitis is the most common hepatobiliary manifestation of inflammatory bowel disease. While more common in ulcerative colitis, it is prevalent in patients with colonic Crohn's disease and may be under diagnosed.

18c) **Describe the management.**

Induction of remission is the first objective. This is most commonly achieved with oral **corticosteroids**. It is wise to have a standard reducing course, to avoid excessive cumulative dosing through *ad hoc* fluctuations in therapy. The Oxford regimen for the past 30 years has been to use prednisolone 40mg/day for 1 week, then 30mg/day for 1 week, then 20mg/day for a month, before decreasing by 5mg/day each week. Others start at 40mg/day and reduce by 5mg/day each week. There is no case for maintenance corticosteroids in Crohn's disease. If disease relapses just once as corticosteroids are tapered, then immunomodulators (such as azathioprine 2–2.5mg/kg/day) should be added. If corticosteroids cannot be withdrawn within 3 months, there is a case for referral to a specialist centre to consider biological or other therapy.

Corticosteroid **side effects** may be early and dose related. These include mood disturbance, insomnia, dyspepsia, glucose intolerance, cosmetic, weight gain, and acne. Extended use may cause osteoporosis, avascular bone necrosis, hypertension, cataracts, dyslipidaemia, or myopathy, or increase the risk of infection. Rapid withdrawal may lead to acute adrenal insufficiency. Even with gradual tapering, corticosteroid-induced pseudorheumatism may occur. Corticosteroid-related side effects are less common when corticosteroids with low systemic bioavailability are used. **Budesonide** is recommended for Crohn's disease of the terminal ileum and ascending colon, but is slightly less effective than prednisolone. It is also ineffective at maintaining remission.

Biological therapies (principally anti-TNFα antibodies such as **adalimumab, infliximab**, or **certolizumab pegol** in some countries, including the USA) are a major advance in the treatment of active Crohn's resistant to or relapsing after corticosteroids. Anti-TNF therapy can help avoid corticosteroids altogether, although it is always a balance between risks and benefit.

Maintenance of remission and **prevention of long-term complications** are secondary goals of therapy. Patients with mild Crohn's disease, not thought to be at risk of long-term complications, may be observed to see if they relapse after initial corticosteroid therapy. Mesalazine was commonly used in the past, but this had little benefit in Crohn's disease, either as induction or maintenance therapy. It is not recommended in current European guidelines. The main role for **azathioprine** is corticosteroid sparing, to maintain remission. Azathioprine should be started if a patient has a relapse within 12 months of treatment with corticosteroids. Azathioprine (or its metabolite mercaptopurine) may also be used for primary prophylaxis, since it is associated with a 50% reduction in the need for corticosteroids over 18 months. Thiopurines (azathioprine/mercaptopurine) have in the past been introduced late in the course of Crohn's disease. Methotrexate is an alternative to azathioprine and probably no less effective, but is generally used only when thiopurines cannot be tolerated. Methotrexate is teratogenic and contraindicated in pregnancy.

Identifying patients at high **risk of developing complications** is potentially possible at diagnosis. Young age at diagnosis, perianal disease, stricturing disease, or the severity of disease at diagnosis (measured by the amount of weight loss, or the need for corticosteroids at diagnosis) are factors to be taken into account. When three of these factors are present, then up to 90% will have a poor outcome within 5 years, necessitating two or more resections, a definitive stoma, or developing complex perianal disease. It is particularly important to consider this in young people, because debilitating disease strikes at the most important years of their lives with respect to education, development of relationships, procreation, career development and economic activity. **Early use of biological therapy** helps reduce hospitalization and surgery: since the future pattern of disease may conceivably be identified at presentation, this should be an impetus for early referral to a specialist centre. Such decisions are complex and merit discussion with the patient.

Anti-TNFα-therapy with adalimumab, certolizumab pegol (not available in Europe), or infliximab (the first such therapy) are effective for induction and maintenance. Anti-TNFα therapy is not without drawbacks. It is expensive and carries risks including infection (including tuberculosis), infusion reactions, or possibly lymphoma when used in combination with azathioprine. The absolute risk of all these events is low, with <0.1 malignancies per 100 patient-years of treatment. Nevertheless, anti-TNF therapy has been the most substantive advance in the treatment of

Crohn's disease in the past decade, and is often introduced at too late a stage when irreversible bowel damage has occurred. Discussion at an early stage with an IBD specialist is appropriate.

Our patient was started on oral prednisolone at the time of diagnosis. Since she had extensive disease with involvement of the proximal and distal small bowel, ileal, and colonic disease, primary prophylaxis with azathioprine was started. Smoking cessation was strongly advised (see below). She responded rapidly and has not needed corticosteroids since.

The optimal **duration of azathioprine** therapy is unresolved. Evidence supports the continuation of therapy for at least 3.5 years. Even after this period, relapse occurs after withdrawal of azathioprine in 14% after 1 year, 36% after 2 years, and 53% after 3 years. Remission is usually achieved on resumption of therapy. The risk of lymphoma during azathioprine therapy is a theoretical concern, but even if the risk is increased 2–4 fold, the number-needed-to-harm (i.e. patients treated before one lymphoma occurs) exceeds 4000 <30 years of age. The general approach is to withdraw azathioprine after 5 years of therapy, based on the individual course of disease, and to reintroduce it if relapse occurs.

18d) **How does smoking and potential pregnancy affect the condition?**

The risk of developing Crohn's disease is higher in active smokers. Smoking is also associated with the location of the Crohn's disease, since smokers with Crohn's disease appear more likely to have disease in the ileum. **Smokers** have a higher incidence and prevalence of complicated disease, with more strictures and fistulas, more often requiring treatment with corticosteroids and immunosuppressants, and more often needing surgery. Smoking cessation may bring rapid improvement in the course of the disease. Interestingly, patients with colonic disease appear to be less prone to the harmful effects of smoking. Female patients with Crohn's disease are more severely affected by smoking than their male counterparts. Perineal complications of Crohn's disease do not seem to be affected by smoking.

It is important to consider that our patient is a young woman in her reproductive years (see Case 23). Patients with Crohn's disease have an increased rate of **voluntary childlessness** (18%), compared with the general population (9%). They also tend to have fewer children. **Involuntary childlessness**, however, is no higher in patients with Crohn's disease. Quiescent disease is associated with normal fertility, but active disease, previous surgery, involvement of fallopian tubes or ovaries, and perianal disease with resulting dyspareunia are associated with decreased fertility. Oral contraceptive medication has no effect on disease course, but the evolution of Crohn's disease during pregnancy is related to the level of activity at the time of conception. Quiescent disease at conception remains so in two out of three patients during pregnancy, while active disease at conception remains active in the same proportion. **Conception** is therefore best planned at a time of disease remission.

As far as the **effect of Crohn's disease on the pregnancy** outcome is concerned, data are conflicting. Increased rates of prematurity, low birth weight, spontaneous abortion, and still birth are associated with poor disease control. This underlines the need for good disease control during pregnancy. Congenital abnormalities do not appear to be increased.

The safety of medication during pregnancy is always a concern. **Corticosteroids** and **azathioprine** are considered safe, despite poorly conceived and inadequately powered studies that have failed to separate disease activity from drug administration. The advantage of well-controlled disease probably outweighs the risk of any unconfirmed increased risk of adverse outcome. Recent data show that azathioprine cannot be detected in breast milk, so **breast-feeding** is usually possible while continuing azathioprine. **Anti-TNFα therapy** with adalimumab or infliximab is probably safe in pregnancy, but data are limited. Once again risk and benefit should be assessed, and a drug should be administered only if indicated (i.e. active disease not responding to conventional immunomodulators).

Regarding the **mode of delivery**, patients with perianal Crohn's disease should generally be advised to have a caesarian section, to protect the anal sphincter. Patients with quiescent disease and without perianal involvement may have normal vaginal delivery, but episiotomy should be avoided due to the risk of developing later perianal disease. All decisions related to pregnancy, delivery, and breast-feeding have high emotive components and concerns, as well as being complex, so are best discussed between IBD and obstetric specialists.

18e) **What is the prognosis?**

At any one time, 55% of Crohn's disease patients are in remission, 15% have mildly active disease, and 30% have significant disease activity. Mortality in patients with Crohn's disease is slightly higher than the general population. Increased mortality is related to disease extent, duration, and female gender. Excess mortality is explained by disease-related deaths, but also by associated hepatobiliary disease, and by lung cancer, attributable to the preponderance of smokers in Crohn's disease patients.

Further reading

Cho JH (2008). The genetics and immunopathogenesis of inflammatory bowel disease. *Nature Rev Immunol*; **8**: 458–66.

Korelitz B (2008). What are the rules when treatment with 6-MP/ASA is started? *Inflamm Bowel Dis*; **14**(Suppl. 2): 262–3.

Katz JA (2008). How long is it advisable to continue maintenance treatment of Crohn`s disease? *Inflamm Bowel Dis*; **14**(Suppl. 2): 264–5.

Etchevers MJ, Aceituno M, Sans M (2008). Are we giving azathioprine too late? The case for early immunomodulation in inflammatory bowel disease. *World J Gastroenterol*; **14**(36): 5512–18.

Mottet C, Juillerat P, Pittet V, Gonvers J-J *et al.* (2007). Pregnancy and breastfeeding in patients with Crohn`s disease. *Digestion*; **76**: 149–60.

Lakatos PL, Szamosi T, Lakatos L (2007). Smoking in inflammatory bowel disease: Good, bad or ugly? *World J Gastroenterol*; **13**: 6134–9.

Rothfuss KS, Stange EF, Herrlinger KR (2006). Extraintestinal manifestations and complications in inflammatory bowel disease. *World J Gastroenterol*; **12**: 4819–31.

Stange EF, Travis SPL, Vermeire S *et al.* for the European Crohn's and Colitis Organisation (ECCO) (2006). European Consensus on the diagnosis and management of Crohn's disease: definitions and diagnosis. *Gut*; **55**(Suppl. 1): i1–i15.

Travis SPL, Stange EF, Lémann M *et al.* for the European Crohn's and Colitis Organisation (ECCO) (2006). European Consensus on the diagnosis and management of Crohn's disease: current management. *Gut*; **55**(Suppl. 1): i16–i35.

Walker D, Orchard T (2008). Do extraintestinal manifestations predict disease course, severity and/or activity in IBD? *Inflamm Bowel Dis* 2008; **14**(Suppl. 2): 200–1.

Case 19

A 35-year-old male financial consultant presented to the emergency department with an extremely painful perianal swelling, fevers, and difficulty walking owing to the perianal pain. He had had two previous perianal abscesses over the past decade, but both had settled with antibiotics. He had had an appendicectomy as a child and a right hemicolectomy 8 years previously for a chronic caecal volvulus.

On examination he had a pulse rate of 90bpm, blood pressure 135/80mmHg, and a temperature of 37.8°C. Examination of the perianal area revealed two discharging sinuses, and cellulitis extending into the buttock.

Investigations showed:

- Hb 14.5g/dL, WCC 15.3 x 10^9/L, platelets 567 x 10^9/L
- Na 141mmol/L, K 4.0mmol/L, creatinine 80μmol/L, urea 6.0mmol/L
- CRP 160mg/L
- ESR 78mm/hour

The emergency department registrar suspected underlying Crohn's disease and was uncertain whether to arrange investigation through the gastroenterologists, or to call the surgeons. In the event, both teams came and an MRI of the pelvis was subsequently carried out after the initial management (Fig. 19.1).

Questions

19a) What initial management would you advise?

19b) What is the differential diagnosis and what further investigations are appropriate?

19c) What does the MRI show and how does this help to classify the disease?

19d) What other imaging modalities could be used?

19e) What treatment should be considered?

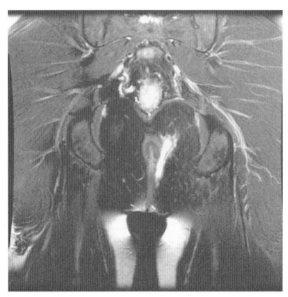

Fig. 19.1 MRI of the pelvis, performed later in the evaluation of the patient, after initial management.

Answers

19a) **What initial management would you advise?**

The priority is to **drain the perianal sepsis**. This is done by an urgent examination under anaesthetic, so the surgeons should be called immediately.

Perianal pain of this nature means that there must be an abscess, which is destructive and will damage the anal sphincter unless drained. Perioperative **antibiotics** (initially intravenous, then oral metronidazole 400–500mg 3 times daily, and a quinolone or cephalosporin for 7–10 days) are advisable in view of the extensive cellulitis. The surgeon should not only drain the abscess, but seek a fistula: a **seton** drain should be inserted at this initial presentation if the fistula tract can be identified. A seton (from the medieval French for a 'bristle') is simply a loop of soft nylon that passes through the skin, fistula track, and anal canal to be tied off outside the body. Its purpose is to prevent further abscess formation by keeping the fistula open until it heals spontaneously or with medical therapy.

Acute perianal pain should be relieved by the examination under anaesthetic, and if pain persists or recurs in the following days, then it must be assumed that there is still undrained sepsis. This is an indication for a **repeat examination under anaesthetic** by an experienced colorectal surgeon. Intraoperative endoanal ultrasound may be helpful in identifying a collection. In our case, two fistulas were identified, setons were inserted and a sigmoidoscopy at the time of the examination under anaesthetic showed evidence of active rectal Crohn's disease. An MRI was subsequently carried out to confirm the internal anatomy of the fistulous tracks.

19b) **What is the differential diagnosis and what further investigations are appropriate?**

Diagnosis of perianal Crohn's disease is not usually difficult (table 19.1), but there is no single method. The current view is that the diagnosis is established by a combination of clinical presentation, endoscopic appearance, radiology, and histopathology.

Perianal abscesses or fistulae may precede the diagnosis by some years, as in this case. Although the diagnosis of Crohn's disease was confirmed by flexible sigmoidoscopy at the initial examination under anaesthetic and subsequent histopathology, full evaluation is needed after recovery,

Table 19.1 Differential diagnosis of perianal Crohn's disease

Cause	Comment
Infection	Tuberculosis usually includes peritoneal involvement and may be indistinguishable from Crohn's disease
Tuberculosis	
HIV	HIV may cause perianal ulceration indistinguishable from Crohn's disease
Syphilis	
Vasculitis	Any vasculitis may cause focal colonic ulceration
• Behçet's	Behçet's may cause perianal ulceration
Lymphoma	Mantle cell lymphoma in elderly males may be indistinguishable from Crohn's colitis at colonoscopy: histopathology should be diagnostic
• Mantle cell lymphoma	
Other	Hidradenitis may present with florid buttock and perianal fistuas and be difficult to discriminate from Crohn's disease
• Hidradenitis suppurativa	
• Rectal mucosal prolapse	Prolapse may cause rectal ulceration that looks (and feels) like Crohn's; disease histology should discriminate

so that a management strategy to induce remission and reduce the risk of relapse can be planned. This includes **pelvic imaging by MRI**, **colonoscopy** (with ileoscopy and serial biopsies), and **small bowel imaging** (by MR-, CT-, or barium enteroclysis).

It turned out that this patient had Crohn's disease limited to the distal colon, but the presentation with perianal disease at a young age (<40 years) puts him in a category with a **poor prognosis** (see Case 18) and high likelihood of needing further surgery or a stoma in the next 5 years. This justifies a proactive approach to medical management.

19c) **What does the MRI show and how does this help to classify the disease?**

The MRI (Fig.19.1) shows complex perianal disease. There is a left transphincteric fistula on a coronal, fat-suppressed (T2) image.

Clinically, the most useful classification distinguishes simple from complex fistulae. (Table 19.2).

There are other classifications, including that of Parks, which is more descriptive and can influence surgical decisions, although complicated to use in routine practice. This describes fistulas in precise anatomical terms, using the external sphincter as the reference point. In this case the fistulas were transphincteric and suprasphincteric, so were categorized as 'complex'.

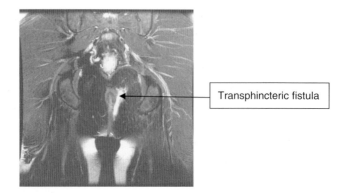

Transphincteric fistula

Fig. 19.1 MRI of the pelvis, performed later in the evaluation of the patient, after initial management.

19d) What other imaging modalities could be used?

MRI of the pelvis is the gold standard for imaging perianal fistulae, but is rarely available immediately. It is appropriate for imaging fistulas when no abscess is suspected. It has an accuracy of 76–100% compared with examination under anaesthetic, and may provide additional information. **Endoscopic ultrasound** is an alternative and has an accuracy of 56–100%, especially when performed by experts in conjunction with hydrogen peroxide enhancement. The choice of technique should depend on the expertise and availability of imaging techniques in each centre. The diagnostic accuracy of fistulography and pelvic CT scanning are too low to be clinically useful.

19e) What treatment should be considered?

Management of perianal Crohn's disease should involve gastroenterologists and colorectal surgeons. The goal is complete healing, although cessation of drainage without healing of the fistulous track is generally the best that medical therapy alone can achieve.

Table 19.2 Classification of fistulae

Simple	Complex
Superficial	Transphincteric
Intersphincteric	Suprasphincteric
	Extrasphincteric

- **Antibiotics**: this patient needed antibiotics because there were signs of systemic sepsis. In the absence of sepsis, antibiotics (metronidazole and ciprofloxacin) are often prescribed for patients with draining fistulas, although there are no controlled trials. Case series report cessation of drainage in about half of patients after 8 weeks, but recurrence is common and antibiotics are best reserved for active sepsis.

- **Azathioprine or mercaptopurine**: 2.0–2.5mg/kg/day of azathioprine, or 1.0–1.5mg/kg/day of mercaptopurine, appear to be effective in both closing and maintaining closure of perianal fistulae. Evidence comes from a meta-analysis of five trials where perianal fistula closure was assessed as a secondary endpoint. Over 50% of patients treated demonstrated fistula healing versus 21% of controls. In this case azathioprine was started as primary prophylaxis to reduce the risk of relapse, because of the poor prognostic features.

- **Infliximab or adalimumab**: infliximab was the first agent shown to be effective in a controlled trial for inducing closure of perianal fistulae, and for maintaining this response. For treatment of simple or complex perianal fistulae, 5mg/kg infusions at weeks 0, 2, and 6 induced complete cessation of all drainage in 69% at 14 weeks. After a year of maintenance infliximab 5mg/kg every 8 weeks, 36% had complete closure compared with 19% on placebo ($p=0.009$), with a reduction in hospitalization and surgery. The combination of medical and surgical management has not been subject to a randomized trial, but case series report around two-thirds achieving complete closure.

This patient had adalimumab at an early stage after drainage of the abscess, because of the poor prognostic features. It was stopped because of practical constraints on availability and he had recurrent fistulae. He needed further examinations under anaesthetic and seton placement, which remained in place over 6 months. He was restarted on adalimumab and is now well, with no evidence of fistulizing disease for over 2 years.

Further reading

Ardizzone S, Maconi G, Cassinotti A, Massari A, Bianchi Porro G (2007). Imaging of perinanal Crohn's disease. *Dig Liv Dis*; **39**: 970–78.

Behm BW, Bickston SJ (2008). Tumor necrosis factor-alpha antibody for maintenance of remission in Crohn's disease. *Cochrane Database Syst Rev*; **1**: CD006893.

Hyder SA, Travis SPL, Jewell DP, George BD (2006). Fistulating anal Crohn's disease: results of combined surgical and infliximab treatment. *Dis Colon Rectum*; **49**: 1837–41.

Kamm MA, Ng SC (2008). Perianal fistulizing Crohn's disease: a call to action. *Clin Gastro Hepatol*; **6**: 7–10.

Parks AG, Gordon PH, Hardcastle J (1976). A classification of fistula-in-ano. *Br J Surg*; **63**: 1–12.

Pearson DC, May GR, Fick GH, Sutherland LR (1995). Azathioprine and 6-mercaptopurine in Crohn's disease. A meta-analysis. *Ann Intern Med*; **122**: 132–42.

Singh B, George BD, Mortensen NJ (2007). Surgical therapy of perianal Crohn's disease. *Dig Liv Dis*; **39**: 988–92.

Case 20

A 36-year-old woman, who worked as a bank teller, was referred with an 18-month history of epigastric pain. The referring family practitioner had checked *Helicobacter pylori* serology, which was positive. Triple eradication therapy had been prescribed and her symptoms had settled for a while, but recurred. Serology for *H. pylori* was again positive. Triple therapy was again given, but symptoms persisted. She was referred for consideration of endoscopy.

She reported epigastric pain made substantially worse by food. Symptoms improved with anti-acids and omeprazole, but not entirely. She complained of nausea, but no vomiting, and there had been no change in bowel habit. She had recently been treated for iron deficiency and had lost weight after dieting, although she remained overweight on examination, with no other abnormality.

In view of weight loss and iron deficiency in the context of persistent dyspepsia, a gastroscopy was requested. This was reported as normal; duodenal biopsies were normal, but gastric biopsies revealed *H. pylori*-associated gastritis.

She was prescribed third-line therapy for *H. pylori* (tetracycline 500mg and bismuth subsalicylate 525mg four times daily, metronidazole 400mg three times daily, and omeprazole 20mg twice daily, all for 2 weeks). On completion of this complex course her symptoms had improved, but not disappeared. A C^{14}-urea breath test confirmed *H. pylori* eradication. Since her pain was worse after meals, a prokinetic drug was added with some effect.

Questions

20a) What is dyspepsia?

20b) How are symptoms of dyspepsia caused when there is no ulcer?

20c) What are the indications for *H. pylori* eradication?

20d) What are the appropriate tests for *H. pylori*?

20e) What is the further management of this patient?

Answers

20a) **What is dyspepsia?**

The term dyspepsia encompasses a heterogeneous group of disorders. It can be **defined** as the presence of epigastric pain after eating. It is generally applied to symptoms thought to be of gastroduodenal origin and should exclude heartburn, or symptoms thought to be originating from the biliary tree or pancreas. For clinical convenience, it can be sub-classified into uninvestigated and investigated. In primary care dyspepsia is extremely common and may affect up to 30% of the population at one time or another.

'**Test and treat**' is a practical initial approach to management. Patients without **alarm signs** of weight loss, vomiting, evidence of gastrointestinal bleeding or anaemia, and not on NSAIDs, can have a non-invasive test for *H. pylori* (see below). If positive, eradication therapy is given and the patient reassessed. Upper gastrointestinal **endoscopy** is appropriate for patients with dyspepsia and alarm symptoms, those with new-onset dyspepsia >50 years of age, and where symptoms persist despite eradication of *H. pylori*. This is indicated to identify peptic ulcer disease, coeliac disease, cancer, or gastro-oesophageal reflux, which are the common causes of **organic dyspepsia**. In the absence of alarm signs, an endoscopy will usually be normal and is unlikely to make any difference to management.

Dyspepsia in the absence of an organic cause is known as **functional dyspepsia**, or non-ulcer dyspepsia. The **Rome III diagnostic criteria** for functional dyspepsia stipulate that the diagnosis can be made where one or more symptoms including bothersome postprandial fullness, early satiation, epigastric pain or epigastric burning, have been present for at least 3 months, with first onset 6 months before diagnosis, in a patient with no structural explanation for their symptoms.

Our patient had a normal endoscopy, with normal distal duodenal biopsies excluding coeliac disease. Her symptoms were predominantly postprandial and, given the time scale, she met the Rome III criteria for a diagnosis of functional dyspepsia. The finding of *H. pylori*-associated gastritis does not explain her symptoms, since functional dyspepsia persists after effective treatment of *H. pylori* in most patients. The interaction between *H. pylori* and dyspeptic symptoms is complex; a positive test does not exclude functional dyspepsia. Nausea may be of central or gastroduodenal origin and does not change the diagnosis of functional dyspepsia in our patient.

20b) **How are symptoms of dyspepsia caused when there is no ulcer?**

Three factors are thought to be involved in functional dyspepsia. These are **delayed gastric emptying** (in about 25%), **impaired gastric fundal relaxation** in response to a meal with resulting impaired accommodation (in about 40%), and **visceral hypersensitivity**, specifically in the duodenum in response to acid or lipids. Basal acid secretion is normal in patients with functional dyspepsia. Smoking, alcohol intake and NSAIDs are not risk factors for developing functional dyspepsia, although once functional dyspepsia has occurred, then patients are more likely to develop symptoms if they use NSAIDs.

The **role of H. *pylori* in functional dyspepsia** remains unclear. It is possible that *H. pylori* infection constitutes a spectrum of illness, from asymptomatic infection with an exaggerated (2-fold increase) gastric acid response to a stimulus, through symptoms of dyspepsia without ulceration (associated with a stimulated increase in gastric acid production of up to 4-fold), to peptic ulcer disease in patients with a marked (6-fold) increase in stimulated gastric acid production. This is likely to be an oversimplification. It does not account for the diversity of patients with asymptomatic, but severe fundal- or pan-gastritis associated with reduced gastric acid production, in contrast to those with antral gastritis who develop peptic ulcer disease. Furthermore, <10% of patients with dyspepsia who are positive for *H. pylori* and undergo eradication therapy have symptom resolution. Nor does it account for those with atrophic gastritis, intestinal metaplasia, and an increased risk of gastric cancer. Psychological factors, especially anxiety, are associated with functional dyspepsia. Whether this is causal or whether it influences health-seeking behaviour, is unclear.

20c) **What are the indications for H. pylori eradication?**

An initial 'test and treat' approach for our patient was appropriate. She was young and at the time of presentation, had no alarm signs. This strategy is cost effective as long as the population prevalence of *H. pylori* is >15%. Below this threshold, there is an increase in false-positive tests, followed by unnecessary treatment with antibiotics. Nevertheless, the number-needed-to-treat is between 12 and 15 (NNT = the number of patients with *H. pylori* and dyspepsia who need to receive eradication therapy in order to achieve symptom resolution in 1 patient).

The general view is that *H. pylori* eradication for **uninvestigated dyspepsia** without alarm signs is recommended and reasonable. This approach in our patient was, however, unsuccessful. She had an upper gastrointestinal endoscopy, because anaemia and some weight loss had occurred, so coeliac disease and other disorders needed excluding. Had she had persistent symptoms after eradication therapy without alarm signs, a breath test would have confirmed whether or not *H. pylori* infection was still present. She was found to have persistent *H. pylori* infection and unexplained iron deficiency anaemia.

Severe *H. pylori*-associated gastritis has been associated with **iron deficiency**, but should not be assumed to be the cause unless other causes, including coeliac disease, have been excluded. Possible mechanisms include occult blood loss from gastritis, reduced availability of ferrous iron for absorption due to reduction in acid production, or bacterial utilization of iron. It is conceivable that *H. pylori* infection may exacerbate iron deficiency due to other causes, or reduce response to replacement therapy, notably in pregnancy or menorrhagia. Consequently *H. pylori* eradication is recommended in patients with iron deficiency, if infected. Investigation of the colon is still mandatory, and *H. pylori* can only be assumed to be the cause of iron deficiency once other causes for blood loss have been excluded. Another indication for eradication therapy is **long-term proton pump inhibitor** therapy. It is possible that proton pump inhibitors in the context of active *H. pylori* infection may accelerate the loss of specialized gastric glands with resulting atrophic gastritis and an increased risk of gastric cancer. It is also established that *H. pylori* is a known gastric carcinogen. Although population screening is not recommended, it is difficult to ignore a positive test. Testing and not treating does not make sense in practice.

20d) **What are the appropriate tests for H. *pylori*?**

Our patient had a serological test for *H. pylori* and was then retested after treatment. This is inappropriate, but all too common in practice, due to misunderstanding basic immunology. **Serology** is simple, widely available and inexpensive, unaffected by proton pump inhibitor (PPI) therapy, but is unable to distinguish between past and current infection. The principal role for serology is at initial presentation: infection is assumed to be current if the antibody is positive and no eradication therapy has been given. It is an IgG antibody test, so will remain positive after eradication.

Confirmation of eradication is best performed by the **urea breath test**, at least 4 weeks after treatment, once the patient has been off PPI therapy for at least 2 weeks. The urea breath test has a sensitivity of 94% and a specificity of 95%. **Endoscopic confirmation** of eradication is only appropriate in those patients who need an endoscopy for other reasons, such as a gastric ulcer that needs re-biopsy, or if antibiotic sensitivity of the *Helicobacter* spp. needs to be determined in refractory disease. At endoscopy, antral biopsies for *H. pylori* should be sent for histopathology or a **rapid urease** test may be performed. Rapid urease testing read within an hour has an accuracy of 90%. The sensitivity improves up to 24 hours at the cost of specificity. For urea breath test and rapid urease testing, PPI therapy can lead to false-negative results so is best stopped 2 weeks before endoscopy if this matters. Our patient had positive *H. pylori* serology, followed by eradication therapy and then (inappropriately) repeat serology. Subsequent biopsies taken at endoscopy confirmed active *H. pylori*-associated gastritis.

As far as treatment is concerned, **first-line eradication therapy** would have been a PPI (e.g. lansoprazole 30mg or omeprazole 20mg), clarithromycin 500mg and amoxicillin 1g or metronidazole 400mg, all twice daily for 1 week. These regimens achieve up to 90% eradication after 7 days, but higher rates of eradication are reported after 14 days' therapy. Macrolide antibiotics in the general population are blamed for resistance to clarithromycin (4% in northern Europe, but up to 20% in southern Europe). Metronidazole resistance is 20–40% in Europe, but as high as 80% in developing nations, due to its extensive use against parasites.

For **second-line therapy**, a repeat course of antibiotics (emphasizing the need for adherence), but exchanging metronidazole for amoxicillin or vice versa) is recommended. Local practice may differ. For **third-line therapy**, the addition of bismuth (as in our case) is recommended, but clarithromycin avoided, unless the strain of *H. pylori* is known to be sensitive. Tetracycline was used as an alternative in our case. **Failure of third-line therapy** is an indication for antral mucosal biopsy for antibiotic susceptibility testing at a specialist centre. No recommendations for fourth-line therapy exist, but levofloxacin and rifabutin have emerged as possible candidates. Fluoroquinolones (such as levofloxacin) are increasingly associated with *Clostridium difficile*-associated diarrhoea, while rifabutin may promote mycobacterial resistance.

20e) **What is the further management of this patient?**

Functional dyspepsia may be divided into a postprandial distress syndrome (**meal-related functional dyspepsia**), characterized by early satiation and/or postprandial fullness and an epigastric pain syndrome (**meal-unrelated functional dyspepsia**). Meal-related symptoms are attributable to dysmotility, whereas meal-unrelated symptoms appear to respond better to acid suppression. There is substantial overlap between the two groups. It follows that once *H. pylori* has been eradicated, persistent meal-related symptoms are appropriately treated with a prokinetic such as domperidone 10mg before a meal. Metoclopramide is an alternative, but crosses the blood–brain barrier and may cause dystonia in a minority. A PPI may be added if postprandial symptoms persist. For meal-unrelated symptoms, PPI therapy is first line, with the later addition of a prokinetic if necessary. To either pattern of symptoms, a tricyclic is the next step. A tiny dose of amitriptyline (10–25mg at night) is often used, but evidence of efficacy is limited.

Further reading

DuBois S, Kearney DJ (2005). Iron-deficiency anaemia and *Helicobacter pylori* infection: A review of the evidence. *Am J Gastroenterol*; **100**: 453–9.

Geeraerts B, Tack J (2008). Functional dyspepsia: past, present and future. *J Gastroenterol*; **43**: 251–5.

Malfertheiner P, Megraud F, O`Morain C, Bazzoli F *et al.* (2007). Current concepts in the management of *Helicobacter pylori* infection: the Maastricht III consensus report. *Gut*; **56**: 772–81.

Megraud F (2007). *Helicobacter pylori* and antibiotic resistance. *Gut*; **56**: 1502.

O'Morain C (2006). Role of *Helicobacter pylori* in functional dyspepsia. *World J Gastroenterol*; **12**: 2677–80.

Tack J, Talley NJ, Camilleri M, Holtman G *et al.* (2006). Rome III *Gastroenterol*; **130**: 1466–79.

Case 21

The gastroenterology registrar was called to see a 38-year-old woman with multiple sclerosis, right upper quadrant pain, and fever. She had had chole-cystitis a week earlier and a laparoscopic cholecystectomy 5 days ago. Histopathology had shown a gangrenous gallbladder with several areas of microperforation. Initially her recovery had been good, but on postoperative day 5 she developed severe right upper quadrant pain, back pain, and fevers. Her only medications were the oral contraceptive pill and interferon treatment for her multiple sclerosis. There was a family history of thrombosis, and pro-phylactic low molecular weight heparin had been given perioperatively.

On examination her pulse was 100bpm and blood pressure 130/70mmHg, with a temperature of 37.9°C. There was no rebound tenderness in the abdo-men, but there was mild tenderness in the right upper quadrant. There was no hepatomegaly, splenomegaly or ascites. Wounds from the laparoscopic surgery did not appear to be inflamed. Rectal examination was normal.

Investigations showed:

- Hb 14.5g/dL, WCC 12.5 x 10^9/L, platelets 360 x 10^9/L
- Na 135mmol/L, K 4.0mmol/L, urea 6.0mmol/L, creatinine 100μmol/L
- Bilirubin 10μmol/L, ALT 60 IU/L, ALP 100 IU/L, GGT 66 IU/L
- Prothrombin time 11.0 sec

Questions

21a) What is the most likely cause of the abdominal pain?

21b) What investigations should be done to confirm the diagnosis?

21c) Why does this problem occur?

21d) What are the possible consequences of the above condition?

21e) How should this patient be managed?

Answers

21a) **What is the most likely cause of the abdominal pain?**

The most likely diagnosis is acute **portal vein thrombosis**. The clinical features of portal vein thrombosis differ according to the stage at which the portal vein thrombosis is discovered. Acute portal vein thrombosis (as in our patient), generally presents with abdominal pain, radiating to, or predominantly in the back. Occasionally there are no symptoms; it depends on the degree of occlusion. High fever may be present in the absence of any infection. Crampy abdominal pain, ileus, rectal bleeding, rebound tenderness, metabolic acidosis, and renal or respiratory failure can occur if there is complete occlusion or any complications. The proportion that progress to chronic portal vein thrombosis and the influence of treatment are unknown. In some patients, portal vein thrombosis can occur silently with non-specific symptoms, and the cause of portal vein thrombosis is often discovered in retrospect, after gastrointestinal haemorrhage occurs.

The differential diagnosis includes a subphrenic collection and bile duct injury from surgery resulting in a biliary leak with secondary biliary peritonitis. Both are less likely on clinical grounds: a tender liver with a sympathetic pleural effusion would be expected in the former and rebound tenderness in the latter.

21b) **What investigations should be done to confirm the diagnosis?**

- Duplex (or colour-flow) **Doppler ultrasonography** is a first-line investigation, because of accuracy, cost, and lack of intervention. It is limited by obesity and overlying bowel gas that prevents imaging of the portal vein. It helps exclude an abdominal (subphrenic) collection (as in our case).

- **Contrast-enhanced CT abdomen**: the portal vein supplies 75% of the blood flow to the liver. Therefore, peak liver contrast enhancement occurs during the portal venous phase, and a decrease in portal flow can be detected.

- **Magnetic resonance angiography** is required only if the anatomy needs to be precisely defined.

21c) **Why does this problem occur?**

- **General thrombogenic factors** are present in approximately 60%

- **Local factors** are present in approximately 40%. This explains why in the course of chronic (although latent) state of thrombophilia, thrombosis develops suddenly in the portal venous system

- **Focal inflammatory lesions**: acute pancreatitis, diverticulitis, appendicitis (*Bacteroides* spp. bacteraemia), cholecystitis, inflammatory bowel disease
  - **Injury to the portal venous system**: splenectomy, colectomy, gastrectomy. As a rule, these operations do not precipitate portal venous thrombosis unless there is an associated thrombogenic state or portal hypertension
  - **Malignancy**: especially lymphoproliferative or haematological disease or (e.g. polycythaemia rubra vera), causing prothrombotic changes or compression
- **Cirrhosis**: advanced disease
- **Multiple factors** are present in 15% of patients
- **No identifiable cause**: in 20% of patients.

21d) **What are the possible consequences of the above condition?**

Portal vein thrombosis is an important condition because of serious long-term complications. The possible consequences of portal vein thrombosis are as follows.

Extension of the thrombus upstream

Ischaemia results from the extension of the thrombus into the mesenteric veins and venous arches. When ischaemia continues for several days, intestinal infarction may follow. Intestinal infarction is responsible for death resulting from peritonitis and multiple organ failure in up to half of those who die from portal vein thrombosis, even when resection of the infarcted gut is carried out. Extensive intestinal resection due to venous thrombosis is a main cause of short bowel syndrome leading to long-term parenteral nutrition (see Cases 33, 49). Small bowel stenosis rarely complicates mesenteric venous ischaemia.

Extension of the thrombus downstream

Unless thrombosis occurs in a patient with underlying cirrhosis, the consequences for the liver are barely discernible. The serum albumin and prothrombin time usually remain at low normal values, while bilirubin is normal. There is also rapid development of collateral veins, often leading to cavernous transformation of the portal vein.

Portal hypertension

Portal pressure is increased to allow portal perfusion through collateral veins. Gastrointestinal bleeding from oesophageal and gastric varices may occur after an unpredictable period. Ascites does *not* occur in isolated portal vein thrombosis, and the presence of ascites or abnormal liver function tests raises the possibility of coexistent hepatic vein occlusion.

21e) **How should this patient be managed?**

This patient needs to be **anticoagulated** to reduce the risk of complications or more extensive thrombosis, initially with therapeutic doses of subcutaneous low molecular weight heparin. A **thrombophilia screen** (below) is appropriate, then warfarin commenced. The duration of warfarin therapy depends on whether thrombogenic factors are found: life long if present, for 6 months if not. The oral contraceptive pill should be stopped.

Thrombophilia should be excluded, even when there is a local cause for portal vein thrombosis. The converse also applies. Comprehensive investigation is recommended (Tables 21.1, 21.2, 21.3) because several thrombogenic factors may occur in the same person. Specialist haematological advice is generally appropriate.

Our patient was found to have protein C deficiency, and life-long anticoagulation was recommended.

Table 21.1 Acquired thrombophilic conditions

Condition	Investigations
Primary myeloproliferative disorders	JAK-2 mutation
	Refer to haematologist for bone marrow biopsy
Paroxysmal nocturnal haemoglobinuria	Blood flow cytometry for CD55 and CD59 deficient cells
Antiphospholipid syndrome	Anticardiolipin ELISA, lupus anticoagulant
Hyper-homocysteinaemia	Serum homocystein concentration after methionine load
Systemic illness, such as ulcerative colitis, Crohn's disease, Behçet's disease	As indicated by symptoms

Table 21.2 Inherited thrombophilic conditions

Condition	Investigations
Antithrombin	Antithrombin concentration
Protein C deficiency	Protein C concentration
Protein S deficiency	Protein S concentration
Factor V Leiden deficiency	Activated protein C resistance/G1691A polymorphism
Factor II gene mutation	G20210A polymorphism
Methyl-tetrahydrofolate reductase mutation	C677T polymorphism

Table 21.3 Risk factors for portal vein thrombosis

Oral contraceptives	Mild increased risk of portal vein thrombosis. Associated cause of thrombophilia common.
Pregnancy	Uncommonly reported in association with portal vein thrombosis

Further reading

Harmanci O, Bayraktar Y (2007). Portal hypertension due to portal venous thrombosis: etiology, clinical outcomes. *World J Gastroenterol*; **13**: 2535–40.

James AW, Rabl C, Westphalen AC, Fogarty PF, Posselt AM, Campos GM (2009). Portomesenteric venous thrombosis after laparoscopic surgery: a systematic literature review. *Arch Surg*; **144**: 520–6.

Primignani M, Mannucci PM (2008). The role of thrombophilia in splanchnic vein thrombosis. *Semin Liver Dis*; **28**: 293–301.

Spaander VM, van Buuren HR, Janssen HL (2007). Review article: The management of non-cirrhotic non-malignant portal vein thrombosis and concurrent portal hypertension in adults. *Aliment Pharmacol Ther*; **26**(Suppl. 2): 203–9.

Thomas RM, Ahmad SA (2009). Management of acute post-operative portal venous thrombosis. *J Gastrointest Surg* Jul 7 [epub ahead of print].

Case 22

A 67-year-old Caribbean woman with chronic renal disease needing dialysis was admitted with diarrhoea. Three months before she had had an episode of antibiotic-associated diarrhoea, resulting from *Clostridium difficile*. She had been treated, the diarrhoea had resolved, and she had no further courses of antibiotics in the interim. She also had psoriasis, had been on prednisolone for many years, and had diverticulosis.

At presentation, she described diarrhoea for 5 days, with loss of continence, preceded by some rectal bleeding 2 days before that. No family members had diarrhoea. The day before presentation, she had developed abdominal pain, which was getting worse. She had collapsed at home, feverish, confused and shaking (possibly a rigor). Her temperature was measured at 38°C.

On examination, she had a pulse rate of 100bpm, respiratory rate of 14/min and a blood pressure of 140/65. Abdominal examination revealed a tender lower abdomen, with guarding and peritonism. Diverticulitis was diagnosed, and she was treated with intravenous coamoxiclav and metronidazole.

Investigations on admission showed:

- Hb 13g/dL, WCC 12.6 x 10^9/L, platelets 172 x 10^9/L
- CRP 159mg/L
- Na 135mmol/L, K 5.0mmol/L, urea 25.4mmol/L, creatinine 526μmol/L
- LFTs normal, albumin 36g/L
- Abdominal radiograph: non-specific bowel gas pattern
- Chest radiograph: no free intraperitoneal air, lungs clear
- CT of the abdomen: enhanced fluid-filled sigmoid and ascending colon, in keeping with colitis. No signs of perforation. No collection (Fig. 22.1).

The following day she had had six diarrhoeal stools over 12 hours, and was pyrexial with a heart rate of 136bpm. Abdominal examination was unchanged apart from distension. Stool examination had detected *Clostridium difficile* toxin (CDT). Coamoxiclav was stopped, oral vancomycin started (125mg four times daily), with intravenous hydrocortisone 100mg four times, and metronidazole 500mg three times daily. Her clinical condition did not improve. She was transferred to gastroenterology and an urgent surgical opinion was requested.

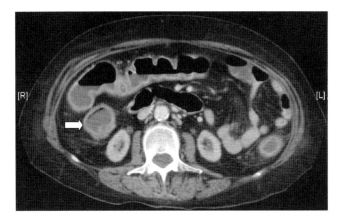

Fig. 22.1 Contrast-enhanced CT scan of the abdomen, showing a fluid-filled colon (arrow), with enhancement of the colonic wall, in keeping with colitis.

Investigations on transfer showed:

- Hb 12.0g/dL, WCC 18.21 x 10^9/L, platelets 203 x 10^9/L
- CRP >160mg/L
- Na 138mmol/L, K 4.5mmol/L, urea 24.5mmol/L, creatinine 418µmol/L
- LFTs remained normal, albumin 23g/L
- Abdominal radiography: dilated colon with a maximum diameter of 11.5cm (caecum). No evidence of free gas (Fig. 22.2).

Questions

22a) Why is *C. difficile* infection becoming more severe?

22b) What is the diagnosis in this patient and how is it best made?

22c) How is severe *C. difficile*-associated diarrhoea best treated?

22d) Discuss the complication that has occurred and its management.

22e) What strategies may prevent outbreaks in hospitals?

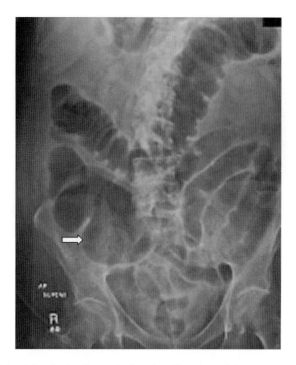

Fig. 22.2 Plain abdominal radiograph showing dilatation of the transverse and descending colon, with marked caecal dilatation, measuring 11.5cm (arrow).

Answers

22a) **Why is C. *difficile* infection becoming more severe?**

Virulence is attributed to an increase in the production of toxins A and B. This appears to be due to mutations in the tcdC regulatory genes, the product of which normally regulates and inhibits production of toxins A and B by tcdA and tcdB genes, respectively. The consequence is a 10-fold increase in production of toxins A and B by the **NAP1/027** strain, relative to the many toxigenic strains that cause milder disease. Non-toxigenic strains do not cause disease. In addition to toxins A and B, NAP1/027 strains produce a third toxin, called binary toxin, unrelated to the gene loci for toxin A or B. Binary toxin is enterotoxic, but its role is currently unclear. NAP1/027 strains have a high level of resistance to fluoroquinolone antibiotics, which has not previously been seen.

The emergence of **resistant strains** is favoured in hospital environments, where fluoroquinolones are commonly prescribed. Some of the increased mortality is related to sicker, more elderly patients in the current hospital environment. It has been recognized, however, that *Clostridium difficile*-associated diarrhoea can affect young people in the community through direct person-to-person contact, peripartum women, and patients with inflammatory bowel disease.

22b) **What is the diagnosis in this patient and how is it best made?**

This patient has **pseudomembranous colitis** and **toxic megacolon**. *C. difficile* infection can broadly be considered as a spectrum from asymptomatic carriage, to *C. difficile*-associated diarrhoea, to pseudomembranous colitis (loosely defined as *Clostridium difficile*-associated diarrhoea with a systemic inflammatory response, sometimes referred to as severe CDAD). Any hospitalized patient with diarrhoea, especially those who have had an antimicrobial within the preceding 8 weeks, should be tested for *C. difficile* toxin. Common culprit antibiotics are cephalosporins and fluoroquinolones. Clindamycin was a particular cause in the past, but is now used much less frequently.

Additional risk factors include immunosuppression, uraemia, age >65 years, burns, chronic pulmonary disease, cancer, proton-pump inhibitor therapy, chemotherapy, post-pyloric tube feeding, and admission to an intensive care unit. Diarrhoea is the hallmark and the most common presentation, but unexplained leucocytosis in a hospitalized patient should prompt a search for *C. difficile* toxin. Diagnosis of CDAD requires demonstration of bacterial toxin in the faeces. The 'gold standard' is the stool cytotoxin assay with a sensitivity of 67–100% and specificity of 85–100%. It takes up to 3 days, and ELISA is faster and cheaper. ELISA is less sensitive if an assay is used that tests only for toxin A. Tests for both toxins (TOX A/B TEST) have a sensitivity of 92–94% and a specificity of 100%. The chance of a false-negative result reduces if the test is repeated three times. Culture alone may isolate *C. difficile*, but does not distinguish between toxigenic and non-toxigenic strains. Flexible sigmoidoscopy with visualization of the mucosa may demonstrate non-specific colitis, but the presence of pseudomembranes is pathognomonic (Fig. 22.3 in the central colour section) and indicates severe disease. Plain abdominal radiography is useful to exclude toxic dilatation (maximum colonic diameter >5.5cm). A CT scan is appropriate for patients with toxic dilatation in preference to endoscopy, to look for early signs of perforation (intramural gas).

22c) **How is severe C. *difficile*-associated diarrhoea best treated?**

Treatment starts with **general fluid resuscitation** and withdrawal (if possible) of any offending antibiotic. Supportive care depends on the severity of disease at presentation, with pseudomembranous colitis being associated with hypotension, acute renal failure, abdominal pain, distension with ileus, marked peripheral leucocytosis, pseudomembranous colitis, or toxic megacolon. Before 2006, two antibiotics were commonly used. Metronidazole used to be as effective as vancomycin (response rate

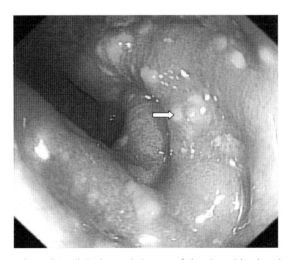

Fig. 22.3 (see colour plate 7) Endoscopic image of the sigmoid colon, in a patient with pseudomembranous colitis. The mucosa exhibits circumferential hyperaemia and oedema. There are discrete pseudomembranes (arrow). Pseudomembranes are characteristic of pseudomembranous colitis, and indicate severe colonic involvement.

90–98%). Since then, the severity of **hospital-acquired *C difficile*** has increased and responsiveness to metronidazole has declined. In our institution, vancomycin is now first-line therapy in all cases. Resistance to vancomycin has not yet been described. **Vancomycin** is significantly more effective than metronidazole in severe disease (98% vs 76%, p=0.02). On the other hand, oral vancomycin cannot be expected to have an equivalent effect in the presence of ileus or toxic megacolon, while intravenous vancomycin is ineffective because it does not reach the intestinal lumen. Consequently (and without much evidence), oral vancomycin and intravenous metronidazole 500mg are often used in severe cases. **Teicoplanin** is an alternative. To this may be added **corticosteroids**, on the basis that the colonic inflammation is toxin driven, rather than infective. Once again, this is empirical therapy, with only anecdotal evidence.

The opinion of an experienced colorectal surgeon should be sought in severe cases, because subtotal colectomy may be lifesaving, although the timing is always difficult to judge. Most patients have resolution of symptoms after 3–5 days. Vancomycin is generally continued for 2 weeks. Shorter courses, especially in the case of recurrent CDAD, may be associated with relapse.

Following resolution of the first episode, **recurrent** CDAD develops in about 20%, irrespective of antibiotic therapy. Recurrence probably results from impaired re-colonization with normal bowel flora, possibly as a consequence of the antibiotic therapy, and not from antibiotic resistance. It typically occurs 4 weeks later. Recurrence of CDAD is generally more severe than the initial infection, possibly because of the weakened state of a patient who often has multiple comorbidities. Passive immunotherapy with **intravenous immunoglobulin** (which contains antibodies to toxins A and B) reduces recurrence, or is effective in severe cases. **Probiotics** (treatment with *Saccharomyces boulardii*, or *Lactobacillus plantarum* GG) may reduce recurrence, but are ineffective as therapy. Therapies aimed at restoring bowel flora have been reported. Administration of donor faeces (from a family member, after filtering), either through a nasogastric tube or at colonoscopy, have been reported to prevent recurrence in case series, but (perhaps not surprisingly!) such therapy remains unpopular. Other non-absorbable antibiotics such as nitazoxinide or rifaximin continue to treat antibiotic-associated diarrhoea with more antibiotics. Tolevamer, an **inert polymer** that binds toxins A and B, but has no antimicrobial activity, is promising. Although inferior to current antibiotic regimens, those subjects who responded to tolevamer had fewer recurrences (3% vs 23% after vancomycin and 27% after metronidazole).

22d) **Discuss the complication that has occurred and its management.**

Our patient with recurrent CDAD had a systemic inflammatory response syndrome (SIRS) and colonic dilatation >5.5cm. This represents **toxic megacolon** and is a medical emergency whatever the cause. Paradoxically, diarrhoea may subside because of colonic dilatation and ileus, but tachycardia, abdominal pain, tenderness or hypotension and leucocytosis should alert the clinician to the need for (or to repeat) plain abdominal radiography. **Toxic megacolon** is defined as a colonic diameter >5.5cm in a patient with SIRS, or any three of the following signs: fever (>38°C), tachycardia (>120bpm), peripheral leucocytosis (>10.5 x 10^9/L), anaemia *plus* dehydration, altered mental status, or electrolyte disturbance. Risk factors for severe CDAD in our patient include recurrent CDAD and comorbidity (chronic renal disease needing dialysis). The lack of clinical response to treatment prompted surgical consultation. Observation for a further 2 days saw no improvement, so a subtotal colectomy was carried out. It is important to recognize the limited physiological reserve of sick, **elderly patients**, so a decision to (or not to) operate should be made at an early stage by an experienced colorectal surgeon. Even timely surgery in these severely ill patients is associated with a mortality of 30%. The procedure of choice is a subtotal colectomy. Less extensive colectomy has been associated with a high mortality. Our patient made a full recovery following her surgery. Pathology of the resected colon confirmed pseudomembranous colitis.

22e) **What strategies may prevent outbreaks in hospitals?**

Rationalization of antibiotic use, with restrictions on cephalosporins and fluoroquinolones, reduces the incidence of CDAD. Antibiotics (even prophylactic doses, prior to certain procedures) should be used only when indicated. *Clostridium difficile* is a spore-forming bacillus. Spores may persist for long periods in the environment and are not killed by standard alcohol-containing hand rubs available in NHS hospitals. **Thorough hand washing** is the only effective way of removing *C. difficile* spores from hands, following contact with a patient. Isolation of patients with proven CDAD may restrict spread in a ward. Of particular importance is access to dedicated toilet facilities for patients with CDAD. Establishment of specific wards to manage patients with CDAD, while in principle attractive, may be logistically impossible. Resources are often unavailable and patients still need to be managed for their primary illnesses.

Further reading

Kelly CP, LaMont JT (2008). *Clostridium difficile* – more difficult than ever. *N Engl J Med*; **359**: 1932–40.

Kuipers EJ, Surawicsz CM (2008). *Clostridium difficile* infection. *Lancet*; **371**: 1486–8.

Jaber MR, Olafsson S, Fung WL, Reeves ME (2008). Clinical review of the management of fulminant *Clostridium difficile* infection. *Am J Gastroenterol*; **103**: 1–9.

Gan SI, Beck PL (2003). A new look at toxic megacolon: An update and review of incidence, etiology, pathogenesis and management. *Am J Gastroenterol*; **98**: 2363–71.

Case 23

A 32-year-old woman with a history of Crohn's disease asked for advice about a planned pregnancy. The history of Crohn's is complex and includes:

- an ileal resection for small bowel Crohn's disease at 23 years of age
- three flares in the past 2 years that had resolved with budesonide and azathioprine
- two perianal fistulae that had required seton insertion a year ago.

She was currently in clinical remission taking azathioprine 125mg/day (weight 65kg). A colonoscopy a year ago had at that time shown aphthoid and serpiginous ulcers in the transverse and descending colon. On examination of her perineum there was scarring, but no active disease or drainage. The seton in a perianal fistula had been removed 6 months previously.

Questions

23a) Will Crohn's disease affect the patient's fertility?

23b) Should the patient's azathioprine be stopped prior to her trying to conceive?

23c) If the patient presents with active disease during pregnancy, what is the best management?

23d) What advice would you give about the mode of delivery?

23e) What advice would you give about breast-feeding and the patient's medication?

Answers

23a) **Will Crohn's disease affect the patient's fertility?**

Given that the patient's Crohn's disease is currently quiescent, her **fertility should be normal**. Patients with IBD have fewer children than the general population, but this is partly due to voluntary childlessness (see Case 18). On the other hand, active Crohn's disease or previous pelvic sepsis can reduce fertility by several mechanisms, including inflammation involving the fallopian tubes or ovaries, and perianal disease causing dyspareunia. Pelvic surgery (but not simple ileal resection) carries a risk of impaired tubal function. Remission is the best time to try for conception, and this also applies to IVF. When conception occurs during a period of remission, about two-thirds remain in remission during pregnancy, which is similar to that in non-pregnant patients with Crohn's disease over a period of 9 months. In contrast, if conception occurs at a time of active disease, two-thirds have persistent activity and of these, two thirds will deteriorate. This underscores the importance of advising patients to conceive at a time when disease is in remission.

23b) **Should the patient's azathioprine be stopped prior to her trying to conceive?**

Medical therapy for Crohn's disease (except methotrexate) should generally **continue during pregnancy**, because the benefits of controlled disease outweigh the risks of medication. Given the patient's history of small and large bowel Crohn's disease and perianal disease, she should be strongly encouraged to continue her azathioprine.

Most of the experience on azathioprine and mercaptopurine in pregnancy comes from the transplant and rheumatology literature. Azathioprine is safe in these populations, with no consistent reports of abnormalities with regard to fertility, prematurity, or congenital defects. The US Food and Drug Administration (FDA), however, currently rates azathioprine/mercaptopurine as 'class D' ('Positive evidence of risk in humans, risk/benefit ratio should be considered'). This **unfortunate advice**, which is in the process of being revised, appears to stem from animal studies using a 10-fold higher dose than is tolerated by humans. There is *no* consistent evidence of harm to pregnant patients with IBD or the fetus, but a substantial risk that stopping the drug will be associated with a relapse with potentially adverse outcomes to the patient or pregnancy.

Active Crohn's disease during pregnancy is associated with a risk of spontaneous abortion, prematurity, or low birth weight. Studies on animals given azathioprine (equivalent to 2.5mg/kg/d) or mercaptopurine (equivalent to 1.5mg/kg/d), report only low birth weights. High doses (10–20mg/kg/day) have been associated with an increased incidence of congenital malformations, prematurity, low birth weight, and chromosomal abnormalities. In humans, a follow-up study on 341 pregnancies during or after treatment with azathioprine or mercaptopurine reported no excess rates of prematurity, spontaneous abortion, congenital abnormalities, or neonatal/childhood infections. The only **prospective cohort** study confirms that the outcome in pregnant patients with IBD treated with thiopurines is no different to the general population. Consequently, despite the FDA rating, most **European IBD specialists** consider that these drugs are safe and best continued during pregnancy, because the benefit/risk ratio is strongly in favour of continued therapy. It may be worth noting (and explaining to the patient) the risks of miscarriage (12%) and fetal abnormality (5–7%) in normal pregnancy. With the exception of methotrexate, the greatest risk to a mother with IBD and fetus during pregnancy is active disease, not the medication used to treat it.

23c) **If the patient presents with active disease during pregnancy, what is the best management?**

- **Prednisolone or budesonide**: corticosteroids cross the placental barrier but are rapidly converted to less active metabolites by placental 11-hydroxygenase, resulting in low fetal blood concentrations. Prednisone or prednisolone are more rapidly metabolized than alternative compounds. Although risks of prematurity, spontaneous abortion, or cleft palate are often cited, these have only been seen in animals.

- No increase in congenital malformations has been found in humans. Enemas and suppositories are considered acceptable until the third trimester. No studies on budesonide during pregnancy are available in humans with IBD, although studies with inhaled budesonide suggest that the drug is safe. Toxic doses of budesonide have demonstrated both teratogenic and embryocidal effects in animals.

- It is important to ask the patient whether she has stopped **azathioprine** and to encourage her to restart this if she has.

- Depending on the severity of the flare and response to corticosteroids, **anti-TNF agents** can be considered. Anti-TNFα antibodies are species-specific. Murine models have failed to show any teratogenicity or embryotoxicity. Post-marketing data of more than 500 pregnancies, of which a third had infliximab during the first trimester, have shown no difference to the general population (75% live births, 14% miscarriage, 11% therapeutic termination). There are fewer, but similar data on adalimumab from a teratology registry that is independent of industry. There is, however placental transfer of infliximab (high serum concentrations have been detected in the baby of a mother who received infliximab 10mg/kg every 8 weeks during pregnancy) and of adalimumab, although it is not yet known whether this induces antibody formation in the baby. The implications of exposure to infliximab or adalimumab on the newborn are unknown, but patients and physicians should be aware that *in utero* exposure occurs, and that treatment may best be avoided in the last weeks of pregnancy if drug circulation in the neonate is to be avoided. Specialist advice is appropriate.

23d) **What advice would you give about the mode of delivery?**

The mode of delivery is primarily dictated by obstetric necessity, but it should be a joint decision with the patient and informed by the views of the gastroenterologist or colorectal surgeon. The **critical considerations are** risks to the anal sphincter and the pelvic floor in patients whose continence may subsequently be impaired after surgery, perianal disease, or active inflammatory bowel disease. The risk of a third-degree obstetric tear is very low with good obstetric practice, but the obstetrician needs to know the **likelihood of colectomy, ileorectal, or pouch anal anastomosis** before a decision to proceed with normal vaginal delivery is made.

Decision making clearly differs between individual patients, and specialist advice is essential. Vaginal delivery is usually acceptable if disease has been readily controlled with medical therapy, the risk of surgery is low, and there has been no perianal disease. Episiotomy should be avoided if possible, because a high rate of perianal involvement has been reported, but is better than an uncontrolled laceration. On the other hand, **Caesarian section** is advisable if there is active (some would include previous) perianal disease, if hospital admission for intensive treatment of inflammatory bowel disease has been necessary (since this is associated with the need for colectomy), or if the patient has had medically refractory disease. Treatment with azathioprine is a marker of the latter, but decisions should be tailored to the individual.

23e) **What advice would you give about breast-feeding and the patient's medication?**

Tiny amounts of **azathioprine/mercaptopurine metabolites** (nanomolar concentrations of methyl mercaptopurine and thiouric acid) appear in breast milk, but these are undetectable in the baby. Three studies have examined this in a small number of patients, but all are consistent.

◆ Consequently, the **benefits of breast-feeding** outweigh the theoretical risks of exposure through breast milk to the baby. This should of course be discussed with the mother, paying particular attention to the fact that the drug information sheet may advise *against* breast-feeding while on azathioprine of mercaptopurine. These information sheets were written before the studies were available.

Further reading

Caprilli R, Gassull MA, Escher JC *et al.* (2006). European evidence-based Consensus on the diagnosis and management of Crohn's disease: special situations. *Gut*; **55**(Suppl. 1): i36–58.

Christensen LA, Dahlerup JF, Nielsen MJ, Fallingborg JF, Schmiegelow K (2008). Azathioprine treatment during lactation. *Aliment Pharmacol Ther*; **28**: 1209–13.

Goldstein LH, Dolinsky G, Greenberg R *et al.* (2007). Pregnancy outcome of women exposed to azathioprine during pregnancy. *Birth Defects Res A Clin Mol Teratol*; **79**: 696–701.

Case 24

An 85-year-old retired schoolteacher was referred with a 1-month history of abdominal swelling and worsening back pain, which disrupted her sleep. Over that period she had become weak and spent most of her day in a chair. At presentation, she was in a wheelchair.

She had no constitutional symptoms, such as weight loss, fever, or night sweats, and no nausea, vomiting, or dyspepsia. Her bowel habit was unchanged. She had a history of ischaemic heart disease and took diclofenac for her back pain.

On examination, she had ankle oedema, with abdominal distension and shifting dullness, thought to be due to ascites. In the left flank there was a mobile, firm, non-pulsatile mass. It was possible to palpate above the mass, but it could not be further characterized. Vital signs were normal and there was no jaundice, signs of chronic liver disease, or lymphadenopathy. She was admitted for investigation.

Questions

24a) Describe the clinical approach to a mass in the left flank.

24b) What investigations would you request?

24c) What is the differential diagnosis, based on the clinical findings and CT scan?

24d) How would you confirm the diagnosis?

24e) Discuss factors influencing the management of this case.

Answers

24a) **Describe the clinical approach to a mass in the left flank.**

Location: a left flank mass may be a spleen, a kidney, or arise from any other anatomical structure in that location (colon, mesentery, lymph nodes). Palpation above the mass effectively excludes an enlarged spleen. Clinical signs are important when interpreting subsequent CT scan reports. A (very) enlarged spleen is characteristically dull to percussion, has a palpable notch, and descends obliquely throughout inspiration. A palpable kidney typically is not dull to percussion due to overlying bowel, may be balotable and descends only at the end of inspiration.

Mobility of a mass suggests that it does not adhere to surrounding structures, unlike a tumour that has infiltrated surrounding structures. An invading small bowel tumour may still be mobile if attached to a mobile mesentery.

Associated pain or tenderness: pain in the back that wakes a patient up at night commonly indicates pathology. It suggests inflammation or malignancy involving a retroperitoneal structure or organ. Structures in the retroperitoneum include the pancreas, lymph nodes, duodenum, kidneys, and blood vessels. Tenderness is consistent with an inflammatory process or abscess.

Consistency: fluctuation suggests contained fluid (cyst or abscess, the latter being tender). A firm mass suggests organ enlargement or tumour.

Pulsatility: a pulsating mass implies an arterial aneurysm. Note that arterial pulsation should be expansile, since pulsation may be transmitted.

Our patient had a firm, non-pulsatile, non-tender, mobile mass in the left flank associated with back pain. Clinical signs excluded a spleen (able to palpate above the mass) or a kidney (palpable, rather than balotable). This implies a **retroperitoneal lesion** or **tumour**, so both the choice and interpretation of investigations should reflect this.

24b) **How would you investigate?**

Urine dipstix: microscopic haematuria associated with an abdominal mass suggests a renal tumour. A urine dipstix was normal.

Imaging: a CT scan of the abdomen and pelvis is the procedure of choice. CT scanning images the retroperitoneum and provides anatomical cross-sectional images that can be reviewed by radiologists, physicians, or surgeons, for management decisions. Ultrasound scan avoids exposure to radiation, but provides poor views of the retroperitoneum, is a dynamic investigation that is difficult to review on static images, and may still need to be followed by a CT scan before management decisions are made.

CT of the abdomen and pelvis: see Fig. 24.1.

24c) **What is the differential diagnosis based on the CT results and clinical findings?**

The differential diagnosis includes small intestinal adenocarcinoma, lymphoma, gastrointestinal stromal tumour (GIST), or non-steroidal-induced inflammation.

   Adenocarcinoma of the small bowel is rare, with an incidence of 6 cases per million, and represents 2% of all gastrointestinal tumours, but it is the most common primary small bowel malignancy, making up 40% of the total. More than half occur in the duodenum, with 15–20% in the jejunum and 10–15% in the ileum. It is more common in patients of African origin, and in men. Adenocarcinoma develops in pre-existing adenomas or from dysplastic epithelium. Risk factors for adenocarcinoma of the small bowel include familial adenomatous polyposis, hereditary non-polyposis colon cancer (see Case 17), Peutz–Jeghers syndrome, Crohn's disease, enteric duplication cysts, Meckel's diverticula, and coeliac disease.

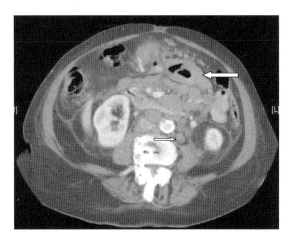

Fig. 24.1 There is extensive retroperitoneal lymphadenopathy (small arrow) with marked thickening of the mid small bowel loops (large arrow). A scan of the chest showed extensive mediastinal lymphadenopathy and there was a small amount of free free fluid in the pelvis.

Patients are typically elderly, presenting in their 7th decade. More than 80% occur >50 years of age. Small tumours are typically asymptomatic and may lead to iron deficiency resulting from chronic blood loss. Non-specific symptoms with loss of appetite and weight loss are common. Pain and obstructive symptoms occur at a late stage. Lesions of the terminal ileum may cause intermittent intussusception, with episodic obstructive symptoms.

Surgical resection is the treatment of choice. The benefit of postoperative chemotherapy remains unproven. The prognosis is poor. Following resection of disease localized to the small bowel, 5-year survival is ~50%. This drops to ~30% once regional nodes are involved and to <5% with distant metastases.

Primary small bowel lymphoma is the second most common, primary malignant tumour of the small intestine, accounting for up to 25% of all small bowel tumours. The small intestine is the most common primary extranodal site for lymphoma, making up ~10% of extranodal lymphomas. Primary small bowel lymphoma is typically focal in the bowel and localized to bowel and regional lymph nodes. Palpable peripheral lymphadenopathy is usually absent. Mediastinal lymph nodes are not seen on chest radiography, and the liver and spleen are not enlarged. Primary small bowel lymphoma is slightly more common in men and in people of European decent. Patients typically present in their 7th decade. **Immunoproliferative small intestinal disease** (IPSID) occurs in young people, especially in Iran, and is distinct from primary small bowel lymphoma in that it displays a diffuse growth pattern. Risk factors for primary small bowel lymphoma include coeliac disease, primary immunodeficiency, AIDS, chronic immunosuppressive therapy and (possibly) Crohn's disease.

Abdominal pain is the presenting symptom in more than two thirds and weight loss is reported in half. Less commonly, patients report fatigue and night sweats. Obstruction of the small bowel is evident in 10% at presentation. Acute gastrointestinal haemorrhage or perforation with an acute abdomen may also occur. Up to 50% of patients have a palpable abdominal mass.

Primary small bowel lymphoma most commonly occurs in the ileum, followed by the jejunum and then the duodenum. Regional lymph nodes are affected half the time. Most primary small bowel lymphomas are B cell lymphomas, of which diffuse large cell lymphoma is the most common, followed by **MALT-lymphoma**. **Enteropathy-associated T cell lymphoma** is typical of coeliac disease. Small non-cleaved cell lymphoma

(Burkitt) occurs in a minority of cases (5%) of small intestinal lymphomas. The treatment of choice is surgical resection. If disease cannot be adequately resected, chemotherapy may be offered. Chemotherapy alone carries a risk of bowel perforation (up to 15%). Primary small bowel lymphoma localized to the bowel has a 5-year survival of <60%. Once regional lymph nodes are involved, 5-year survival drops to 20%.

Malignant **gastrointestinal stromal tumours (GIST)** (20–25% of all GISTs) make up about 12% of all malignant small bowel tumours. Conversely, about 30% of all GISTs (benign or malignant) occur in the small bowel. Most patients are in the 6th decade at the time of diagnosis. Malignant GISTs are most commonly >5cm in diameter. Histopathologically they consist of spindle-shaped cells, thought to originate from the interstitial cells of Cajal. This assumption is based on the fact that they express CD117 and CD34, which are also expressed on Cajal cells. More than 90% of GISTs express CD117, which is a product of the *c-kit* gene and a receptor for stem cell growth factor. Most malignant GISTs show a mutation in this gene on chromosome 4, which leads to unregulated activation of the tyrosine kinase associated with CD117. This presents an opportunity for therapy.

Tumours >5cm in diameter are either palpable or present clinically, with bleeding in more than half of patients. Patients with ileal tumours often present with intussusception. Patients may also present with partial obstruction, with abdominal pain, nausea and vomiting, and with weight loss in a third of all cases.

The treatment of choice for a malignant GIST is resection. Unfortunately tumours often recur after resection. Conventional chemotherapy does not work, but **imatinib mesylate**, a tyrosine kinase inhibitor, initially shown to induce remission in patients with chronic myeloid leukaemia, is often effective in patients with unresectable or metastatic GIST. Up to 40% of patients with a GIST of the small bowel will present with liver metastases. Lymph node metastases are *not* typical. Metastatic and unresectable disease carries a poor prognosis. Imatinib prolongs survival, is orally administered, and is the standard of care for patients not eligible for surgery. Even so, tumour resistance eventually leads to tumour progression.

Malignancies of enterochromafin cells are called **carcinoid tumours**. Three quarters of these tumours are in the gastrointestinal tract and are most common in the appendix, followed by the small bowel. Small bowel tumours occur in the ileum in almost 90% and are usually <2cm in size and not palpable. Chronic, non-specific abdominal pain over a long period (>2 years) is characteristic. It is best distinguished from other causes of long-standing abdominal pain by its episodic nature. Patients are frequently asymptomatic until tumours are locally advanced or have metastasized. Liver metastases may be associated with a carcinoid syndrome (flushing, diarrhoea, and wheeze), and may include valvular lesions of the right heart.

Other tumours found in the small intestine include Kaposi sarcoma, schwannomas, ganglioneuromas, and metastatic tumours. Melanoma is the most common metastatic tumour to the small bowel (about a third), but primaries from other sites that spread to the small bowel include carcinomas of ovary, cervix, testes, stomach, colon, kidney, liver, and lung.

Based on the symptoms, the palpable mass and lymph node involvement on CT, the most likely tumour in our patient was thought to be a primary small bowel lymphoma.

24d) **How would you confirm the diagnosis?**

CT enteroclysis is the investigation of choice to image the small bowel and identify extramural extension or lymph node involvement. If this is unavailable, separate small bowel radiology after an abdominal and pelvic CT scan is appropriate (after the scan, because barium contrast interferes with the scan image). An abdominal CT scan is also the first investigation for patients presenting with an acute abdomen or suspected perforation. Barium studies are absolutely contraindicated where perforation is suspected. Tumours of the duodenum and the terminal ileum may be accessible to conventional endoscopy. Double-balloon **enteroscopy**, where available, may access tumours beyond the reach of conventional endoscopes for biopsy. **Surgical resection**, prior to histopathological diagnosis, may be necessary if there is haemorrhage or perforation, where enteroscopy is unavailable, or where tumours are inaccessible to enteroscopy.

24e) **Discuss factors influencing the management of this case.**

The first difficulty in this case was that the lesion was not within reach of conventional endoscopy, preventing a histopathological diagnosis. It was further complicated by the patient's advanced age, poor performance status (Performance Status 3 – more than 50% of her day in a chair), and local lymph node involvement, which made for a very poor prognosis. Surgical resection risked a high mortality and low likelihood of cure. Chemotherapy would similarly be poorly tolerated with a low performance status.

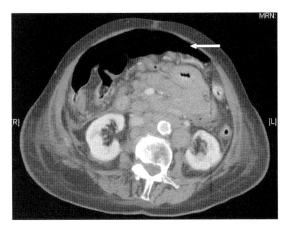

Fig. 24.2 A second CT scan, done 7 days later showing free intraperitoneal air (arrow) in keeping with spontaneous perforation of the tumour.

Consequently our patient was initially managed with inpatient enteral nutritional support and analgesia. The poor outlook was discussed with her family. Unfortunately she developed an acute abdomen within a week of admission and a repeat CT scan showed free intraperitoneal air, indicating spontaneous tumour perforation (Fig. 24.2). She underwent emergency resection of the tumour, but deteriorated following surgery and died. Histopathology of the resection specimen showed an aggressive, diffuse large B cell lymphoma (Fig. 24.3 in the central colour section).

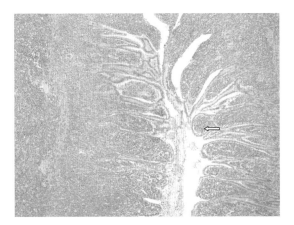

Fig. 24.3 (see colour plate 8) Photomicrograph showing sheets of uniform cells (lymphocytes) infiltrating and expanding small intestinal villi (arrow). Immuno-histochemistry showed monoclonal cells of B cell origin.

Further reading

Banks PM (2007). Gastrointestinal lymphoproliferative disorders. *Histopathology*; **50**: 42–54.

Koniaris LG, Drugas G, Katzman PJ, Salloum R (2003). Management of gastrointestinal lymphoma. *J Am Coll Surg*; **197**(1): 127–41.

Siddiqui MA, Scott LJ (2007). Imatinib: a review of its use in the management of gastrointestinal stromal tumours. *Drugs*; **67**(5): 805–20.

Case 25

A 62-year-old divorced defence lawyer presented with confusion and ascites. His daughters reported that ascites had been present for about a year. Apparently he had stopped drinking alcohol 6 months previously, but he had drunk about 20 units of alcohol per day for 30 years. Mild confusion had been present for 3 months, but it had become worse in the 2 weeks before admission. Medication at the time of presentation included lactulose, frusemide 80mg/day, and spironolactone 100mg/day. Intravenous 5% dextrose was administered on presentation to the emergency department.

On examination he was disorientated in time and place. Asterixis was present, but he was afebrile with a pulse rate of 66bpm, and blood pressure 115/60mmHg. There were multiple spider naevi and moderate muscle wasting. The liver was palpable 4cm below the costal margin and there was a moderate amount of ascites. Rectal examination revealed melaena.

Investigations showed:

- Hb 12.8g/dL, WCC 5.8 x 10^9/L, platelets 100 x 10^9/L
- Na 129mmol/L, K 3.6mmol/L, creatinine 86μmol/L, urea 6mmol/L
- Bilirubin 59μmol/L, ALP 137 IU/L, ALT 33 IU/L, albumin 24g/L
- Prothrombin time 19.8 sec
- CRP <8mg/L
- 'Liver disease screen' normal or negative (see Case 1)
- Cranial CT scan showed cerebral and cerebellar atrophy with a small chronic subdural haemorrhage. The CT appearance was similar to a CT carried out 6 months previously.
- Abdominal ultrasound showed a small shrunken liver, gross ascites, patent portal and hepatic veins; no focal liver lesions; normal sized spleen.

Questions

25a) What is the cause and pathophysiology of the disorientation?

25b) What is the immediate management?

Initially the patient improved, but he deteriorated with similar symptoms 3 weeks later. The patient was unable to return home, because he remained too confused.

25c) What further treatment would you suggest?

Answers

25a) **What is the cause and pathophysiology of the disorientation?**

This patient almost certainly has cirrhosis (excessive alcohol in the past, spider naevi, hypoalbuminaemia, increased prothrombin time, thrombocytopenia, ascites, shrunken liver) and the most likely cause of the disorientation and confusion is **hepatic encephalopathy**. Non-hepatic causes should always be considered, including intracranial haemorrhage and Wernicke's encephalopathy. Although there was significant brain atrophy seen on the CT, this correlates poorly with mental state.

Theories to explain hepatic encephalopathy in patients with cirrhosis include:

- Disorder of astrocyte function with Alzheimer type II astrocytosis
- Changes in gene expression in the brain that up-regulate or down-regulate transport proteins
- Ammonia hypothesis
- GABA hypothesis
- Neurosteroids.

Astrocytes play a key role in the regulation of the blood–brain barrier, and the detoxification of chemicals (including ammonia), and it is possible that neurotoxic substances, including ammonia and manganese, gain entry to the brain in liver failure. These neurotoxic substances may then contribute to morphological changes in astrocytes. Astrocytes may undergo Alzheimer type II astrocytosis in cirrhosis, although this is not observed in fulminant hepatic failure.

Genes coding for transport proteins, for example the peripheral-type benzodiazepine receptor, may be up-regulated and others down-regulated in cirrhosis and fulminant hepatic failure. This may impair neurotransmission.

Hyperammonaemia may affect cognitive function. **Ammonia** is produced in the gastrointestinal tract by **bacterial degradation** of amines, amino acids, purines, and urea. Ammonia is also produced by enterocytes, which contain glutaminase to convert glutamine to glutamate and ammonia that is normally detoxified in the liver by conversion to urea. In cirrhosis, the decreased functioning hepatocyte mass reduces detoxification of ammonia by these processes. Portosystemic shunting also diverts ammonia-containing blood away from the liver, and both factors contribute to hyperammonaemia.

Ammonia is also consumed by the conversion of glutamate to glutamine by glutamine synthetase by normal skeletal muscle, even though cells do not possess the enzymatic machinery of the urea cycle. Muscular **glutamine synthetase** activity increases in cirrhosis and portosystemic shunting, but when muscle wasting occurs in advanced cirrhosis, this potentiates hyperammonaemia. Glutamine synthetase is also expressed in the kidneys and cerebral astrocytes. The kidney plays a key role in ammonia excretion, but astrocytes are unable to up-regulate glutamine synthetase activity, so the brain is vulnerable to hyperammonaemia. Ammonia has multiple **neurotoxic effects**. It alters the transit of amino acids, water, and electrolytes by astrocytes and neurons, impairs amino acid metabolism, energy utilization, and inhibits both excitatory and inhibitory postsynaptic potentials. Treatments that decrease blood ammonia are associated with improvement in hepatic encephalopathy, but serum ammonia is normal in 10% of patients with encephalopathy. Furthermore, many patients with cirrhosis have elevated ammonia levels without evidence for encephalopathy, and infusion of ammonia does not induce the electroencephalographic changes associated with hepatic encephalopathy when it is administered to patients with cirrhosis. There is little role, therefore, for measuring ammonia concentrations in hepatic encephalopathy.

GABA (gamma-aminobutyric acid) is a neuroinhibitory substance produced in the gastrointestinal tract. Of all brain nerve endings, 24–45% may be GABAergic, which generate inhibitory postsynaptic potentials. It was previously thought that encephalopathy was related to excess GABA and stimulation of endogenous benzodiazepine receptors, since flumazenil improved cerebral function in some patients. However, further work has demonstrated no change in brain GABA and it now appears that flumazenil improves mental function in only a small percentage of patients with cirrhosis.

The neuronal GABA receptor complex also contains a binding site for **neurosteroids**, which have been implicated in encephalopathy since elevated levels of allopregnanolone, the neuroactive metabolite of pregnanolone, has been found in the brains of cirrhotic patients dying of hepatic encephalopathy.

25b) **What is the immediate management?**

- **Airway support**: tracheal intubation for patients with severe encephalopathy may be necessary.

- **Discontinue 5% dextrose** infusion, since this is likely to exacerbate hyponatraemia (Na 129mmol/L). If the patient needs intravenous volume expansion, 20% albumin should be considered, especially if there is renal impairment (see Case 11).

- **Stop diuretics**, since there is both hyponatraemia and gastrointestinal bleeding. The gastrointestinal bleeding may provoke pre-renal failure, so renal function needs to be optimized by appropriate volume expansion.

- **Oral and rectal lactulose** at a dose that produces 2–3 loose bowel motions per day is required. If the patient is deteriorating, 30mL orally, rectally or by nasogastric tube, may be required every 1–2 hours to induce a rapid laxative effect. Lactulose inhibits intestinal ammonia production by a number of mechanisms. Lactulose is converted to lactic acid, which acidifies the gut lumen, inhibits ammoniagenic coliform bacteria, and promotes non-ammoniagenic lactobacilli. Lactic acid also favours the conversion of NH_4^+ to NH3 and promotes the passage of NH3 from tissues into the lumen. Lactulose conceivably works as a laxative, reducing colonic bacterial load, but this is debatable. Care should be taken, because lactulose overdose may cause ileus, severe diarrhoea, electrolyte disturbance, and hypovolaemia.

- **Do not restrict dietary protein**, especially in advanced disease, since these patients are usually markedly malnourished. A protein intake of 1–1.5g protein/kg/day is recommended.

- **Active management of the precipitating event** (Table 25.1) should be the focus of treatment.

Blood in the upper gastrointestinal tract increases ammonia production and nitrogen absorption from the gut. A **gastroscopy** should be performed as soon as it is felt safe to do so, in case variceal banding is necessary (see Case 5). **Sepsis**, including spontaneous bacterial peritonitis, should be excluded, since infection may predispose to impaired renal function and to increased tissue catabolism, both of which increase blood ammonia levels. It is crucial that multiple blood cultures, a urine sample, and a diagnostic ascitic tap are carried out. **Renal impairment** leads to decreased clearance of urea, ammonia, and other nitrogenous compounds. **Drugs** that act on the central nervous system are best avoided, including opiates, benzodiazepines, antidepressants, and antipsychotic agents, since these may worsen encephalopathy. **Constipation** increases intestinal production and absorption of ammonia. **Hepatocellular carcinoma** needs to be considered and excluded (see Case 14). **Diuretic therapy** can lead to decreased serum potassium levels and alkalosis, which may facilitate the conversion of NH_4^+ to NH3.

Table 25.1 Precipitants of hepatic encephalopathy

- Gastrointestinal bleeding
- Sepsis
- Electrolyte disturbance
- Renal impairment
- Dehydration
- Drugs
- Constipation
- Progression of underlying liver disease
- Hepatocellular carcinoma
- Diuretic therapy
- Dietary protein overload (rare)

In the **absence of a readily identifiable precipitant**, infection should be assumed, so our patient was started on broad-spectrum intravenous antibiotics (a third-generation cephalosporin). Initially the patient improved, but he deteriorated with similar symptoms 3 weeks later. The patient was unable to return home, because he remained too confused.

25c) **What further treatment would you suggest?**

For chronic encephalopathy (unresponsive to therapy), consider the following treatments.

- **Imaging of splanchnic vessels** to identify large spontaneous portal-systemic shunts potentially amenable to radiological occlusion.

- **Neomycin** or other non-absorbable antibiotics such as rifaxamin, in an effort to decrease the colonic concentration of ammoniagenic bacteria. Neomycin is reserved as a second-line agent, after initiation of treatment with lactulose, because it risks ototoxicity and nephrotoxicity from some systemic absorption. Rifaxamin, unavailable in the UK but widely used in Europe, is better tolerated and may be as effective as lactulose at improving hepatic encephalopathy.

- **Treatment to increase ammonia clearance**: L-ornithine L-aspartate (LOLA) is a stable salt of the constituent amino acids. L-ornithine stimulates the urea cycle, with resulting loss of ammonia. Both L-ornithine and L-aspartate are substrates for glutamate transaminase, which increases glutamate and then consumes ammonia in the conversion of glutamate to glutamine by glutamine synthetase. LOLA was found to be effective in treating hepatic encephalopathy in a number of European trials. Oral zinc administration has the potential to improve hyperammonaemia by increasing the activity of ornithine transcar-bamylase, an enzyme in the urea cycle.

- Occlusion of TIPSS or surgical shunts if a patient has had a procedure to reduce portal hypertension.

- Experimental therapy with AST-120 carbon microspheres, which has been shown to reduce encephalopathy in preliminary trials.

- Referral for **liver transplantation**.

This patient was referred and listed for liver transplantation for chronic hepatic encephalopathy. He made a slow recovery post-transplant, but is now well, with no confusion 7 years post-transplant. The explant liver showed no evidence of recent alcohol use.

Further reading

Häussinger D, Schliess F (2008). Pathogenetic mechanisms of hepatic encephalopathy. *Gut*; **57**: 1156–65.

Morgan MY, Blei A, Grüngreiff K *et al.* (2007). The treatment of hepatic encephalopathy. *Metab Brain Dis*; **22**: 389–405.

Wright G, Jalan R (2007). Management of hepatic encephalopathy in patients with cirrhosis. *Best Pract Res Clin Gastroenterol*; **21**: 95–110.

Case 26

A 47-year-old South African man was admitted with right flank and right iliac fossa pain, of 1 month's duration. The pain was constant, but exacerbated by eating. He described weight loss, night sweats, and an intermittent non-productive cough on direct questioning.

On examination his pulse rate was 96bpm, and blood pressure 121/90mmHg. He was apyrexial. His weight was 62kg, 8kg less than he last recalled. The abdomen was tender in the right iliac fossa, with no abdominal masses and no peritonism. He was still well nourished and did not have lymphadenopathy, but was pale and had finger clubbing. After 48 hours in hospital he developed diarrhoea and fever up to 39°C.

Investigations showed:

- Hb 10.8g/dL, MCV 82 fL, WCC 7.9 x 10^9/L
- CRP 110mg/L
- Albumin 18g/L
- Chest radiograph showed right upper lobe and left mid-zone infiltration. The left cardiac border was indistinct. Small cavities were visible in both infiltrates (Fig. 26.1)
- Colonoscopy showed several small ulcers, scattered around the caecum; stenosed terminal ileum with several large ulcers (Fig. 26.2 in the central colour section), and intensely hyperaemic, nodular and friable mucosa in between. Proximal to these lesions the mucosa was normal. Multiple biopsies were taken for histopathology and microbiology.

Questions

26a) Name and discuss this disease.

26b) How is the diagnosis made?

26c) Discuss the clinically relevant issues.

26d) Describe the management.

26e) What messages does this case carry for doctors practising in developed countries?

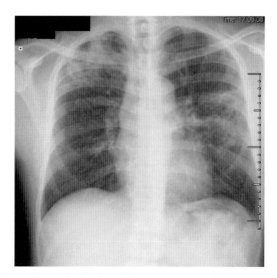

Fig. 26.1 A chest radiograph showing right upper lobe and left mid-zone (lingula) infiltrates. There is cavitation in both areas.

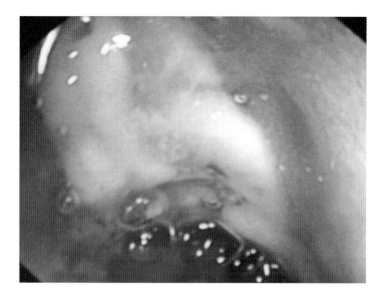

Fig. 26.2 (see colour plate 9) An endoscopic view of the terminal ileum, showing a large ulcer, surrounded by inflamed mucosa.

Answers

26a) **Name and discuss this disease.**

The diagnosis is **intestinal tuberculosis**. Tuberculosis (TB) is on the increase, with statistics from 2004 indicating an incidence of 8.9 million cases per year. The disease accounts for 1.7 million deaths per year. *Mycobacterium tuberculosis*, the responsible agent, is the most common mycobacterium in the *M. tuberculosis* complex. Another member of this complex, *M. bovis*, is traditionally responsible for some cases of intestinal tuberculosis, but has become much less common since milk pasteurization. *M. bovis* typically causes intestinal disease through the ingestion of milk and is not associated with pulmonary disease. In contrast, respiratory infection is by far the most important portal of entry for disease caused by *M. tuberculosis*.

Infection occurs through inhalation of infectious droplets from a person with active pulmonary TB. Tiny droplets (<10μm) from coughing or sneezing remain suspended in the air, and when inhaled find their way to the most distal airways. Bacilli are then phagocytosed by alveolar macrophages, but the bacillus can evade lysosomal degradation and multiply, eventually rupturing the macrophage. The risk of infection depends on exposure, but the risk of developing active disease depends on the host's immune response. Only 10% of people infected will develop active TB. Primary infection in childhood in developing countries is associated with haematogenous spread of TB bacilli throughout the body, whether active disease develops at that stage or not. These bacilli remain dormant and most never reactivate.

Secondary, or **reactivated infection**, may occur years later and presents differently. Although secondary TB in an immunocompetent host is usually confined to the lungs, about 15% of cases are extrapulmonary. In order of frequency, extrapulmonary TB involves lymph nodes, the genitourinary system, bones and joints, meninges, gastrointestinal tract, and pericardium. This list excludes miliary TB, which may be present in multiple organs simultaneously, through haematogenous spread. It is worth noting that tuberculosis can affect any organ in the body.

Abdominal TB (11–16% of cases of extrapulmonary TB) may involve the intestine (from the mouth to the anus), abdominal lymph nodes, peritoneum, or solid organs. **Intestinal TB** is most commonly (50–55%) ileocaecal in immunocompetent patients. This may be due to relative stasis, lack of digestive activity, or phagocytosis of *M. tuberculosis* by the M-cells on Peyer's patches. Similar conundra apply to the common ileocaecal location of Crohn's disease. A useful practice point is that if intestinal TB affects a region distant from the ileocaecal valve, then immunocompromise (such as HIV infection) should be suspected.

Intestinal infection is usually caused by swallowing infected sputum in people with pulmonary TB, but may occur from reactivation of primary TB. In one series, almost half of patients with pulmonary TB had intestinal involvement, often without abdominal symptoms. However, only 50–60% of people with intestinal TB have overt pulmonary TB. The frequency of lesions is broadly inversely proportional to the distance from the ileocaecal valve. Oesophageal TB is rare and accounts for 0.2% of cases, while gastric tuberculosis occurs in 1% of abdominal TB. Duodenal TB is often isolated, without evidence of pulmonary TB in 80%. Tuberculosis of the colon may be segmental, rectal, or less frequently diffuse. Tuberculosis of the anus may present as fistulating disease. The clinical mimicry of Crohn's disease is striking and potentially a major diagnostic pitfall in the developed world.

26b) **How is the diagnosis made?**

The **clinical** presentation of abdominal TB is non-specific. Abdominal pain is the most common symptom, present in >90%. Fever may occur in two-thirds. Half have night sweats and weight loss, with diarrhoea in only 10–15%. Radiographic imaging by ultrasound, barium studies, CT or MRI does not make a definitive diagnosis. This also applies to endoscopic appearances, but endoscopic biopsies are the mainstay of (eventual) diagnosis.

The diagnosis of TB depends on the demonstration of TB bacilli in samples of body fluid (most commonly sputum) or tissue. **Microscopy** of sputum, although able to deliver a rapid diagnosis, is insensitive, since it is positive in only 40–60% of cases of pulmonary TB. It is even less sensitive in abdominal TB since 40% will not have pulmonary involvement. Definitive diagnosis relies on **culturing** *M. tuberculosis* or by amplifying DNA through the **polymerase chain reaction (PCR)** in body fluid or tissue. The drawback of culture is the 4–8 weeks required for growth. Culture in liquid media is faster and may deliver results within 2–3 weeks. PCR is more rapid, and stool specimens may be positive in up to 90% of cases of intestinal TB. Positive PCR on formalin-fixed, paraffin-embedded intestinal mucosal biopsies has been reported in up to 75% of cases of intestinal TB.

In the Western world, **failure to suspect the diagnosis** is a cause of diagnostic delay. When tissue has been obtained from a lesion, biopsies should be formalin-fixed for histopathology and also sent in saline to microbiology for culture. Caseating granulomas and acid-fast bacilli are seen only in a minority of endoscopic mucosal biopsies from patients with intestinal TB. While granulomas may be seen in 40%, only a quarter of these (i.e. 10% of all cases) have caseation. The yield of biopsy culture is also low <20%, but has the useful potential for determining antibiotic sensitivity.

Tuberculin skin testing and **interferon-γ-release assays** (e.g. ELISPOT®, QuantiFERON®-TB) both measure an immune response to mycobacterial antigens (see Case 35 for more detail). They are both useful for screening for latent tuberculosis in areas of low incidence and prevalence. They are unable, however, to distinguish between latent and active tuberculosis. A positive tuberculin skin test may be caused by vaccination with Bacille Calmette-Guérin (BCG), which also limits its usefulness. Neither test is useful in areas of high incidence, where exposure of the population to TB is extensive.

Histopathology is usually (but by no means always) diagnostic. **Epithelioid cell granulomas, with central caseous necrosis** are typical of TB. This reflects the dominant cell-mediated immune response, with macrophages and T-lymphocytes (CD_4 cells of the T_H1 phenotype) being most important. T-lymphocytes play a central role in activating macrophages through production of cytokines (especially IFNγ and TNFα). Macrophages aggregate around the site of primary infection, forming granulomas, which contain the infection. Delayed-type hypersensitivity (type IV immune response) plays a lesser role. It represents a reaction to mycobacterial antigens and leads to destruction of macrophages and caseation. Delayed hypersensitivity also inhibits mycobacterial growth and is responsible for the tissue damage seen in tuberculosis.

In our patient, demonstration of acid-fast bacilli in the terminal ileal biopsies was sufficient to diagnose intestinal TB. Biopsies from the caecum and terminal ileum showed multiple epithelioid cell granulomas in the lamina propria. Granulomas in the ileal biopsies showed caseation. Ziehl–Nielsen stain showed acid-fast and alcohol-fast bacilli at both sites. (Figs 26.3 and 26.4 in the central colour section). Although the chest radiograph was consistent with TB, the patient had no sputum, so the diagnosis was made on microscopy of intestinal mucosal biopsies obtained at colonoscopy. Stool samples were sent only after the diagnosis of TB, to exclude acute bacterial infection as a cause for diarrhoea. Therapy was started. Tissue culture subsequently showed *M. tuberculosis* sensitive to all four first-line antituberculous drugs.

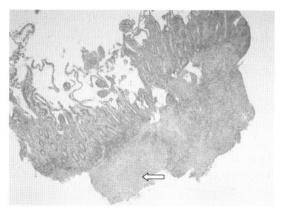

Fig. 26.3 (see colour plate 10) Mucosal biopsy from the terminal ileum, showing a large epithelioid cell granuloma with central caseation (arrow).

26c) **Discuss the clinically relevant issues.**

The clinical, radiological and histological picture is characteristic of secondary (reactivation) of pulmonary TB with concomitant ileocaecal **TB in an immunocompetent host**. This implies a degree of containment of the infection. Our patient tested negative for HIV. Tuberculosis in the **HIV-positive host**, especially when advanced, presents differently. Lung lesions more closely resemble those of primary TB, and microscopy of mucosal biopsies do not reveal granulomas (consider the pathogenesis, above). There may be numerous neutrophilic micro-abscesses and numerous acid-fast bacilli, in contrast to few acid-fast bacilli in those with

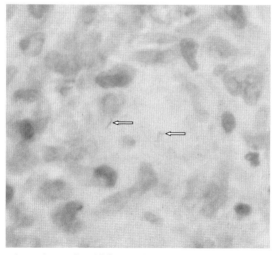

Fig. 26.4 (see colour plate 11) Acid-fast and alcohol-fast bacilli (arrows) in a mucosal biopsy.

well formed granulomas in immunocompetent hosts. Extrapulmonary TB occurs more frequently in HIV-positive patients (in half or more cases).

Intestinal TB may be complicated by **stricturing**, which may resolve rapidly on treatment, although an appreciable minority may require stricture-plasty or resection to relieve obstructive symptoms. **Malabsorption** may be due to stasis proximal to strictured bowel, with subsequent bacterial overgrowth (see Case 10). A more serious complication is that of **spontaneous perforation** of the terminal ileum. In India, TB of the terminal ileum is second only to typhoid as a cause of terminal ileum perforation.

Finally, digital clubbing in our patient implies a **suppurative lung** complication. This includes lung abscesses in a pre-existing cavity, although our patient had no evidence of an abscess on chest radiography. Secondary bronchiectasis may also lead to clubbing, from chronic suppuration. Our patient had no evidence of a lung tumour or cardiac cause for clubbing. Uncomplicated TB does not cause clubbing.

26d) **Describe the management**

Standard therapy means treatment for 6 months, using four drugs for 2 months and two drugs for 4 months. This is curative in most patients, provided the organism is sensitive. **Rifampicin** 5mg/kg, **isoniazid** (INH) 10mg/kg, **ethambutol** 15mg/kg and **pyrazinamide** 20mg/kg are given for the first 2 months. This is the bactericidal stage and is followed by a 4-month continuation (sterilization) stage, in which rifampicin and isoniazid are given. At least one randomized trial has shown that a 6-month course of therapy with this regimen had a cure rate of 99%, compared with 12 months of isoniazid and ethambutol alone, which had a cure rate of 94%. Rifampicin and isoniazid may both cause a hepatitis, which may lead to fulminant hepatic failure (see Case 1). Should hepatitis (ALT >3-fold elevated) develop, both need to be stopped and reintroduced one-by-one, to identify the culprit.

Pyridoxine (vitamin B_6) is advocated if isoniazid is administered, to prevent the development of peripheral neuropathy. It should be remembered that pyridoxine can itself cause peripheral neuropathy if administered in excess of the recommended daily requirement. Ethambutol may cause optic neuritis and pyrazinamide can precipitate gout. Specialist advice is best sought when managing intestinal TB, because management includes contact tracing and monitoring compliance with therapy, which are facilitated by a multidisciplinary team.

Drug resistant TB is becoming a global problem as the result of monotherapy and/or non-compliance to drug regimens. **Multi-drug resistant (MDR) tuberculosis**, prominent since the 1990s, is defined as *M. tuberculosis* resistant to at least rifampicin and isoniazid. **Extensively drug resistant (XDR) tuberculosis** implies resistance to rifampicin, isoniazid, any fluoroquinolone and at least one of the injectable second line drugs (amikacin, capreomycin, or kanamycin). The spread of MDR and XDR tuberculosis can only be stemmed by appropriate infection control measures and ensuring patient compliance with therapy, such as through **directly observed treatment**. Compliance with therapy is a more appropriate term than adherence in these circumstances, because of the implications for public health that may merit enforcement.

26e) **What messages does this case carry for doctors practising in developed countries?**

Although 80% of new cases of TB occur in developing regions of the world, it also occurs in industrialized countries among migrants, marginalized communities, and immunocompromised patients, including chronically debilitated or elderly patients. Because the incidence of intestinal TB is very low in developed countries, the **index of suspicion** is also low and the diagnosis delayed. In contrast, Crohn's disease is common in developed countries. For the gastroenterologist this is particularly important, since both are chronic granulomatous diseases with a similar distribution. The clinical presentation with abdominal pain, weight loss and diarrhoea is also similar, as is the endoscopic appearance. If the chest radiograph is normal, other imaging may not adequately distinguish between the two. Microscopy of tissue samples may not reveal acid-fast bacilli, and granulomas may be of very similar appearance.

The **diagnostic differentiation** is extremely important. If Crohn's disease is mistaken for TB, therapy may be delayed and potentially harmful antituberculous drugs may be prescribed inappropriately. On the other hand, TB is usually curable with a 6-month course of chemotherapy, and diagnostic delay may lead to institution of therapy when it is too late. Furthermore, misdiagnosis of TB as Crohn's disease may lead to the administration of corticosteroids or anti-TNF therapy, with dire consequences.

The clinician needs to focus on factors that put the **likely diagnosis in context**. The pros and cons of each possibility are best listed, so that the less likely diagnosis is rejected. Such factors include a family history of inflammatory bowel disease, or a history of TB contacts, and these should be obtained. Diarrhoea is more common in Crohn's disease. Fever is more common in TB. Radiologically, ileocaecal TB destroys the ileocaecal valve and caecum, which is not typical of Crohn's. Although ulceration of the terminal ileum is seen in both conditions, radial, circumferential ulcers, with intensely inflamed surrounding mucosa are more typical of TB. Ulceration in Crohn's disease is more often longitudinal, with normal mucosa in between. Aphthoid ulcers are uncommon in TB, but the findings remain subjective and there is considerable overlap. The typical granulomas of TB are often multiple, large, and confluent, with caseous necrosis. Crohn's granulomas are usually single and do not show caseation.

If uncertain, initial therapy will be guided by the prevalence in the particular area. If in doubt, the possibility of TB should be treated first, because of the dire consequences of treating TB with immunomodulators for Crohn's disease. Surgical resection of the area, if localized, should be considered, since this may be diagnostic as well as therapeutic.

Further reading

Epstein D, Watermeyer G, Kirsch R (2007). Review article: the diagnosis and management of Crohn's disease in populations with high-risk rates for tuberculosis. *Aliment Pharmacol Ther*; **25**: 1373–88.

Gan HT, Chen YQ, Ouyang Q *et al.* (2002). Differentiation between intestinal tuberculosis and Crohn's disease in endoscopic biopsy specimens by polymerase chain reaction. *Am J Gastroenterol*; **97**(6): 1446–51.

Khan R, Abid S, Jafri W, Abbas Z *et al.* (2006). Diagnostic dilemma of abdominal tuberculosis in non-HIV patients: An ongoing challenge for physicians. *World J Gastroenterol*; **12**: 6371–5.

Jassal M, Bishai WR (2009). Extensively drug-resistant tuberculosis. *Lancet Infect Dis*; **9**: 19–30.

Pettengell KE, Larsen C, Garb M, Mayet FG *et al.* (1990). Gastrointestinal tuberculosis in patients with pulmonary tuberculosis. *Q J Med*; **74**: 303–8.

Sharma MP, Bhatia V (2004). Abdominal tuberculosis. *Indian J Med Res*; **120**: 305–15.

Case 27

A 27-year-old male teacher presented with a 2-year history of intermittent dysphagia for solids, which occurred about once every three meals. There was no regurgitation, bolus obstruction, odynophagia, or chest pain. His weight was stable and there was no history of melaena or haematemesis. He had reflux, which caused intermittent heartburn, but symptoms were controlled with omeprazole. This had not made any difference to the dysphagia.

The only other medical history was childhood asthma. There was a family history of Crohn's disease, but no other family history of gastrointestinal disease.

On examination, he was fit and well, with a body mass index of 25kg/m². His hands, skin, and abdomen were normal, with no tremor, normal speech, no goiter, and no abdominal findings.

Investigations showed:

- Barium swallow: there was no structural abnormality in the hypopharynx or oesophagus and no stricture. There was transient hold up of a swallowed marshmallow. The gastro-oesophageal junction opened normally.
- Gastroscopy: oesophagus, stomach and duodenum looked normal. Oesophageal, gastric and duodenal biopsies were taken.

Questions

27a) What is the differential diagnosis?

27b) By examining the oesophageal biopsy (Fig. 27.1 in the central coloured section), what is the diagnosis?

27c) What changes could be present on endoscopy in this condition?

27d) What is the treatment of this condition?

27e) What is the prognosis?

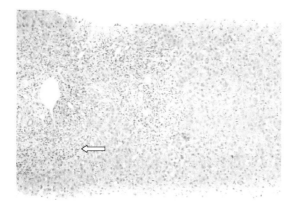

Plate 1 (see Fig. 2.1, p12) A low-power magnification image of a liver biopsy, showing a severe inflammatory infiltrate at the interface between the portal triad and lobule (arrow).

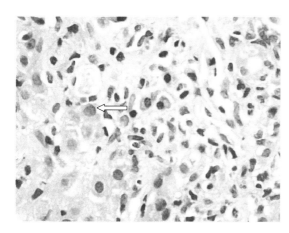

Plate 2 (see Fig. 2.2, p12) A higher magnification showing distinct plasma cells (arrow).

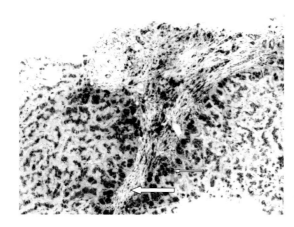

Plate 3 (see Fig. 6.1, p37) Photomicrograph of a liver biopsy stained with Prussian blue (Perl's stain) showing features of parenchymal iron deposition (small arrow) and advanced fibrosis (large arrow).

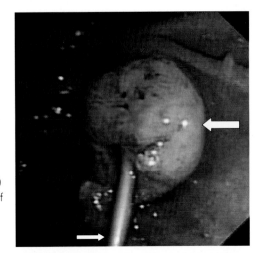

Plate 4 (see Fig. 9.4, p60) Endoscopic photograph of the tumour (large arrow) after stent (small arrow) insertion.

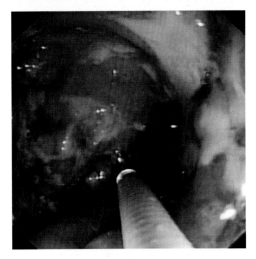

Plate 5 (see Fig. 18.1, p111) An endoscopic view of the terminal ileum showing inflammation and ulceration.

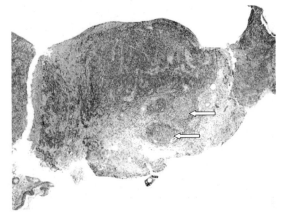

Plate 6 (see Fig. 18.2, p111) A photomicrograph showing non-caseating granulomas (arrows) in a biopsy from the terminal ileum.

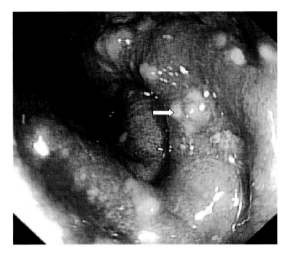

Plate 7 (see Fig. 22.3, p143) Endoscopic image of the sigmoid colon, in a patient with pseudomembranous colitis. The mucosa exhibits circumferential hyperaemia and oedema. There are discrete pseudomembranes (arrow). Pseudomembranes are characteristic of pseudomembranous colitis, and indicate severe colonic involvement.

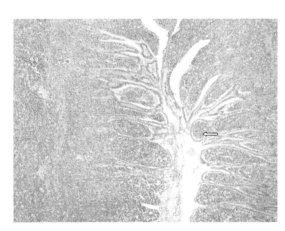

Plate 8 (see Fig. 24.3, p159) Photomicrograph showing sheets of uniform cells (lymphocytes) infiltrating and expanding small intestinal villi (arrow). Immunohistochemistry showed monoclonal cells of B cell origin.

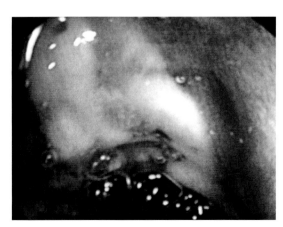

Plate 9 (see Fig. 26.2, p168) An endoscopic view of the terminal ileum, showing a large ulcer, surrounded by inflamed mucosa.

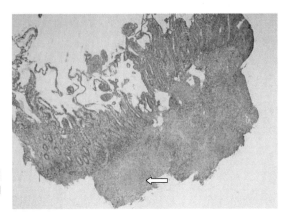

Plate 10 (see Fig. 26.3, p173) Mucosal biopsy from the terminal ileum, showing a large epithelioid cell granuloma with central caseation (arrow).

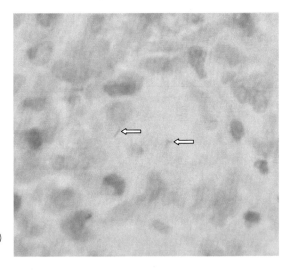

Plate 11 (see Fig. 26.4, p173) Acid-fast and alcohol-fast bacilli (arrows) in a mucosal biopsy.

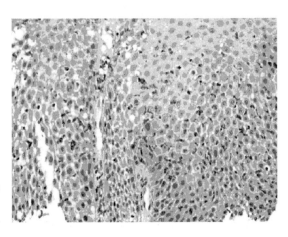

Plate 12 (see Fig. 27.1, p181) Mid-oesophageal biopsy from a patient with dysphagia and a normal oesophagus at endoscopy.

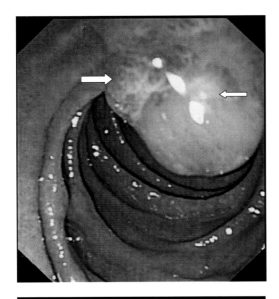

Plate 13 (see Fig. 29.4, p19) Papilla at ERCP. Mucin extruding (small arrow) from the distorted papilla (large arrow).

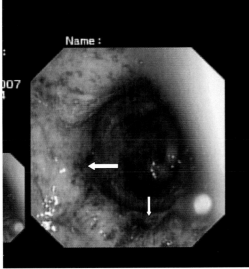

Plate 14 (see Fig. 31.1, p216) Photograph of mucosal appearance in the sigmoid colon: patchy erythema (large arrow), with some ulceration (small arrow) and haemorrhagic patches.

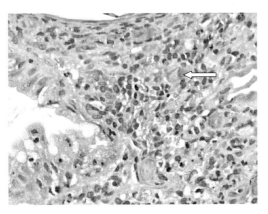

Plate 15 (see Fig. 31.2, p217) Haematoxylin and eosin staining of mucosal biopsy showing classic 'owl's eye' inclusion bodies (arrow).

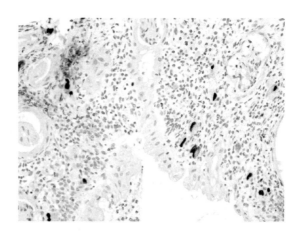

Plate 16 (see Fig. 31.3, p217) Positive immunohistochemistry for CMV.

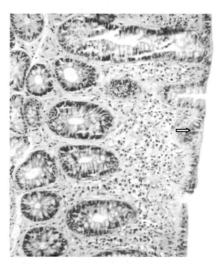

Plate 17 (see Fig. 36.1, p248) Photomicrograph showing chronic inflammatory cells in the lamina propria, and intraepithelial lymphocytosis (arrow), consistent with lymphocytic colitis.

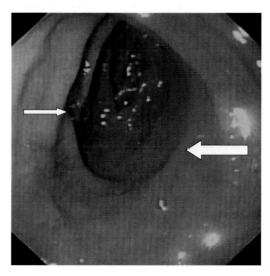

Plate 18 (see Fig. 38.1, p261) An endoscopic photograph of this patient's duodenum, showing a paucity of folds (large arrow) with fissuring (small arrow), although endoscopy in coeliac disease is commonly normal.

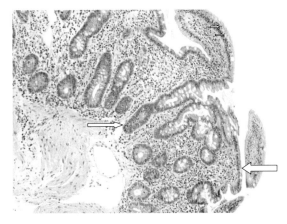

Plate 19 (see Fig. 38.2, p261) A photomicrograph showing subtotal villous atrophy, with blunting of the villi (large arrow), crypt hyperplasia (small arrow), and increased intraepithelial lymphocytes (tiny arrows).

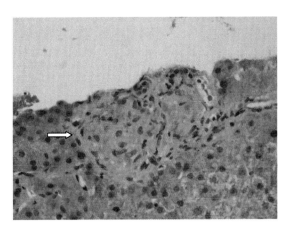

Plate 20 (see Fig. 42.1, p286) A needle biopsy of the liver (haematoxylin and eosin stain) showing a granuloma (arrow).

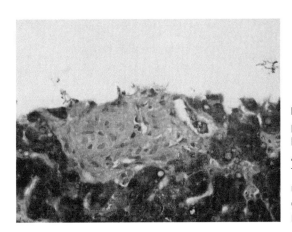

Plate 21 (see Fig. 42.1, p287) The same biopsy using a Periodic Acid Schiff stain. The granuloma does not contain stored glycogen, so is PAS-negative.

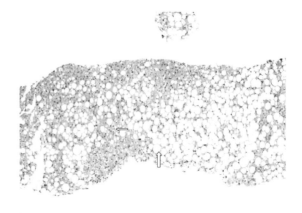

Plate 22 (see Fig. 45.1, p305) Liver biopsy in non-alcoholic fatty liver disease (low power) showing steatosis (large arrow) and interface hepatitis (small arrow).

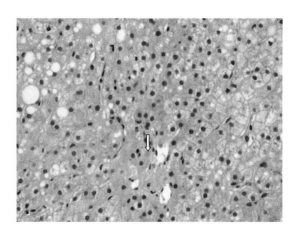

Plate 23 (see Fig. 15.2, p306) Liver biopsy in non-alcoholic fatty liver disease (high power) showing Mallory's hyaline (arrow).

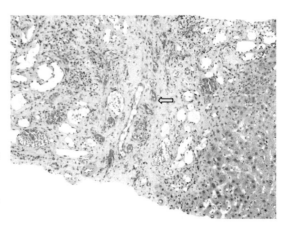

Plate 24 (see Fig. 48.2, p326) Angiosarcoma of the liver. Vascular channels are identifiable (arrow), but not the characteristic spindle-shaped cells at this magnification.

Answers

27a) **What is the differential diagnosis?**

The differential diagnosis is:

- Eosinophilic oesophagitis
- Peptic stricture from gastro-oesophageal reflux
- Achalasia
- Muscle disorders
  - Muscular dystrophies
  - Hyper or hypothyroidism
  - Myasthenia gravis
- Oesophageal involvement in systemic conditions (e.g. scleroderma)
- Oesophageal spasm.

Intermittent dysphagia in a young adult over many years (particularly with an episode of food impaction), should raise the possibility of **eosinophilic oesophagitis**. This becomes more likely with a personal or family history of allergic disorders. It should always be considered in the differential diagnosis of chronic unexplained dysphagia, but has been recognized only relatively recently. The barium swallow is usually normal, but strictures of varying length and diameter can occur.

Distinguishing eosinophilic oesophagitis from **gastro-oesophageal reflux** disease can be difficult, but the latter only causes food impaction if a mechanical stricture (which should be visible on barium swallow) is present. It is notable that a proton pump inhibitor relieved reflux symptoms in this patient, but did not relieve dysphagia. Dysphagia due to severe oesophagitis without a stricture is not that uncommon, but the sensation is relieved by acid suppression.

Achalasia should be considered, but several features make the diagnosis unlikely. Patients with achalasia tend to have dysphagia for both solids and liquids. Furthermore, chest pain occurs in up to half of patients, and 60–90% describe regurgitating undigested foods during or shortly after a meal. The barium swallow might also be expected to show features of achalasia given the 2-year history. The typical feature of achalasia on barium swallow is the 'bird's beak' appearance of the gastro-oesophageal junction, due to the non-relaxing sphincter, and sometimes associated with a dilated oesophagus. Fluoroscopy during the swallow may reveal decreased peristalsis. At endoscopy, there may be a transient resistance to the passage of the endoscope through the gastro-oesophageal junction that is recognized by an experienced endoscopist alert to the potential diagnosis.

Muscular disorders must not be overlooked, but often are at first presentation. There are three categories to consider. The first is muscular dystrophy: two uncommon forms of muscular dystrophy involve the striated muscles of the pharyngo-oesophageal region. **Dystrophia myotonica** is a familial disease characterized by myopathic facies, myotonia, swan neck, muscle wasting, frontal baldness, testicular atrophy, and cataracts. **Oculopharyngeal dystrophy** is a syndrome that presents later in life with ptosis and dysphagia, with a dominant pattern of inheritance. The second category is **hyperthyroidism** or **hypothyroidism**, which can also affect striated musculature. The third muscle disorder is **myasthenia gravis**, which is a disorder of the motor end plate, affecting the striated oesophageal musculature with clinical manifestations that resemble the myopathies. The characteristic feature is fatigue during repeated effort, with successive attempts to swallow (pharyngo-oesophageal transfer) causing more symptoms as the meal progresses.

Systemic conditions such as scleroderma, polymyositis, or mixed connective tissue disease can involve the oesophagus. Other findings such as sclerodactyly, telangiectases or weakness, are generally detected in conjunction with symptoms of dysphagia.

Oesophageal spasm generally presents with retrosternal chest pain, with episodes lasting for minutes or hours. Intermittent dysphagia occurs in 30–60% of patients. A barium swallow can reveal a 'corkscrew

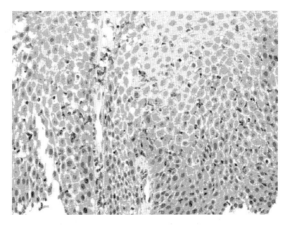

Fig. 27.1 (see colour plate 12) Mid-oesophageal biopsy from a patient with dysphagia and a normal oesophagus at endoscopy.

oesophagus', due to dysfunctional circular muscle contractions that in extreme situations trap barium between powerfully contracted segments. The endoscopic appearance is normal.

27b) **By examining the oesophageal biopsy (Fig. 27.1 in the central colour section) what is the diagnosis?**

The diagnosis is **eosinophilic oesophagitis**. The diagnosis hinges on histopathological evidence of eosinophils infiltrating the oesophageal mucosa. It is well recognized that other diseases are associated with eosinophilic infiltration of the oesophagus, including gastro-oesophageal reflux, but with a lesser degree of eosinophilic infiltrate. For diagnosis of eosinophilic oesophagitis, the eosinophilic infiltration in the squamous epithelium should exceed 20 eosinophils/high power field at x400 magnification. Mid-oesophageal biopsies should be the standard of care for patients with dysphagia and a normal endoscopy.

27c) **What changes could be present on endoscopy in this condition?**

Typical endoscopic findings of eosinophilic oesophagitis include mucosal longitudinal linear furrows, a corrugated appearance or plaque-like exudates, friability of the oesophageal mucosa ('crêpe-paper' mucosa), and strictures of variable length. Most patients appear to have a normal oesophagus at endoscopy, so the endoscopist should be encouraged to take biopsies.

27d) **What is the treatment?**

Corticosteroids, either topical or systemic, are generally effective. Initial treatment should be swallowed fluticasone (220μg dose x four puffs, swallowed with a minimal amount of water twice daily, instructing patients not to eat or drink for 2 hours after each dose). Continue therapy for 6 weeks, if there is a response. Recurrent symptoms are best treated with the same dose, but for a longer period. If there is no initial response, systemic corticosteroids (prednisolone 40mg/day, tapered over 6 weeks) should be considered.

Elimination diets: although eosinophilic oesophagitis appears likely to be an allergic disorder, identifying the triggering allergens (food or environmental) is labour intensive and unproductive. Patients may have multiple allergies, making it difficult to comply with allergen-avoidance or food restriction. Paediatric patients are often treated with an elimination or liquid diet and improve, but they comply with food restriction better than adults.

Oesophageal dilatation: patients with eosinophilic oesophagitis are at increased risk for mucosal tears and perforation after oesophageal dilatation. Medical treatment of eosinophilic oesophagitis decreases the risk of strictures. Dilatation should be carried out only in patients who fail medical therapy and have severe dysphagia.

New therapies such as anti-IL5 monoclonal antibody therapy are evolving.

27e) **What is the prognosis of this condition?**

Untreated, patients with eosinophilic oesophagitis may develop strictures, with weight loss, food impaction, or even perforation. After patients are successfully treated, it is likely that 25–40% will have relapse of their symptoms. The long-term outcome for patients with eosinophilic oesophagitis who have been treated and the proportion that require multiple courses of treatment is unknown. There have been no cases of oesophageal malignancy observed in association with eosinophilic oesophagitis.

Further reading

Attwood SE, Lamb CA (2008). Eosinophilic oesophagitis and other non-reflux inflammatory conditions of the oesophagus: diagnostic imaging and management. *Best Pract Res Gastro*; **22**: 639–60.

Basavaraju KP, Wong T (2008). Eosinophilic oesophagitis: a common cause of dysphagia in young adults? *Internat J Clin Pract*; **62**:1096–107.

Ferguson DD, Foxx-Orenstein AE (2007). Eosinophilic esophagitis: an update. *Dis esophagus*; **20**: 2–8.

Case 28

A 44-year-old French woman presented to the emergency department with severe, acute right upper quadrant pain, and was referred to the gastroenterology registrar on call. The pain had developed shortly after her evening meal, was constant, and radiated through to her back. She had vomited once. On specific questioning it appeared that she had had some back pain in the preceding days.

She was being treated for autoimmune liver disease with prednisolone 40mg/day. This had been started 3 days before, when her ALT increased. She had a 30-pack/year smoking history, but rarely drank alcohol.

At the time of referral she had already had intravenous morphine for the pain. Her pulse was 104bpm, blood pressure 127/82mmHg, temperature 36.1°C, and respiratory rate 36/min. Her abdomen was at that time tender in the right upper quadrant, but nowhere else. There was no tenderness on percussion, but there was generalized involuntary guarding. She could not lie flat, because this exacerbated the pain.

Investigations showed:

- Hb 14g/dL, WCC 13.82 x10^9/L, platelets 179 x10^9/L
- Na 134mmol/L, K 4.0mmol/L, creatinine 84 μmol/L
- Bilirubin 25μmol/L, ALT 260 IU/L, ALP 508 IU/L, albumin 41g/L
- CRP 5mg/L
- Amylase 73 IU/L.

Questions

28a) What is the differential diagnosis? Consider the factors that complicate the patient's assessment.

28b) What common conditions need excluding, and what uncommon medical conditions should be kept in mind?

28c) What investigations should be requested on admission?

28d) Discuss the medical management of the underlying condition.

28e) Discuss potential complications and the further management of this patient.

Answers

28a) **What is the differential diagnosis? Consider the factors that complicate the patient's assessment.**

The differential diagnosis includes

- Biliary colic (and associated complications)
- Peptic ulcer (and associated complications)
- Mesenteric ischaemia
- Acute pancreatitis with a normal amylase
- Peritonitis with features obscured by corticosteroids
- Ruptured ectopic pregnancy.

The patient has presented with acute, postprandial, right upper quadrant (RUQ) pain, localized tenderness, and generalized guarding, *without* percussion tenderness. Postprandial pain is characteristic of **biliary colic** due to passage of a stone into or through the cystic duct, peptic ulcer, and mesenteric ischaemia. Guarding is not a feature of any of these conditions if they are uncomplicated. Vomiting commonly occurs with biliary colic, but our patient had had an ultrasound scan 6 months before, which had shown no gallstones. **Acalculous cholecystitis** is very rare; RUQ tenderness (Murphy's sign) with a thickened gallbladder wall in the absence of stones is suggestive. **Acute cholangitis** is characterized by RUQ abdominal pain, jaundice, and fever usually with rigors (**Charcot's triad**). Our patient had neither jaundice nor fever. **Mesenteric ischaemia** is unlikely in a young patient, but characteristically presents with severe pain and a paucity of signs. Our patient had no risk factors for arterial thromboembolism. **Acute pancreatitis** presents with upper abdominal pain that may radiate to the back, and may be associated with peritonism. Acute pancreatitis with a (relatively) normal amylase can occur in patients with chronic pancreatitis and little glandular function, commonly caused by alcohol. Our patient had no risk factors for pancreatitis.

Acute symptoms justify an anatomical approach to differential diagnosis, but the generalized guarding indicates **peritonitis**. Perforation of a hollow organ is the usual cause. **Peptic ulcer perforation** usually leads to instantaneous pain and peritonism, due to acid in the peritoneal cavity. The chemical irritation caused by acid causes pain, before bacterial peritonitis supersedes. In contrast, peritonitis which develops (for example) after iatrogenic perforation during colonoscopy may take hours to develop, because the colonic pH is neutral. Diverticulitis or appendicitis are other potential causes, but perforation is usually preceded by a typical clinical syndrome. Small bowel tumours or diverticula may also perforate, but are rare. In any woman in their reproductive years, an **ectopic pregnancy** needs to be considered. Localized pain may be followed by rupture, with ensuing peritonitis. This is usually associated with hypotension and anaemia, due to haemorrhage. A pregnancy test should be carried out. Other gynaecological causes include pelvic inflammatory disease, which may cause RUQ pain if complicated by the Fitz–Hugh–Curtis syndrome, and **ovarian torsion**, which presents with abdominal pain (albeit lower abdominal pain) and vomiting. Acute renal colic generally presents with pain at the renal angle, which radiates to the groin, is severe, and is associated with vomiting.

The assessment of this patient was complicated by the fact that she had received an opioid analgesic just before referral, which masked signs of peritonism. She was also on high-dose corticosteroids, which can also mask signs of peritonitis. The underlying autoimmune hepatitis was a red herring and not responsible for her acute symptoms. It does not cause acute liver distension to provoke capsular pain.

28b) **What common conditions need excluding and what uncommon medical conditions should be kept in mind?**

Three common medical conditions causing severe abdominal pain (including peritonism) are **diabetic ketoacidosis, lower lobe pneumonia**, and an **acute coronary syndrome**. All can cause abdominal pain, are treatable, and carry serious consequences for the patient if missed.

Uncommon medical causes of acute abdominal pain are acute porphyria, familial Mediterranean fever, acute angio-oedema, and heavy metal poisoning. Addison's disease, although it can cause chronic abdominal pain, does not present as an acute abdomen. These should be suspected if initial investigations do not reveal the cause.

The **acute porphyrias** include acute intermittent porphyria, variegate porphyria and hereditary coproporphyria. They are caused by genetically determined deficiencies in various enzymes involved in the synthesis of heme. In the UK, acute intermittent porphyria is the most common type. A deficiency in hydroximethylbilane synthetase (HMB-synthetate) underlies the condition. People affected by this condition are heterozygous for the affected gene and have half-normal levels of HMB-synthesate. Acute attacks are precipitated by substances that induce the rate-limiting (hepatic) enzyme, involved in heme synthesis, aminolaevulinic acid synthetate (ALA-synthetase). This enzyme is the first in the heme-biosynthetic pathway, upstream of HMB-synthetase. The list of precipitant drugs that should be avoided is long and may be found in the British National

Formulary or on the **European Porphyria Initiative** website (www.porphy-ria-europe.org). Steroid hormones seem to be particularly important, because attacks do not occur before puberty. Hormonal contraceptives should be avoided. Premenstrual attacks are similarly related to endogenous progesterone, but surprisingly, pregnancy usually poses no problem, indicating a beneficial metabolic factor.

Acute attacks of porphyria may also be precipitated by a reduction in caloric intake, as with acute illness, dieting or fasting. Abdominal pain is the most prominent manifestation. The pain is usually diffuse and constant. Fever and abdominal tenderness are unusual, and inflammatory markers are usually normal. Other features of an acute attack include constipation, mental symptoms of anxiety, confusion, paranoia, depression, and hallucination. Sympathetic over-activity manifests with tachycardia or dysrrhythmias. Peripheral neuropathy is not universally present in acute attacks, and skin lesions do *not* occur. The **diagnosis** of an acute attack is made by demonstrating elevated levels of urinary porphobilinogen. Normal urinary porphobilinogen during an acute attack effectively excludes acute intermittent porphyria as the cause of acute symptoms. Faecal porphyrins are usually normal (in contrast to variegate porphyria and hereditary coproporphyria). Urinary ALA is increased, although levels may be normal in the absence of an acute attack. In these circumstances the diagnosis is based on detecting HMB-synthesase deficiency in erythrocytes.

Acute porphyria is managed in the first instance symptomatically with opioid analgesia, antiemetics, and sedatives. Intravenous **glucose** (300g/day) may be effective in milder cases but intravenous **haematin** is more effective and should be started without delay and continued for 4 days. Haem arginate or haem albumin may also be used. In the long term there is an increased risk of hypertension, renal disease, and hepatocellular carcinoma.

Familial Mediterranean fever (FMF) is the prototype of the hereditary periodic fever syndromes and is especially common in people of Jewish, Italian, Turkish, Armenian, or Arab decent. Acute attacks start early in life, are always associated with a fever, and are accompanied by abdominal pain in 90%. Abdominal pain may vary from mild generalized pain, to severe pain with peritonism and ileus. Amyloidosis (AA) is a late complication, which occurred commonly before colchicine was shown both to prevent this and reduce the frequency of attacks. **Acute angioedema** is bradikinin mediated. and may be due to a hereditary

C1 esterase deficiency or due to the development of autoantibodies (acquired) against C1 esterase. Attacks of colicky abdominal pain with episodes of laryngeal oedema are characteristic. Urticaria is *not* a feature. Therapy with attenuated androgens is effective as prophylaxis. In some settings ε-aminocaproic acid is also used. **Heavy metal poisoning** with arsenic, lead, mercury or cadmium may all be associated with abdominal pain. A thorough occupational history is important. In the acute setting a urine heavy metal assay is the investigation of choice. Chelating agents are available for all but cadmium.

28c) **What investigations should be requested on admission?**

Urine dipstix helps exclude diabetic ketoacidosis. An **erect chest radiograph** and **abdominal radiograph** are mandatory. The chest radiograph may indicate pulmonary consolidation and should reveal intraperitoneal air if present. An abdominal radiograph (which need not be an erect film) may show the distended bowel loops of an ileus. Pancreatic calcification (indicating underlying chronic pancreatitis) should be sought. Calcified gallstones are present in only 10% of patients with gallstones, so gallstones are rarely seen on plain radiography. In contrast, most renal stones are radio-opaque and may be visible on plain radiography. Our patient's pain, however, was not typical of renal colic. An **ECG** is necessary to exclude myocardial ischaemia.

Blood tests including biochemistry, inflammatory markers, and full blood count will reveal electrolyte abnormalities, liver function derangement (due to the passage of a gallstone), evidence of inflammation or infection, and may show changes of underlying chronic disease. Our patient had a normal CRP, with a mildly elevated leucocyte count. Mild leucocytosis may result from underlying infection, although the CRP is usually markedly elevated. It is worth noting that if done early, the CRP may be normal, because there is a lag in CRP response. Mild leucocytosis may be caused by the prednisolone therapy in this patient, or result from pain, which causes demargination of leucocytes in the periphery, through catecholamine release. Metabolic stress (as with diabetic ketoacidosis) can cause a leucocytosis, even without underlying infection. Liver function tests were unhelpful in our patient, as they were already elevated because of the autoimmune hepatitis. Acute pancreatitis (in the absence of a chronic component) was effectively excluded by the normal serum amylase. The normal serum albumin and haemoglobin are consistent with an acute event.

A chest radiograph showed lucency under the right hemi-diaphragm (Fig. 28.1). A lateral decubitus abdominal radiograph was requested (carried out after the patient had been positioned on her left side for 10 min), which showed a locule of air above the liver (Fig. 28.2). A surgical opinion was sought. At the time of surgical review, the opioid analgesia had worn off and the patient clearly had peritonism. A CT scan of the abdomen revealed free air above the liver and in the porta hepatis (Fig. 28.3). The site of visceral perforation was not evident, but peptic ulcer perforation was thought to be the most likely diagnosis. The patient was taken to theatre and a small **perforated duodenal ulcer** was identified and treated with simple closure using an omental patch.

28d) **Discuss the medical management of the underlying condition.**

While gastric acid secretion plays a central role in peptic ulcer disease (PUD), because ulceration occurs during increased acid secretion and healing occurs during acid suppression, pepsin contributes to ulceration. Impairment of mucosal protection mechanisms, including disruption of the integrity of the mucous gel layer, reduced bicarbonate production, impaired blood flow, and mucosal repair also contribute. *Helicobacter pylori*, NSAID use, and acid-hypersecretory states are the main risk factors for the development of PUD. Zollinger–Ellison syndrome, due to a gastrinoma with excess gastrin secretion, may cause multiple ulcers, but is very rare. *H. pylori* stimulates acid and pepsin production; both *H. pylori* and NSAIDs impair mucosal defence. NSAIDs do so partly through

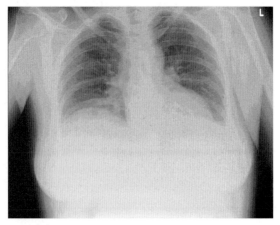

Fig. 28.1 This erect chest radiograph shows elevation of the right hemidiaphragm, with subtle subdiaphragmatic radiolucency (arrow). The gastric air bubble is clearly visible on the left. Note that this is a poor inspiratory film, and lung fields should be interpreted with caution.

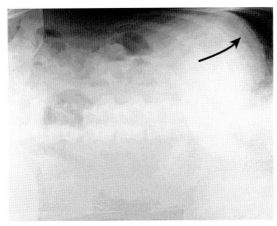

Fig. 28.2 A lateral decubitus film of the abdomen showing a locule of air above the liver (arrow) and the same lucency over the liver, further to the right, below the diaphragm.

inhibition of prostaglandin synthesis. Other risk factors that contribute to the development of PUD are psychological stress, smoking, other drugs such as potassium chloride, bisphosphonates, corticosteroids or mycophenolate mofetil, and advancing age with concomitant decline in prostaglandin levels. Certain chronic conditions are associated with an

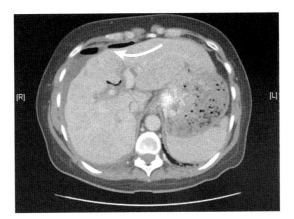

Fig. 28.3 A CT scan at the level of the porta hepatis showed a small amount of free gas anterior to the liver (large arrow) and gas locules in the porta hepatis (small arrow). There is free intra-abdominal fluid, mainly in the perihepatic region, which tracked inferior to the porta hepatis, right paracolic gutter, and pelvis on further sections. Note the irregular liver contour, in keeping with chronic liver disease.

increased risk of PUD, including chronic lung disease, renal failure, and liver cirrhosis.

Duodenal ulceration is the most common form of PUD in the West and is associated with *H. pylori* in >95%. **Gastric ulceration** may also be associated with *H. pylori* in up to 70% of cases in early studies, but is now more commonly caused by NSAID ingestion. Although most PUD may be explained by either *H. pylori* or NSAIDs, recent series from the USA report that neither *H. pylori*, nor a history of NSAID use could explain up to a third of gastric and duodenal ulcers. The reliability of this finding may be affected by inaccurate history taking related to NSAID use and/or unreliable testing procedures for *H. pylori*. Even so there is a subset of PUD in which a cause is not found. Before the first effective antisecretory therapy with H_2 blockers, the mainstay of therapy for recurrent or complicated PUD was surgery. Gastric surgery for PUD has almost vanished since the advent of proton pump inhibitor (PPI) therapy and the discovery of *H. pylori*.

Eradication of *H. pylori* is indicated if found in a patient with PUD. **Eradication of H. pylori** alone (Table 28.1) effectively heals and prevents recurrent *H. pylori*-associated PUD. Treatment with an antisecretory drug alone heals, but does not prevent recurrence unless treatment is continued. The combination of eradication therapy and acid suppression is superior to acid suppression alone in healing duodenal ulcers, but not necessarily with gastric ulcers.

The main benefit of *H. pylori* eradication therapy is to **prevent recurrent ulceration**. Following *H. pylori* eradication, recurrence of PUD is reduced

Table 28.1 *Helicobacter pylori* eradication therapy for *low-risk* patients*

First-line – 7 days treatment
>90% eradication rate. Usual reason for failure is poor adherence and not bacterial resistance

Omeprazole 20mg or lansoprazole 30mg twice daily	Amoxicillin 1g twice daily or (if penicillin allergic) metronidazole 400mg twice daily	Clarithromycin 500mg twice daily

Second-line – 14 days treatment (if failure of first-line)

Omeprazole 20mg or lansoprazole 30mg twice daily	Amoxicillin 1g twice daily or (if penicillin allergic) clarithromycin 500mg twice daily	Metronidazole 400mg twice daily

*Patients with dyspepsia in the community, or gastritis at endoscopy with no ulceration or other complications.

to <10%, compared with 60–70% if eradication therapy is not given. Maintenance therapy with a PPI is indicated for those patients who have to use long-term NSAIDs (rheumatological diseases, or aspirin for ischaemic heart disease). Misoprostil, a prostaglandin E analogue, is effective at reducing recurrence of NSAID-induced gastric ulceration. At a dose of 800μg/day, the recurrence rate was 4% at 12 weeks with continued NSAID therapy, compared with 65% on placebo in one study. This compares favourably with a PPI, but misoprostil is associated with more side effects.

Another strategy to manage patients with **PUD who need long-term NSAIDs** is to use a different analgesic. Selective COX-2 inhibitors are associated with a lower incidence of gastrointestinal side effects, although several agents have been withdrawn from the market because of increased cardiovascular side effects. Other novel NSAIDs include cyclo-oxygenase-inhibiting nitric oxide donators, which maintain mucosal blood flow while inhibiting cyclo-oxygenase, and are under development.

Following the diagnosis of a peptic ulcer, most often by endoscopy, **standard treatment** includes acid suppression for 4 weeks (esomeprazole 40mg, lansoprazole 30mg, daily omeprazole 20mg, or pantoprazole 40mg) for duodenal ulcers and 8 weeks for gastric ulcers, together with eradication therapy (Tables 28.1 and 28.2). Medication is best taken 30 min before breakfast to ensure maximal acid suppression, since this coincides with the time of maximal number of active binding sites. At the time of endoscopy, biopsies for *H. pylori* should be taken. Before PPI therapy has been started, a rapid urease test can be carried out on mucosal biopsies. If the patient is already on a PPI, histopathological examination of biopsies is necessary. Empirical eradication therapy for *H. pylori* can be justified in the case of duodenal ulceration, since these are almost always associated with infection. A positive test result for any ulcer allows confirmation of *H. pylori* as the cause and is best practice in view of the possibility of a non-*H. pylori* ulcer and the small percentage of alternative aetiologies.

Patients with *H. pylori* can be classified into low risk and high risk groups.

Low risk

- Dyspepsia in the community
- Antral or body gastritis at endoscopy, with no ulceration or other complications.

Table 28.2 *Helicobacter pylori* eradication therapy for *high-risk* patients*

1st line – 7 days treatment			
As above for low risk patients			
2nd line – 14 days treatment (after failure of 1st line)			
Omeprazole 20mg or lansoprazole 30mg twice daily	Metronidazole 400mg twice daily	Amoxicillin 1g twice daily or (if allergic to penicillin) clarithromycin 500mg twice daily	De-Noltab® 2 twice daily
3rd line – 14 days treatment (after failure of 1st and 2nd line)			
Omeprazole 20mg or lansoprazole 30mg twice daily	Metronidazole 400mg twice daily	Tetracycline 500mg three times daily	De-Noltab® 2 twice daily
4th line – 14 days treatment (generally reserved for patients with a MALT lymphoma on specialist advice			
Omeprazole 20mg or lansoprazole 30mg twice daily	De-Noltab® 2 twice daily	Plus TWO antibiotics not used before e.g. rifabutin, tetracycline or levofloxacin. Contact microbiology for patient specific advice	

*History of PUD; patients who continue to need NSAIDs, have peptic ulcers, or MALT lymphoma.

High risk

- Low-risk patients who continue to need NSAIDs
- Peptic ulcers, particularly if bleeding
- MALT lymphoma.

A second endoscopy to confirm ulcer healing is only necessary for gastric ulcers, 8 weeks after diagnosis. Multiple biopsies should be taken at the edge of the ulcer or healed area to exclude underlying malignancy, which may be present in 1% of gastric ulcers. Duodenal ulcers are almost never malignant, and require neither biopsy nor repeat endoscopy.

28e) **Discuss the potential complications and further management of this patient**

Complications of PUD include haemorrhage, perforation, and gastric outlet obstruction. The most common of these is haemorrhage. 15% of peptic ulcers bleed, and the risk increases with age. **Haemorrhage** may occur without preceding symptoms in 20% of cases. The risk of recurrent haemorrhage is reduced by eradication of *H. pylori*. Testing for *H. pylori* in acute upper gastrointestinal haemorrhage is hampered by a high false-negative rate for the rapid urease test. The urea breath test is inappropriate in the circumstances. Management of a bleeding ulcer first involves appropriate resuscitation, then endoscopic therapy (injection of adrenaline, heater probe application, or endoscopic clipping). Two modalities are best used: adrenaline injection plus one other. Successful endoscopic haemostasis is only then followed by high-dose intravenous therapy with a PPI. The Hong Kong regimen of **intravenous omeprazole** 80mg followed by 8mg/hour for up to 72 hours, reduces the rate of re-bleeding. The mechanism may be related to inhibition of thrombolysis at a higher gastric pH, with the formation of stable clot. Failure to establish haemostasis endoscopically requires surgical intervention, or radiographic embolization of a bleeding vessel.

Perforation of a peptic ulcer is the most common complication after haemorrhage. Up to 7% of peptic ulcers perforate. Penetration refers to direct extension of an ulcer into an adjacent organ, as opposed to free intraperitoneal perforation. A perforated peptic ulcer requires surgery. With the availability of acid suppression and eradication therapy, an omental patch (simple closure of the defect) is the procedure of choice. Eradication of *H. pylori* is highly effective at preventing recurrent duodenal ulcer perforation, and makes long-term acid suppression unnecessary. The most important prognostic factor determining outcome is time to diagnosis and appropriate surgery.

Delayed diagnosis (>24 hours) is associated with significant reduction in survival and a high index of suspicion needs to be maintained, especially for patients on corticosteroids or of advanced age, when clinical features of peritonitis may be masked. Any acutely ill elderly patient without a clinically identifiable explanation for their condition needs thorough evaluation of the abdomen, with appropriate radiological imaging. Conversely, it is worth noting that cocaine may be associated with duodenal ulcer perforation, which should be considered when perforation presents in young patients.

Gastric outlet obstruction occurs in up to 2% of patients with PUD. It may be inflammatory, presenting acutely with oedema in the duodenal bulb obstructing the gastric outlet, which may resolve with medical therapy. More commonly it is chronic, due to recurrent ulceration with fibrosis, causing a fixed stenosis of the gastric outlet. This is an indication for pneumatic (balloon) dilatation in conjunction with appropriate medical therapy (acid suppression and eradication therapy). If unsuccessful, a definitive surgical procedure is warranted.

PUD is occasionally refractory to medical therapy. A **refractory ulcer** is defined as an ulcer of >5mm that does not heal after appropriate PPI therapy (above). Missed *H. pylori* infection, continued NSAID ingestion and Zollinger–Ellison syndrome need to be considered.

Our patient had a diagnosis of visceral perforation made within 4 hours of presentation, and was appropriate for surgery, which was successful. Eradication therapy was prescribed, but since it was thought to be associated with prednisolone for her autoimmune liver disease, PPIs were continued long term. Confirmation of successful eradication of *H. pylori* would normally be achieved by a breath test 4 weeks after cessation of therapy, but because of the need to continue PPI therapy, a repeat endoscopy and mucosal biopsy for histopathology was arranged 8 weeks after surgery.

Further reading

Behrman SW (2005). Management of complicated peptic ulcer disease. *Arch Surg*; **140**: 201–8.

Kocer B, Surmeli S, Solak C, Unal B *et al.* (2007). Factors affecting mortality and morbidity in people with peptic ulcer perforation. *J Gastroenterol Hepatol*; **22**: 565–70.

Medicines Advisory Committee. Oxford Radcliffe Hospitals (2009). Adult guidelines: 1) Prescribing proton pump inhibitors, 2) *Helicobacter pylori* eradication. *Medicines information leaflet*. Oxford Radcliffe Hospitals NHS Trust; **2**(6).

Yuan Y, Padol IT, Hunt RH (2006). Peptic ulcer disease today. *Nat Clin Pract Gastroenterol Hepatol*; **3**: 80–9.

Case 29

A 50-year-old male university science lecturer presented for follow up with his gastroenterologist. He had previously had recurrent acute pancreatitis with four episodes over a period of 3 years, each with a marked increase in serum amylase. The last attack was a year ago. He denied drinking any alcohol. A cholecystectomy had been carried out after his second attack of pancreatitis. He reported some postprandial fullness and 4kg weight loss. He had no other medical history and was on no medication. Examination was normal.

Investigations showed:

- Hb 14.0g/dL, WCC 5.6 x 10^9/L, platelets 145 x 10^9/L
- Na 135mmol/L, K 4.1mmol/L, urea 3.5mmol/L, creatinine 75µmol/L
- Bilirubin 15µmol/L, AST 40 IU/L, ALT 40 IU/L, ALP 60 IU/L, GGT 35 IU/L, albumin 40g/L
- Amylase normal
- CA 19.9 normal
- A CT of the abdomen carried out 2 years previously had shown a pseudocyst in the head of the pancreas. Follow-up CT of the abdomen is illustrated (Fig. 29.1 and 29.2).
- An endoscopic ultrasound (Fig. 29.3) was carried out to characterize the lesion. This showed a very large cystic dilatation of the main pancreatic duct. There were multiple papillary projections. The main pancreatic duct was grossly dilated. A 'fish-mouth' papilla was also seen (Fig. 29.4 in the central coloured section).

Questions

29a) What are the causes of recurrent acute pancreatitis?

29b) What is the differential diagnosis of the above lesion? Describe how to differentiate between these diagnoses.

29c) How would fine-needle aspiration assist in diagnosis of this lesion?

29d) How should this patient be managed?

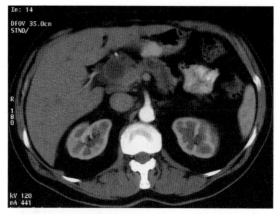

Fig. 29.1 CT scan.

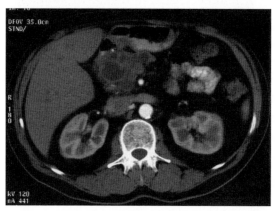

Fig. 29.2 CT scan.

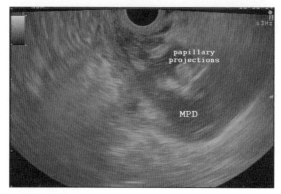

Fig. 29.3 Endoscopic ultrasound.
MPD: main pancreatic duct

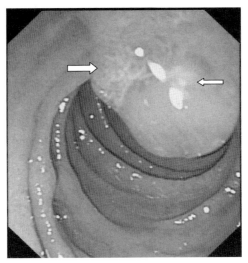

Fig. 29.4 (see colour plate 13) Papilla at ERCP.
Mucin extruding (small arrow) from the distorted papilla (large arrow).

Answers

29a) **What are the causes of recurrent acute pancreatitis?**

Any cause of acute pancreatitis may lead to further episodes if it is not corrected. The history and conventional diagnostic tests including blood tests for calcium and triglycerides, abdominal ultrasound to look for gallstones, MRCP, and CT scan of the abdomen, generally detect the cause of recurrent episodes of pancreatitis in 70% of cases. Endoscopic ultrasound may detect small stones in the common bile duct missed at ultrasound or MRCP. In view of the potential complications from ERCP (see Case 9), ERCP is now rarely an appropriate *diagnostic* investigation, although may be an appropriate *therapeutic* intervention.

Causes of recurrent pancreatitis are shown in Table 29.1.

29b) **What is the differential diagnosis of the above lesion? Describe how to differentiate between these diagnoses**

Based on the CT and endoscopic ultrasound findings, the main differential diagnoses in this case are:

- Pancreatic cystic neoplasm:
  - Mucin-producing tumours: intraductal papillary mucinous neoplasm (IPMN) and mucinous cystic neoplasm (MCN)
  - Serous cystadenoma (SCA)
- Inflammatory pseudocyst, secondary to previous pancreatitis
- Cystic adenocarcinoma.

Although inflammatory pseudocysts are more commonly associated with episodes of acute pancreatitis, it is important to exclude non-inflammatory cystic lesions that can cause acute pancreatitis, because they can have a risk of malignant transformation.

This lesion is most likely to be **intraductal papillary mucinous neoplasm** (IPMN). IPMN is a cystic neoplasm arising from the pancreatic duct, with mucin-producing epithelium. The CT scan and endoscopic ultrasound (Figs 29.1–29.3) show that the main pancreatic duct is markedly dilated and has papillary-type projections. Solid nodules in the wall of the pancreatic duct and the 'bright' sonographic features of mucin were seen. A 'fish-mouth' papilla, with mucin extruding from the ductal orifice, is characteristic of intraductal papillary mucinous neoplasm (Fig. 29.4). These lesions have a high risk of malignant transformation and can present with acute pancreatitis that is often recurrent. They are commonly **misdiagnosed** as the far more common 'pseudocysts'.

Table 29.1 Causes of recurrent pancreatitis

Mechanical

Congenital
Pancreatic divisum, annular pancreas

Acquired
- Gallstones (most frequent aetiological factor)
  - Microlithiasis (<2mm in diameter and usually seen at endoscopic ultrasound and ERCP)
  - Gallbladder sludge (usually seen on ultrasound)
  - Common bile duct macrolithiasis
- Sphincter of Oddi dysfunction (third most common cause of recurrent acute pancreatitis after gallstones and alcohol)
- Benign and malignant tumours of the pancreatic ductal systems
- Strictures of the pancreatic duct
- Choledochocele

Toxic
- Alcohol (very common cause)
- Organophosphates

Drug-induced (dose-dependent or idiosyncratic reactions)
- Examples – azathioprine, oestrogens, metronidazole, corticosteroids

Metabolic
- Hypertryglyceridaemia
- Hypercalcaemia

Familial and inherited
- Cystic fibrosis transmembrane regulator (CFTR) gene mutation
- Trypsinogen gene mutation

Miscellaneous
- Vasculitis
- Viral (mumps coxsackie) or parasitic infection
- Tuberculosis

Idiopathic (<10% of cases if investigated in detail)

As for differentiating an intraductal papillary mucinous neoplasm from other pancreatic cysts, Table 29.2 summarizes the characteristics of four common cystic lesions. A post-inflammatory pseudocyst is by far the most common.

29c) **How would fine-needle aspiration assist in the diagnosis of this lesion?**

Endoscopic ultrasound-guided, fine-needle aspiration yields fluid for cytology and chemical analysis. **Cytology** can be obtained in up to 80% of pancreatic cystic lesions (Table 29.2). **Cyst fluid** should be analysed for amylase (indicating communication with the pancreatic duct), and tumour markers such as CEA. Interpretation remains difficult and specialist advice is appropriate. A prospective study of 112 cysts reported a CEA <5ng/mL

Table 29.2 Differentiating pancreatic cystic lesions

Clinical	Morphology	Cystic fluid	Cytology	Malignant potential
Intraductal papillary mucinous neoplasm				
Equal gender distribution 6–7th decade Recurrent pancreatitis or abdominal pain occasionally found	Macrocyctic-and microcystic with dilatation of pancreatic duct	Viscous, transparent, with mucin	Mucinous columnar cells with atypia Fluid stains positive for mucin	Yes
Mucinous adenocarcinoma				
Females in 5th decade, especially from Asia, Often coincidentally detected, but can cause pain if large	Macrocystic or septated, may have thickened walls Peripheral calcification, with a solid component, No communication with pancreatic duct	Viscous, transparent, with mucin	Unique ovarian- like stroma	Yes
Serous cystadenoma				
Females in 7th decade	Microcystic or honeycomb lesion 20% are macrocystic	Thin, non-mucinous, haemorrhagic	Monomorphic cuboidal cells with clear, PAS-positive cytoplasm	No
Post-inflammatory pseudocyst				
History of acute pancreatitis	Unilocular, thick walled Septations are unusual	Glutinous, dark and opaque	Inflammatory cells, without mucin or epithelial cells	No

consistent with a serous cystadenoma, but when >192ng/mL indicated a mucinous adenocarcinoma (sensitivity 75%, specificity 85%). No other tumour markers (including CA 19.9) are accurate enough to provide a definitive diagnosis. When morphological criteria, cytology, and CEA >192ng/mL were combined, endoscopic ultrasound could differentiate mucinous from serous lesions with 91% sensitivity and 31% specificity.

The aspirate of this lesion had a high amylase resulting from communication with the pancreatic duct. Cytology showed columnar cells with atypia, and a CEA of 230ng/mL. This was consistent with an intraductal papillary mucinous neoplasm.

29d) **How should this patient be managed?**

Main duct mucin-producing tumours should, in general, be considered for resection. Endoscopic ultrasound helps predict potential malignancy on the basis of cyst wall thickness, intramural nodules, cystic dilatation of the main pancreatic duct and intracystic compartments >10mm. Intraductal papillary mucinous neoplasms are often multifocal, with a recurrence rate of 10% after surgery. Surveillance by ultrasound or MRCP may be appropriate and should be discussed with the patient. This is in contrast to mucinous cystic neoplasms, which do not recur after resection.

Before surgery, it is important to consider:

- symptoms
- age and life expectancy
- degree of surgical risk
- location and size of lesion.

Current mortality for patients undergoing pancreaticoduodenectomy is <2% in established centres. Specialist advice is appropriate.

This patient underwent a pancreaticoduodenectomy (Whipple's procedure). Histopathology confirmed an intraductal papillary mucinous carcinoma. The common bile duct and main pancreatic duct were free of tumour at the resection margin.

Further reading

AGSE guideline (2005). the role of endoscopy in the diagnosis and the management of cystic lesions and inflammatory fluid collections of the pancreas. *Gastrointest Endosc*; **61**: 363–70.

Brugge WR, Lauwers GY, Sahani D, Fernandez-del Castillo C, Warshaw AL (2004). Cystic neoplasms of the pancreas. *N Engl J Med*; **351**: 1218–26.

Brugge WR, Lewandrowski, Lee-Lewandroxski E *et al.* (2004). The diagnosis of pancreatic cystic neoplasms: a report of the cooperative pancreatic cyst (CPC) study. *Gastroenterology*; **126**: 1330–6.

Tanaka M, Chari S, Adsay V *et al.* (2006). International consensus guidelines for management of intraductal paillary mucinous neoplasms and mucinous cystic neoplasms of the pancreas. *Pancreatology*; **6**: 17–32.

Case 30

A 70-year-old woman was referred for assessment of loss of appetite, nausea, and weight loss of 12kg over the preceding 12 months. She had an iron-deficient, microcytic anaemia.

Her past medical history included pernicious anaemia, common variable immune deficiency, and bronchiectasis. On examination she had crackles generally heard across her lung fields, together with hepatomegaly.

Questions

30a) What is pernicious anaemia?

30b) What other diseases are associated with pernicious anaemia?

30c) Discuss the differential diagnosis and appropriate investigations

30d) Discuss the causes and features of the diagnosis.

30e) How is pernicious anaemia treated?

Answers

30a) **What is pernicious anaemia?**

Pernicious anaemia is the consequence of **vitamin B12 deficiency** resulting from autoimmune destruction of the gastric parietal cell mass and consequent absence of **intrinsic factor**. The type of gastritis is termed **chronic atrophic gastritis Type A** (as opposed to type B, due to *Helicobacter pylori*). Type A gastritis predominantly affects the gastric corpus, causing mucosal atrophy, achlorhydria, and secondary hypergastrinaemia. Gastrin concentrations may approach those seen in Zollinger–Ellison syndrome (ZES) from gastrin-secreting tumours. In contrast to ZES, hypergastrinaemia is secondary to achlorhydria, with a high antral pH; it is therefore not associated with excessive gastric acid production or gastroduodenal ulceration. Destruction of chief cells leads to low serum levels of pepsinogen I.

Pernicious anaemia is more common in people of northern European decent, and the prevalence in the UK is estimated at 120 per 100,000. It is slightly more prevalent in women, with a ratio of 1.6:1. Ninety percent of cases develop >40 years of age, with a peak at 60 years of age.

Patients are generally asymptomatic before severe corpus atrophy has occurred. Once the disease is advanced and vitamin B12 (cobalamin) concentrations are reduced, patients often develop **non-specific symptoms** of fatigue, nausea, or weight loss. Mucosal consequences of B12 deficiency manifest with a **sore tongue** which is beefy red. A *megaloblastic anaemia* with marked macrocytosis is characteristic, but neurological symptoms are the most worrying. A **myelopathy** affecting the posterior columns of the spinal cord manifests as **loss of proprioception**, and a **peripheral neuropathy** develops. A useful clinical clue is an extensor plantar response in the absence of ankle tendon reflexes. Psychiatric disturbances with paranoia ('megaloblastic madness') may occur, but advanced cases are now uncommon. Without cobalamin replacement the course is fatal.

Advanced gastric atrophy is visible at endoscopy, with loss of rugal folds and visible submucosal vessels. Biopsies should be taken to confirm severe atrophy of the corpus, with sparing of the antral mucosa. Intestinal metaplasia may be present. An earlier stage of type A gastritis has been described (a so-called 'proliferative stage'), with hyperplasic polyps secondary to the hypergastrinaemia. Type A autoimmune gastritis should be suspected in people who have multiple gastric polyps in the absence of long-term therapy with a proton pump inhibitor.

30b) **What other diseases are associated with pernicious anaemia?**

Pernicious anaemia is associated with **other autoimmune diseases**, including adrenal insufficiency, hypothyroidism, Grave's disease, type 1 diabetes, myasthenia gravis, vitiligo, alopaecia, and coeliac disease. This association is sometimes referred to as **polyglandular autoimmune syndrome type II**. Polyglandular autoimmune syndrome type II is inherited in a polygenic fashion, with an onset in adulthood, and is more common in females. The autosomal recessive polyglandular autoimmune syndrome type I has its onset in childhood and may also include pernicious anaemia. Pernicious anaemia is also associated with premature greying of hair, blue eyes, blood group A, HLA B8 and DR3, and **common variable immunodeficiency** (as in our patient).

Pernicious anaemia is a well documented risk factor for **gastric adenocarcinoma**. It is possible that common variable immunodeficiency increases this risk. Nevertheless, there is no recommended protocol for endoscopic screening of these patients. It is unclear whether the risk is related to a combination of autoimmune (type A) gastritis and *Helicobacter pylori*-associated (type B) gastritis. An increased incidence of gastric mucosal carcinoid tumours has been reported, due to hyper-gastrinaemia. Carcinoid syndrome is not associated more often than by chance. Pancreatic and oesophageal malignancies may occur more frequently.

30c) **Discuss the differential diagnosis and appropriate investigations.**

Before considering the specific clinical circumstances in the current patient, a brief comment about **uncomplicated pernicious anaemia** is appropriate. The condition is so common in older people that treatment of B12 deficiency is generally started without further investigation. Investigation of a low serum vitamin B12 in **younger patients** includes measurement of gastric parietal cell and **intrinsic factor antibodies**. False-negative results are common in older people. **Thyroid function** should be checked, because of the association with autoimmune thyroid disease. Addison's disease should be considered as a potential cause of persistent fatigue in a patient with pernicious anaemia. Folate concentrations should be measured to exclude concomitant folate deficiency as a cause of a macrocytic anaemia. Terminal ileal disease (such as Crohn's) should be considered, but rarely causes B12 deficiency unless a long segment (>100cm) is affected or resected. **Upper gastrointestinal endoscopy** is appropriate if there is doubt about the diagnosis, to obtain biopsies from the body and antrum of the stomach; it is wise to take distal duodenal biopsies to exclude small intestinal villous atrophy at the same time. The Schilling test uses isotopes of cobalamin to test absorption of an oral dose with and without intrinsic factor; it is now obsolete. Measurement of serum gastrin or serum pepsinogen is unnecessary.

For this particular patient, nausea and loss of appetite are non-specific, but our patient had hepatomegaly, which makes malignancy more likely. Metabolic disturbance (hyponatraemia, hypercalcaemia), drugs and intracranial pathology should also be considered. The weight loss and iron deficiency call for urgent assessment, although achlorhydria can decrease iron absorption.

Weight loss should not simply be ascribed to a loss of appetite and reduced food intake. Underlying **malignancy** and **gastric carcinoma** in association with pernicious anaemia tops the list, with hepatomegaly from metastases. Malabsorption, from coeliac disease associated with pernicious anaemia, or villous atrophy associated with common variable immunodeficiency is possible, but would not explain the hepatomegaly. Endomysial or tissue transglutaminase antibodies are of no diagnostic value in immunodeficiency, owing to low IgA and IgG concentrations. **Non-Hodgkin lymphoma** associated with common variable immuno-deficiency could account for the systemic symptoms and hepatomegaly. Finally, bronchiectasis with chronic airways infection may cause weight loss. Hepatomegaly might conceivably be due to **amyloidosis** of the AA type, although this usually presents with renal disease before organo-megaly is evident.

An upper gastrointestinal endoscopy is the investigation of choice to identify a gastric carcinoma, or obtain small intestinal biopsies. This patient had a gastroscopy which revealed a large gastric tumour involving the posterior wall of the stomach, extending from the upper body to the pre-pyloric antrum. Histopathology revealed a gastric adenocarcinoma. A staging CT scan of the abdomen and pelvis was requested (Fig. 30.1) and this revealed a large gastric tumour with locally advanced disease extending through the wall of the stomach into the lesser omentum, lymph node enlargement at the porta hepatis and coeliac axis, and multiple focal liver lesions suggestive of metastases. Stage T3N2M1.

30d) **Discuss the causes and features of the diagnosis.**

Gastric adenocarcinoma has declined worldwide since the 1930s. Even so, gastric cancer remained the second most common cause of cancer-related death worldwide in 2002. The decline only applies to antral (non-cardia) gastric tumours, probably from better food preservation following

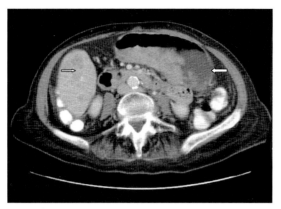

Fig. 30.1 CT scan showing a large gastric tumour (large arrow) extending through the wall of the stomach into the lesser omentum, with lymph node enlargement at the porta hepatis and coeliac axis, and multiple focal liver lesions (small arrow) consistent with metastases.

the advent of refrigeration, and a reduction in *H. Pylori* infection. *H. pylori* is classified as a class I carcinogen by the WHO. The incidence of gastric cancer remains high in the Far East (Japan and China), thought to be due to the consumption of high volumes of raw and preserved fish with a high nitrate content. Bacteria convert nitrates to carcinogenic nitrites. *H. pylori*-associated (type B) chronic gastritis may lead to gastric atrophy, intestinal metaplasia, dysplasia, and cancer. Chronic autoimmune gastritis (type A) may cause gastric cancer via the same sequence of events, and the common factor appears to be the chronic inflammation. Both type A and B gastritis are associated with **intestinal type** tumours, as opposed to the **diffuse type** responsible for linitis plastica.

Gastric cancers typically present late. Tumours localized to the mucosa, which have the best chance of cure when completely resected, are usually asymptomatic, and found incidentally or in association with a screening programme. These '**early gastric cancers**' are more commonly encountered in Japan than in the UK, although it is difficult to demonstrate that this is because of ready access to endoscopy. Symptoms usually herald spread of the tumour. Direct transmural extension involves adjacent organs. Lymphatic spread occurs relatively early. Distant metastases most commonly involve the liver. Metastatic involvement of the supraclavicular nodes on the left (Virchow–Trossier), a periumbilical nodule (Sister Mary Joseph nodule), or transperitoneal spread with malignant ascites, all imply advanced disease.

As for all cancers, a histopathological diagnosis is essential and tissue is readily obtained through endoscopic biopsies. Gastric cancer is generally staged according to the TNM classification, and may also be categorized into stages I–IV. Our patient already had distant metastases (M1), which made her disease stage IV, regardless of the depth of tumour invasion into the gastric wall (T3) or lymph node involvement (N2).

30e) **How is this condition treated?**

Once distant metastases are present, gastric cancer is unresectable, and median survival is <1 year. Large tumours that adhere to adjacent organs and involve regional lymph nodes without distant metastases, although potentially resectable, carry a 5-year survival of <10%. Non-adherent invasive gastric cancer, with or without lymph node involvement, carries a 5-year survival of <30% after resection. Tumours that invade the sub-mucosa and do not affect nodes have a 60% 5-year survival after resection.

Resection of distal gastric cancer involves a subtotal gastrectomy. Diffuse or proximal tumours require total gastrectomy. There has been much debate between Japan and the West about the extent of lymph node clearance. Lymph node resection involves removal of nodes along the lesser curve, the greater curve (N1/D1), the left gastric artery, the hepatic artery, the coeliac artery, and the splenic artery (N2/D2). **D1 resection** involves removal of the affected part of the stomach or the whole stomach along with the lesser and greater omentum. **D2 resection** includes the omental sac, part of the transverse mesocolon, clearance of nodes surrounding the above mentioned arteries, and partial resection of adjacent organs (spleen and pancreatic tail). Extended (D2) lymph-adenectomy adds to the surgical complications without a significant survival benefit, so D1 resection is usually recommended.

Adjuvant chemotherapy adds no clinically significant survival benefit, but perioperative chemotherapy with platinum-based regimens, seems to improve survival. One trial has shown that 3 cycles of preoperative and 3 cycles of postoperative combination therapy with epirubicin, cis-platin and 5-fluorouracil (ECF regimen) was associated with a 5 year survival of 36%, compared with 23% for those having surgery alone; this was confirmed in a subsequent study.

Two-thirds of gastric cancers diagnosed in the West are unresectable or have metastasized at the time of diagnosis. Depending on the patient's health, **palliative chemotherapy** may be given. The choice of chemo-therapy is large, which suggests that none show particular advantage, so

specialist advice is appropriate. **Post-operative chemoradiation** is prac-
tised in the USA. The standard of care in the UK is ECF, which offers a
small survival benefit. Oxaliplatin and capcytabine may be substituted
for cisplatin and 5-fluorouracil (EOX regimen). Docetaxel may be substituted for epirubicin, and may have some benefit over ECF at the cost
of more frequent neutropenia. Irinotecan with 5-fluorouracil (IFL
regimen) has also been tested and may be better than cisplatin and
5-fluorouracil, the latter being a commonly used regimen in the USA.
Targeted therapies with **monoclonal antibodies** to the epidermal growth
factor receptor (cetuximab), and vascular endothelial growth factor
(bevacizumab) and tyrosine kinase inhibitors (erlotinib and gefitinib)
are under investigation. The matrix metalloproteinase inhibitor mari-
mastat did not fulfil early promise.

It needs to be remembered that the current chemotherapeutic regimens are toxic and offer a small survival benefit. Our patient opted for
palliative radiotherapy for symptom control.

Further reading

Bonenkamp JJ, Hermans J, Sasako M *et al.* (1999). Extended lymph-node dissection for
gastric cancer. *N Engl J Med*; **340**: 908–14.

Foukakis T, Lundell L, Gubanski M, Lind PA (2007). Advances in treatment of patients
with gastric adenocarcinoma. *Acta Oncologica*; **46**: 277–85.

Karlson B-M, Ekbom A, Wacholder S *et al.* (2000). Cancer of the upper gastrointestinal
tract among patients with pernicious anaemia: A case-cohort study. *Scand J
Gastroenterol*; **35**: 847–51.

Orlando LA, Lenard L, Orland RC (2007). Chronic hypergastrinaemia: causes and
consequences. *Dig Dis Sci*; **52**: 2482–9.

Peter S, Beglinger C (2007). *Helicobacter pylori* and gastric cancer: The causal relationship.
Digestion; **75**: 25–35.

Case 31

A 60-year-old retired female secretary who had had two renal transplants for adult polycystic kidney disease, presented unwell with 5 weeks of profuse, watery (non-bloody) diarrhoea and 9kg weight loss. She had had her first transplant in 1992, which failed in 1997 because of rejection. The second transplant was in 2000 and this was functioning well. She also had Type 2 diabetes mellitus, gout, and epilepsy (no seizures for 3 years). Daily medications were sodium valproate 400mg, frusemide 250mg, allopurinol 100mg, doxazosin 8mg twice daily, loratidine 10mg, mycophenolate 2g, prednisolone 5mg, atorvastatin 10mg, aspirin 75mg, and colchicine or codydramol, as needed.

She looked unwell, with a pulse rate of 90 beats per minute, a temperature of 37.8°C, and blood pressure 140/75mmHg, with a 15mmHg postural drop. There was no local tenderness in the abdomen, and the transplanted kidney was palpable in the left iliac fossa.

Investigations showed:

- Hb 13.4g/dL, WCC 10.7 x 10^9/L, platelets 355 x 10^9/L
- Na 138mmol/L, K 3.7mmol/L, urea 21.5mmol/L, creatinine 182 μmol/L (stable for this patient)
- Bilirubin 3μmol/L, ALT 40 IU/L, ALP 191 IU/L, GGT 50 IU/L, albumin 41g/L
- Abdominal radiograph: normal, with no colonic dilatation.

Questions

31a) What are the possible causes of the diarrhoea?

31b) What investigations should be done and what treatment administered while waiting for these investigations?

31c) Describe the findings on the sigmoidoscopy photograph and the histology (Figs 31.1–31.3 in the colour section).

31d) What is the diagnosis and describe different methods for diagnosis?

31e) What is the treatment for the above condition?

Answers

31a) **What are the possible causes of the diarrhoea?**

The possible causes of the diarrhoea are best categorized as infective, medication related, and 'other'.

Infective

Bacterial:

- *Salmonella* spp (*Campylobacter* sp or *Shigella* spp usually cause bloody diarrhoea).

- *Clostridium difficile* (pseudomembranous colitis) commonly presents as watery diarrhoea, low grade fever, and crampy abdominal pain, although it is often bloody. Symptoms usually begin during, or up to 6 weeks after, antibiotic therapy. *C. difficile* colitis is more likely to occur in the absence of antibiotics in transplant recipients. Severe pseudomembranous colitis can cause toxic megacolon, which is fatal in up to 60% of patients, largely because of comorbidity (see Case 22).

Viral and parasitic:

- CMV, rotavirus: the anti-CMV response is predominantly cell mediated. Calcineurin inhibitors (tacrolimus or cyclosporin) suppress T-cell proliferation, thereby predisposing transplant recipients to CMV colitis. Risk factors for CMV infection include: CMV-negative recipient receiving organ from CMV-positive donor, use of monoclonal antibody to treat rejection (OKT3), and older recipients (>55 years). CMV disease most frequently manifests as a non-specific syndrome of fever, myalgia, malaise, leucopenia, and/or thrombocytopenia. CMV in the gut generally presents as fever, diarrhoea, and abdominal pain. Gastrointestinal bleeding may also complicate severe CMV enteritis or colitis. There are rare instances of perforation resulting from CMV colitis and megacolon.

Microsporidia, cryptosporidia, and parasites:

- Should be considered in immunocompromised individuals.

Medication-related

- Immunosuppressive agents (especially mycophenolate, ciclosporin, tacrolimus, and sirolimus). Questions regarding recent changes of medication are important

- Non-immunosuppressive agents (e.g. antiarrhythmics, antibiotics, antihypertensives, diuretics, diabetic medication, laxatives, proton pump inhibitors, protease inhibitors).

Other

- **Post-transplant lymphoproliferative disorder**: this can vary from a low grade, indolent process to an aggressive neoplasm. Clinical features suggesting this diagnosis include lymphadenopathy, unexplained fever, and systemic features, such as weight loss
- **Colon cancer**: unlikely, because of acute onset
- **Bacterial overgrowth**: commonly presents with abdominal pain, diarrhoea, bloating, weight loss, or weakness. There is usually a history of small bowel diverticula, dysmotility, strictures, or surgically formed blind loops
- **Lactose intolerance**: the main symptoms are bloating, flatulence, abdominal cramps and diarrhoea. It is unlikely to cause weight loss.
- **Colonic ischaemia**: possible, given the age and comorbidity, but this usually presents with sudden-onset, crampy, abdominal pain, an urgent desire to defecate, and passage of bright red or maroon blood mixed with the stool, within 24 hours. Mild to moderate abdominal tenderness is often present over the involved segment of bowel.
- New presentation of inflammatory bowel disease or flare of pre-existing inflammatory bowel disease: this is unlikely given the sudden onset.

31b) **What investigations should be done and what treatment administered while waiting for these investigations?**

Investigations that should be requested are:

- Stool microscopy/cytology/sensitivity, ova/cysts/parasites, and *C. difficile* toxin assay
- Flexible sigmoidoscopy to obtain biopsies
- Check CMV status of patient and donor
- Colonoscopy is best avoided in the acute stage as bowel preparation exacerbates the physiological disturbance caused by severe diarrhoea.

Treatment should be oral and intravenous fluids to support renal graft function. Oral intake can be continued. Intravenous hydrocortisone is best started on admission, while waiting for stool cultures and mucosal biopsy results to return, because acute ulcerative colitis is a diagnostic possibility. It is better to **treat both** the possibility of acute ulcerative colitis and infective colitis, rather than either alone. Vancomycin (to cover *C. difficile*) and ciprofloxacin or azithromycin (to cover Gram-negative pathogens) are appropriate antibiotics.

31c) **Describe the findings on the sigmoidoscopy photograph and the histopathology**

The sigmoidoscopy picture reveals patchy mucosal erythema, with some ulceration and haemorrhagic patches. Standard haematoxylin and eosin staining revealed classic 'owl's eye' inclusion bodies (Fig. 31.2); CMV immunohistochemistry was positive (Figs 31.1, 31.2, 31.3).

31d) **What is the diagnosis and describe different methods for diagnosis?**

The diagnosis is **CMV colitis**. Positive immunofluorescence on tissue biopsy has a 100% positive predictive value, but sensitivity is variable. Clinically significant CMV colitis can usually be identified, however, on haematoxylin and eosin staining. Quantification of IgM and IgG antibodies to CMV are unreliable and conventional CMV cultures have a sensitivity of about 50%. The CMV rapid antigen test has a high positive predictive value (100%), but can only be carried out on cellular specimens. Amplification by PCR has the highest negative predictive value (100%), but the positive

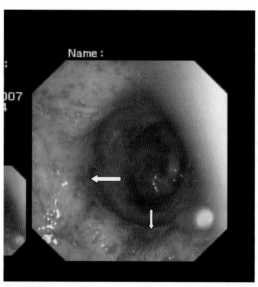

Fig. 31.1 (see colour plate 14) Photograph of mucosal appearance in the sigmoid colon: patchy erythema (large arrow), with some ulceration (small arrow) and haemorrhagic patches.

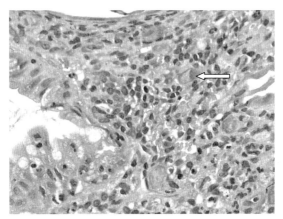

Fig. 31.2 (see colour plate 15) Haematoxylin and eosin staining of mucosal biopsy showing classic 'owl's eye' inclusion bodies (arrow).

predictive value is only 60%. Reactivation of CMV in a previously infected recipient tends to be less clinically severe than *de novo* infection.

31e) **What is the treatment for the above condition?**

CMV colitis is treated if the colitis is causing serious symptoms with high-dose intravenous ganciclovir, but not for positive PCR alone. Viral resistance has been described. Other therapies include a CMV hyper-immune globulin and foscarnet. Specialist advice is appropriate.

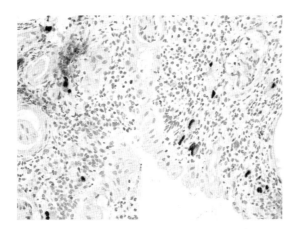

Fig. 31.3 (see colour plate 16) Positive immunohistochemistry for CMV.

4

Further reading

Altiparmak MR, Trablus S, Pamuk ON *et al.* (2002). Diarrhoea following renal transplantation. *Clin Transplant*; **16**: 212–16.

Ayre K, Warren BF, Jeffrey K, Travis SPL (2009). The role of CMV in steroid-resistant ulcerative colitis: a systematic review. *J Crohn's & Colitis*; **3**: 141–148.

Kaufman H S, Kahn A C, Iacobuzio-Donahue C *et al.* (1999). Cytomegaloviral enterocolitis: clinical associations and outcome. *Dis Colon Rectum*; **42**: 24–30.

Rubin RH (2001). Gastrointestinal infectious disease complications following transplantation and their differentiation from immunosuppressant-induced gastrointestinal toxicities. *Clin Transplantation*; **15**(Suppl. 4): 11–22.

Case 32

A 42-year-old mother of three presented to her family practitioner with increased bowel frequency, loose stools, and urgency, but without rectal bleeding. She had recently returned from a trip to Malaysia. A stool sample was sent, and culture revealed *Campylobacter sp*. She was treated with a course of antibiotics.

Two months later she was reviewed by her family practitioner. She still passed frequent, poorly formed stools and had intermittent abdominal pain, although sometimes had constipation. She complained of abdominal bloating and was tired all the time. Avoidance of dairy products had made no difference. A repeat stool sample was negative. At this point, she was referred to a gastroenterology clinic.

She was seen 3 months later. She reported frequent passage of semi-formed/ loose stools, without blood or mucus. She had some urgency, especially on waking in the morning, but had no nocturnal diarrhoea. Her stools flushed away easily and were not greasy. Defaecation was preceded by lower abdominal pain, which settled temporarily on opening her bowels.

Investigations:

- Hb 12.7g/dL, WCC 6.23 x 10^9/L, platelets 267 x 10^9/L, MCV 89fL
- CRP <6mg/L
- U&E and LFT normal
- EMA negative, IgA normal
- TSH normal
- Colonoscopy normal
- Histology of colonic mucosa normal.

Questions

32a) What is the likely diagnosis?

32b) What are the risk factors for development of this syndrome?

32c) How does it develop?

32d) How should it be managed?

32e) What is the long-term outlook for this patient?

Answers

32a) **What is the likely diagnosis?**

A history of abdominal pain for >3 months that improves on defaecation and is associated with a change in bowel frequency or stool consistency is highly suggestive of irritable bowel syndrome (IBS). The most commonly used criteria are the Rome criteria, most recently updated in 2006 (Table 32.1).

In our patient, persistent symptoms had been preceded by infectious diarrhoea and had not abated following antibiotic therapy, with subsequent negative stool samples. A diagnosis of **post-infective irritable bowel syndrome** was therefore made. A diagnosis of post-infective IBS must be preceded by an episode of infective gastroenteritis with two or more of the following criteria: fever, vomiting, diarrhoea, and a positive stool culture. In 1962 Chaudry and Truelove described a cohort of 130 cases of 'irritable colon syndrome'. They reported that 26% of patients in their cohort associated the onset of their symptoms with an episode of acute dysentery. This was the first clear description of post-infective IBS. The largest study has involved 840 patients with *Campylobacter jejuni* infection. Of these, 794 were studied, and 103 or 14% met criteria for post-infectious IBS. The predominant symptom was loose stools. A third study reported 169 students with travellers' diarrhoea, of whom 10% developed post-infective IBS with predominantly diarrhoeal symptoms.

32b) **What are the risk factors for development of the syndrome?**

The risk factors are similar to IBS of any aetiology, not preceded by infection. Pre-existing psychological disorders of anxiety and depression are more frequent in patients with post-infective IBS, but such a history is less common in post-infective IBS than other forms of IBS. Female gender and an age <30 years have been shown to confer a greater risk of developing post-infective IBS. Nevertheless, the duration of the precipitating infection is one of the strongest risk factors. When the initial illness lasts >3 weeks, the risk of developing post infective IBS increases 11-fold compared with a duration <1 week. Specific bacteria may also increase the risk, possibly due to an increased severity of mucosal damage and longer duration of infection. Infection with *Campylobacter* or *Shigella* species carries an increased risk of developing post-infective IBS compared with *Salmonella* sp. Vomiting in the course of the illness has been shown to reduce the risk of post-infective IBS.

Table 32.1 International criteria (Rome III: 2006) for the diagnosis of IBS

ROME III diagnostic criteria	ROME II diagnostic criteria
Irritable Bowel Syndrome	**Irritable Bowel Syndrome**
*Diagnostic criterion**	At least 12 weeks, which need not be consecutive, in the preceding 12 months of abdominal discomfort or pain that has *two out of three* features:
Recurrent abdominal pain or discomfort** at least 3 days/month in last 3 months associated with *two or more* of the following:	
• Improvement with defaecation • Onset associated with a change in frequency of stool • Onset associated with a change in form (appearance) of stool	• Relieved with defaecation • Onset associated with a change in frequency of stool • Onset associated with a change in form (appearance) of stool.
* Criterion fulfilled for the last 3 months with symptom onset at least 6 months prior to diagnosis.	Symptoms that cumulatively support the diagnosis of Irritable Bowel Syndrome:
**'Discomfort' means an uncomfortable sensation not described as pain.	• Abnormal stool frequency (for research purposes 'abnormal' may be defined as >3 bowel movements/day and <3 bowel movements/week)
In pathophysiology research and clinical trials, a pain/discomfort frequency of at least 2 days a week during the screening evaluation is recommended for subject eligibility.	• Abnormal stool form (lumpy/hard or loose/watery stool) • Abnormal stool passage (straining, urgency, or feeling of incomplete evacuation) • Passage of mucus • Bloating or feeling of abdominal distension

32c) **How does it develop?**

Serotonin (5-hydroxytryptamine or 5HT) is found in enterochromafin cells in the gut. These **enterochromafin cells** have been shown to be increased in the rectal mucosa of patients with post-infective IBS when compared with patients with other types of IBS. Consistent with this observation, postprandial levels of plasma **serotonin** are increased in patients with post-infective IBS. Serotonin affects gastrointestinal motility and secretions from enterocytes, as well as **visceral sensation**. Inflammation may play a part in post-infective IBS, illustrated by increased numbers of intraepithelial lymphocytes and lamina propria lymphocytes, which persist for at least a year after the acute infection. This has been associated with altered intestinal permeability. Furthermore, an increased level of IL-1β in the rectal mucosa of patients with enteric infection who go on to develop post-infective IBS has been reported when compared with those who make a full recovery. Even so a double-blind placebo-controlled trial of prednisolone in post-infective IBS showed no improvement in symptoms, even though mucosal lymphocytes were reduced. The IL-10/IL-12 ratio is depressed in patients with IBS. IL-10 is an anti-inflammatory cytokine, and IL-12 is pro-inflammatory.

A trial showing improvement in symptoms on the administration of probiotics has shown normalization of the IL-10/IL-12 ratio. This has yet to be replicated, but is suggestive of an inflammatory component in the aetiology of the disorder. A **genetic component** related to increased production of IL-10 has been shown to be less common in patients with IBS. IBS-type symptoms are increasingly recognized in patients with otherwise quiescent inflammatory bowel disease, suggesting an overlap between inflammation and dysmotility, which is not surprising when considered. Another factor that may play a role is bile salt malabsorption after enteric infections. Lactose intolerance, however, is less common in adults than in the paediatric population following enteric infection.

32d) **How can it be managed?**

As for IBS in general, the treatment of post-infective IBS is directed at symptom relief. It follows that IBS is subcategorized, based on the predominant symptom into **constipation-predominant IBS** (C-IBS), **diarrhoea-predominant IBS** (D-IBS) and alternating or **mixed symptoms** (M-IBS). Our patient complained of abdominal pain along with an increased stool frequency.

Lifestyle factors need to be reviewed. Excessive caffeine intake (xanthines stimulate cAMP) and even small amounts of alcohol can cause diarrhoea. Constipation on the other hand is sometimes exacerbated by inactivity, inadequate fluid intake, and a diet low in soluble fibre. **Soluble fibre** supplementation (for instance, with a tablespoon of Golden Linseed daily, mixed with a live yoghourt or a fruit compôte) can improve constipation, but has little effect on pain. **Fermentation of fibre** may increase symptoms of bloating and flatulence. **Specialist dietary advice** to reduce resistant starch intake is often helpful when symptoms of bloating and or diarrhoea predominate. **Resistant starch** is that component of complex carbohydrate (starch) that remains undigested in the small intestine. This then gets fermented by colonic bacteria to cause bloating. Foods high in resistant starches include bread, potatoes and pasta that are processed to prolong their shelf-life. Fibre intake needs to be titrated to the individual if it is to make any difference at all.

Loperamide or codeine slow bowel transit and may be beneficial in patients with increased stool frequency. Loperamide has little effect on pain, while codeine may become habit forming. Colicky pain may be treated with **antispasmodics** such as hyoscine butylbromide or mebeverine. Paediatric doses of antidepressant medication may have a particularly useful role in D-IBS and pain. **Tricyclic antidepressant** compounds like amitriptyline are effective for pain at low doses (10–30mg at night), which would be subtherapeutic for depression. Their anticholinergic effects, which delay bowel transit, may help symptoms of D-IBS. Selective serotonin reuptake inhibitors (SSRIs) may similarly improve pain perception, but may cause diarrhoea. Serotonin receptor modulators have been shown to have good therapeutic effect, but are not commonly used be-cause of their side effects.

Other pharmacological and non-pharmacological approaches may be necessary for refractory symptoms. **Tegaserod**, a partial $5\text{-}HT_4$ agonist, was shown in an initial trial to benefit women with C-IBS. It accelerates bowel transit, increases bowel frequency, and improves abdominal pain. Unfortunately, because of increased cardiovascular events, this drug is not available. **Alosetron**, a $5\text{-}HT_3$ antagonist, was found to be beneficial in D-IBS in women, by increasing small intestinal absorption, slowing colonic transit and improving visceral pain. Complications of severe constipation, ischaemic colitis, and bowel perforation lead to withdrawal or restricted use of this drug. A trial of **colestyramine** or colesevalam, for possible bile-salt malabsorption, is sometimes worth exploring when diarrhoea is troublesome. There is no evidence to support the use of antibiotics for bacterial overgrowth. **Acupuncture** and **hypnotherapy** are complementary approaches that have been subject to randomized controlled trials and may be suggested to patients who do not have adequate symptom relief. Some patients opt for alternative or complementary therapies, for which evidence is lacking, but individual cases may benefit.

32e) **What is the long-term outlook for this patient?**

Patients with IBS, whether post-infective or not, generally have a chronic relapsing and remitting symptom pattern. The likelihood of resolution in the long term is better in patients without significant psychological comorbidity. Similarly, patients with an acute onset of symptoms, achieve resolution more often compared with those with a gradual onset of symptoms. One study showed resolution of symptoms at 6 years of follow-up in 43% of patients with post-infective IBS, compared with 31% in patients with IBS not following an infection. In another study,

80% of patients with post-infective IBS still had some symptoms of IBS after 5 years. This group had had documented *Salmonella sp* infection prior to the onset of symptoms.

Our patient was reviewed 11 months after initial symptom onset. Symptoms were much improved, but still present at this stage.

Further reading

Drossman DA (2006). The functional gastrointestinal disorders and the Rome III process. *Gastroenterology*; **130**: 1377–90.

Du Pont AW (2008). Postinfectious irritable bowel syndrome. *Clin Infect Dis* 2008; **46**: 594–9.

Spiller R, Campbell E (2006). Post-infectious irritable bowel syndrome. *Curr Opin Gastroenterol*; **22**: 13–7.

Spiller RC (2007). Role of infection in irritable bowel syndrome. *J Gastroenterol*; **42**(Suppl. XVII): 41–7.

Spiller R, Aziz Q, Creed F, Emmanuel A *et al.* (2007). Guidelines on the irritable bowel syndrome: mechanisms and practical management. *Gut*; **56**: 1770–98.

Case 33

A 61-year-old British man living in Kazakhstan was well until he developed severe abdominal pain with a fever. A diagnosis of acute diverticulitis, perforation, and peritonitis was made. He underwent an emergency laparotomy, which confirmed a perforated sigmoid diverticulum. The sigmoid colon was resected and a loop ileostomy was formed. His postoperative recovery was good, but 3 weeks after discharge he presented with nausea, decreased appetite, and lethargy. He described emptying his ileostomy bag about 4 times/day, but was unsure of the volume.

On examination the patient looked dehydrated. The wound was clean. The stoma looked healthy and easily admitted a little finger. On rectal examination there was no pus. On sigmoidoscopy there was a healthy rectum.

Investigations showed:

- Hb 15.3g/dL, WCC 10.7 x 10^9/L, platelets 824 x 10^9/L
- Na 119mmol/L, K 6.1mmol/L, urea 41.2mmol/L, creatinine 402μmol/L
- Mg 0.49mmol/L
- Bilirubin 18μmol/L, AST 34 IU/L, ALP 204 IU/L, albumin 49g/L
- ESR 16mm/hour, CRP 4.3mg/L
- CT scan: normal postoperative appearances, with no abscess formation.

Questions

33a) What problem has this man developed? Which non-gastroenterological condition has similar clinical features?

33b) What are the possible causes of 33a? What is the most likely cause in this case and why?

33c) What is the initial management?

33d) If the patient does not respond to the initial management, what is the next step?

33e) If the patient has been nil by mouth, what is the best way of reintroducing oral intake?

Answers

33a) **What problem has this man developed? Which non-gastroenterological condition has similar clinical features?**

This man has **ileostomy dysfunction** (a high output stoma syndrome), which has clinical and biochemical features similar to Addison's disease. The dehydration and electrolyte disturbance associated with ileostomy dysfunction presents with the clinical and biochemical appearance of Addison's disease (hyponatraemia, hyperkalaemia, lethargy), but the adrenal function is normal. This man also had abdominal pain prior to surgery, and Addison's disease is associated with abdominal pain. However, in this patient, the abdominal pain was explained by the perforated diverticulum.

33b) **What are the possible causes of 33a? What is the most likely cause in this case, and why?**

The possible causes of ileostomy dysfunction are:

- Inappropriate diet (either solid or liquid components)
- Bacterial overgrowth
- Partial obstruction (strictures, or a parastomal hernia)
- Prestomal ileitis
- Infection
- Short bowel syndrome
- Gastric acid hypersecretion
- Coincidental undiagnosed disease.

Hyperosmolar or hypo-osmolar fluids from an inappropriate diet will promote fluid flux into the intestinal lumen, and if the sodium content of the jejunal fluid is <90mmol/L, then there is no net water absorption. This is not important where there is functioning distal ileum or colon, but in the absence of either, dehydration and sodium depletion occur rapidly.

Bacterial overgrowth may cause ileostomy dysfunction, but is unlikely in this case because there was no small intestinal resection; it is the loss of the ileocaecal valve when re-anastomosed to the colon that increases the risk of bacterial overgrowth of the small intestine.

Partial obstruction caused by strictures or parastomal hernia may cause ileostomy dysfunction, but in this case there was no obvious hernia on examination and the stoma readily admitted a little finger.

Prestomal ileitis is more likely to occur if the original resection was for inflammatory bowel disease.

Infection (including small intestinal *Clostridium difficile*) should be excluded and stool should be routinely sent for toxin assay, microscopy, culture, and sensitivity.

Short bowel is commonly considered in ileostomy dysfunction, but is less commonly the cause. In this case no small bowel was resected. The surgical notes should always be scrutinized, and if the remaining small bowel looks <2m in length, it is good practice for the surgeon to measure the length of the remaining gut from the duodenojejunal flexure. In some instances, there is inaccurate estimation of the proportion of small bowel resected, resulting in unexpected short bowel syndrome. In general, the length of the remaining jejunum is of critical importance: patients with a jejunal length of less than 100cm cannot maintain adequate nutrient absorption on oral feeding and will require long-term parenteral nutrition. Patients with a jejunal segment >100cm can usually maintain nutritional balances, but may have stomal losses of fluid, magnesium, and electrolytes that may need regular parenteral crystalloid. The loss of the ileum results in obligatory bile acid and cobalamin (B_{12}) malabsorption. The colon is of paramount importance in maintaining fluid and electrolyte balance. Defining the anatomy of the remaining bowel (both small and large) is of fundamental importance to making strategic management decisions.

The exact mechanism of **gastric acid hypersecretion** is unknown. It may be related to the removal of intestinal peptides that normally inhibit gastric acid secretion and/or gastrin release.

Finally, **coincidental undiagnosed disease** causing malabsorption (e.g. villous atrophy, hyperthyroidism, hypolactasia, pancreatic insufficiency, dysmotility) should not be overlooked.

33c) **What is the initial management?**

The management of high output stoma involves:

- **Rehydration** with intravenous fluids and electrolyte replacement (including **magnesium** in particular) as necessary

- **Measuring stoma output** by asking nursing staff to measure the volume. The output should be <1200ml/day. A patient with an output >1500ml/day will not manage at home without parenteral fluids

- **Dietician review** of oral intake, especially the type of fluid, and quantity of drinks and food

- **Medication review** in particular looking for lactose-containing medication, antidiarrhoeal agents, proton pump inhibitors, and prokinetic agents that may exacerbate high output stoma syndrome

- **Review surgical notes** to determine amount of small bowel remaining
- Trial of empirical therapy:

  - **Dietary adjustments** and isotonic fluids (see below)
  - **Omeprazole 80mg/day** (to inhibit gastric acid hypersecretion, common in short bowel syndrome)
  - **Metronidazole** 400mg three times daily for 1 week (in case of bacterial overgrowth)
  - **Loperamide** in very large doses, starting at 4–10mg four times daily (use tablets or capsules, because the elixir contains lactose).

33d) **If the patient does not respond to the initial management, what is the next step?**

If the patient does not respond to empirical therapy, that is if the output remains above 1500ml/day, then establish **basal output** by making the patient nil by mouth and administering intravenous fluids for 48–72 hours. Electrolytes (Na, K, Mg) need to be monitored daily. If the basal output is >1200ml/day, then it is very unlikely that the patient will ever manage without intravenous fluids at home. Advice from a specialist centre with expertise in high output stomas is usually appropriate.

33e) **If the patient has been nil by mouth, what is the best way of reintroducing oral intake?**

The best approach to reintroducing oral fluids is to establish the effect of **isotonics** alone by mouth for 24–48 hours. This is the simplest 'challenge' to small intestinal function, since net water absorption by the jejunum only occurs at a luminal [Na]>90mmol/L. It is important to involve the dietician to educate the patient and nursing staff how isotonic fluids are constituted (the **WHO oral rehydration solution** is made by adding 3.5g NaCl, 2.9g trisodium citrate (or 2.5g $NaHCO_3$), 1.5g KCL and 20 g glucose to 1L of water), or 500mL Lucozade Sport® plus 1 teaspoon salt. Commercial 'isotonic' drinks do *not* contain enough sodium and should be avoided. The ileostomy output should be measured whilst on isotonic fluids. If the output is <1200ml/day, the patient can establish the effect of solid food, under supervision by an experienced dietician. It should be recognized that general dieticians (let alone general surgeons!) often do not have sufficient experience to advise in this area and specialist advice from an intestinal failure unit is often helpful.

If the output is >1200ml/day, the following medications should be instituted, in succession:

- omeprazole 80mg/day
- plus loperamide 8–12mg, 4 times per day
- plus codeine 60mg, 4 times per day
- consider octreotide 3 times per day. Stop octreotide after 72 hours if the impact on the output is <300mL/d.

If the output <1500mL/day at this stage, polymeric supplements can be introduced. If the output >1500mL/day, a plan for long term intravenous fluids or parenteral nutrition will be necessary, arranged through a specialist centre.

This patient had a good recovery from this episode and went on to have a re-anastomosis 3 months later. He returned to Kazakhstan shortly after this and remains well.

Further reading

Nightingale J, Woodward JM (2006). Small Bowel and Nutrition Committee of the British Society of Gastroenterology. Guidelines for management of patients with a short bowel. *Gut*; **55**(Suppl. 4): iv1–12.

Lochs H, Dejong C, Hammarqvist F, Hebuterne X *et al.* (2006). ESPEN Guidelines on enteral nutrition. *Gastroenterology Clin Nutr*; **25**: 260–74.

Abu-Elmagd KM. Intestinal transplantation for short bowel syndrome and gastrointestinal failure: current consensus, rewarding outcomes, and practical guidelines. *Gastroenterology* 2006; **130**(Suppl 1): S132–7.

Case 34

A 28-year-old Caucasian woman, who worked for the military, presented with a 12-month history of passing blood per rectum. Bright red blood was mixed in with the stool at almost every bowel motion. There was no blood on the paper or otherwise in the pan. Over the same period, her bowel habit had started alternating between being loose and constipated. She also reported occasional colicky abdominal pain, not related to opening her bowels. She had not lost any weight. She had no relevant past medical history or family history.

Examination of the abdomen was unremarkable. A digital rectal examination and proctoscopy revealed no abnormalities and no source of bleeding.

Investigations showed:

- Hb 7.7g/dL, MCV 58fL, platelets 485 x 10^9/L, ESR 29mm/hr
- Colonoscopy: a concentric, stenosing tumour at the hepatic flexure
- Histopathology showed a moderately differentiated adenocarcinoma with a large mucinous component and surrounding inflammatory infiltrate.

She was referred to a colorectal surgeon and oncologist for further investigation and appropriate management.

Questions

34a) Should rectal bleeding always be investigated?

34b) What is the best investigation for this patient?

34c) What should you tell the patient to expect regarding further investigation and management?

34d) What effects and side effects can the patient expect from adjuvant chemotherapy?

34e) Should family members be screened?

Answers

34a) **Should rectal bleeding always be investigated?**

Bright red blood per rectum is a common symptom. In a survey of the general population in the UK, 20% of people between 20 and 80 years of age reported blood loss per rectum within the preceding 6 months. The most common cause is haemorrhoids, although this does not, of course, exclude more proximal pathology. Patients >50 years of age should best have full colonic imaging, either by colonoscopy or CT scanning (below).

The management of younger patients is subject to some debate. The American Society for Gastrointestinal Endoscopy guidelines (2000) state that colonoscopy is 'generally indicated' for patients with visible rectal bleeding. This is not universally accepted and practice varies, because the judicious allocation of resources needs to be balanced against the possibility of missing serious pathology.

A prospective cohort study of colonoscopy for investigating a history of visible rectal bleeding in 622 patients from Italy confirmed that colonic malignancy is very rare in patients <50 years of age. In the group of 312/622 patients <40 years of age, only 2/312 (0.6%) had a colonic malignancy (both were distal to the splenic flexure and in reach of a flexible sigmoidoscope). Diverticular disease was found in 11/312 (3.5%), and 10 (3.2%) had ulcerative colitis, both easily diagnosed by flexible sigmoidoscopy. Malignancy of the colon does, however, sometimes occur in young people. Diagnosis may be delayed as a consequence of a low index of suspicion, and this may be associated with a worse outcome. Concomitant iron deficiency anaemia in this young patient influences the choice of investigation (below). It is probable that tumour biology is different and more aggressive at a younger age.

34b) **What is the best investigation for this patient?**

It is clear that the risk of colorectal cancer in a 28-year-old patient without a family history of the condition is extremely low. There are, however, clinical points of note. The rectal bleeding was constant, with almost every bowel motion, mixed in with stool and not otherwise noticed in the bowl or on the toilet paper. This is not typical of anal canal bleeding. The fact that the blood was described as 'bright red' is an unreliable indicator of the distance of pathology from the anus. Furthermore, the patient reported intermittent colicky abdominal pain. Of most note, however, our patient had a profound microcytic anaemia. The elevated platelet count can be assumed to indicate either significant chronic blood loss, or an acute phase response, both of which indicate serious pathology. The elevated ESR is more difficult to interpret, because red blood cells tend to sediment more quickly in the presence of anaemia.

Bright red rectal bleeding with normal proctoscopy, colicky abdominal pain, and microcytic anaemia requires thorough examination of the colon to confirm or exclude significant organic pathology. It is debatable whether the patient should have an upper gastrointestinal endoscopy as well to exclude villous atrophy associated with coeliac disease: this should generally be routine in patients with iron deficiency anaemia (see Case 38), but in the present case the rectal bleeding gives clear evidence of colonic pathology. **Colonoscopy** is the procedure of choice in this patient, because she is young and should be spared unnecessary radiation associated with CT colonography. Colonoscopy has the added benefit of enabling mucosal biopsy for histopathological diagnosis.

Colorectal imaging has, however, undergone a revolution in the past 5 years and colonoscopy should not be assumed always to be the default investigation.

The optimal technique depends on:

- Purpose of the investigation
- Most likely pathology (carcinoma, polyps, IBD, or telangiectasia)
- Age of patient, comorbidity, and available resources (waiting times).

Barium enema and flexible sigmoidoscopy

- *Advantages*: reliably images caecum; may be more available than colonoscopy; flexible sigmoidoscopy images the sigmoid colon.
- *Limitations*: colonoscopy still needed if a potential polyp is identified; adequate separation of sigmoid loops cannot always be achieved (hence need to be combined with flexible sigmoidoscopy). Barium enema may still miss polyps >1cm, although reliably (96%) identifies colorectal cancer. CT techniques and colonoscopy have made barium enema virtually obsolete in developed countries.

Flexible sigmoidoscopy

- *Advantages*: simple, safe procedure; usually performed without sedation after a phosphate enema without full bowel preparation; allows biopsies to be taken. Initial **procedure of choice** for assessing inpatients with diarrhoea (bloody or otherwise) and out-patients with distal colonic bleeding.
- *Limitations*: does not image the proximal colon.

Colonoscopy

- *Advantages*: gold-standard for colonic imaging at all ages except for the elderly or frail; allows therapeutic intervention.
- *Limitations*: lack of capacity to meet demand in many hospitals; potentially incomplete examination (caecal intubation rate may be 85–90%); risk of perforation (about 0.1%); need for bowel preparation (risk of potentially serious metabolic disturbance in elderly).

CT colon (also called minimal or long preparation CT colonography)

- *Advantages*: minimal preparation. Bowel preparation only needs a few millilitres of gastrograffin contrast over 3 days prior to procedure. Sensitivity is 85–90% for colorectal cancer. Initial colonic imaging **procedure of choice for elderly** or frail patients.
- *Limitations*: less sensitive than CT colonography or barium enema.

CT colonograpy (also called virtual colonoscopy/CT pneumocolon)

- *Advantages*: sensitivity as good as colonoscopy in trained hands. Initial colonic imaging **procedure of choice** in many centres for patients >45 years of age when the aim is to exclude cancer; provides some limited additional information from cross-sectional imaging of the whole abdomen; reduces the need for colonoscopy by 10–20%. The major advantage over barium enema is that there is no need for flexible sigmoidoscopy.
- *Limitations*: radiologist time to scrutinize scans (20–30min/scan); extracolonic pathology may not be detected, since intravenous contrast is not given routinely.

34c) **What should you tell the patient to expect regarding further investigation and management?**

Surgical resection is appropriate. She will need a **thoracoabdominal and pelvic CT scan** to stage the tumour and exclude metastases. MR scan of the abdomen is generally only needed as well for patients with rectal cancer, because it better defines pelvic anatomy than a CT scan. If imaging excludes metastases, resection of the primary tumour performed by a specialist colorectal surgeon using a **laparoscopic-assisted** approach, is the next step. Discussion about the surgical technique is done with the specialist colorectal surgeon, if laparoscopic expertise or equipment is not locally available, then a patient this young is usually best referred to a specialist centre. The chance of needing a stoma with a tumour at the hepatic flexure is low.

The resected tumour is then further staged by histopathology. This is the most reliable predictor of long-term outcome. It forms the basis of decisions regarding adjuvant chemotherapy. Staging may be based on the **TNM (tumour-node-metastasis) staging** system or on the older **Dukes'** system (Tables 34.1–34.3). Adjuvant chemotherapy is generally offered to all patients following resection who are found to have stage III (node positive) disease (Dukes' stage C), if they are fit enough for a 6-month course of chemotherapy. Age has to be considered, because survival benefit from chemotherapy must be seen in the context of the patient's population-based life expectancy.

34d) **What effects and side effects can the patient expect with adjuvant chemotherapy?**

There is a modest, but clear survival benefit for patients with Dukes' C carcinoma of the colon who receive adjuvant chemotherapy. The absolute benefit for stage III (node-positive) disease is about 10% over 5 years for **5-fluorouracil** (5-FU)-based chemotherapy. The addition of **oxaliplatin** may add a further 5% absolute survival benefit in this group. Higher risk patients with node-negative disease and transmural (T4, Table 34.1) tumours, or presentation with bowel perforation or obstruction, may benefit more. Chemotherapy for stage II colorectal cancer is less well defined. Patients may have an absolute survival benefit of just 4% from 5-FU-based chemotherapy. Oxaliplatin has not been shown to add any benefit in these patients.

Therapy needs to be tailored to the individual and account taken of their views. 5-FU is usually administered for 5 days out of every 28 for a total of 6 cycles. The drug is given either as a daily bolus or a continuous infusion, and is administered with folinic acid (leucovorin). Side effects from bolus regimens include neutropenia, stomatitis, and diarrhoea, which are less common with continuous infusions. On the other hand, continuous infusions have a higher rate of hand and foot syndrome

Table 34.1 Dukes' classification of colorectal cancer

A	Tumour confined to the mucosa and submucosa
B	Tumour invading the muscularis propria (B_1=T2N0M0; B_2=T3N0M0)
C	With lymph node(s) involvement
D	With distant metastasis

Table 34.2 TNM staging for colorectal cancer

Primary tumour (T)

Tx   Primary tumour cannot be assessed

Tis Carcinoma *in situ*

T1   Tumour invades submucosa

T2   Tumour invades muscularis propria

T3   Tumour invades through the muscularis propria into the subserosa

T4   Tumour directly invades other organs or structures, or perforates visceral peritoneum

Regional lymph nodes (N)

Nx   Regional lymph nodes cannot be assessed

N0   No regional lymph node metastases

N1   Metastases in 1–3 regional lymph nodes

N2   Metastases in 4 regional lymph nodes

Distant metastases (M)

Mx   Presence or absence of distant metastases cannot be determined

M0   No distant metastases detected

M1   Distant metastases detected

(painful erythematous rash of the hands and feet), which is also the major side effect of capecitabine (an orally administered prodrug of 5-FU). Capecitabine has also been associated with severe secretory diarrhoea causing hypomagnesaemia and hypokalaemia. Oxaliplatin may cause paraesthesiae and a cumulative, dose-related peripheral neuropathy, which may be irreversible.

Table 34.3 Stage grouping and 5-year survival

Stage	TNM classification	Approximate 5-year survival (%)
I	T1–2, N0, M0	90
IIA	T3, N0, M0	80–85
IIB	T4, N0, M0	70–80
IIIA	T1–2, N1, M0	65–80
IIIB	T3–4, N1, M0	50–65
IIIC	T1–4, N2, M0	25–50
IV	T1–4, N0–2, M1	5–8

Our patient underwent a laparoscopic-assisted, extended right hemicolectomy. Histopathological staging showed a completely resected tumour with no affected lymph nodes, T3N0M0 (stage IIA, Dukes B$_2$). She received 6 cycles of capecitabine, which was well tolerated. Stage IIA colon cancer (T3N0M0) has a 5-year survival rate of around 80%, after resection with curative intent (Table 34.3).

34e) **Should family members be screened?**

Our patient had colon cancer diagnosed at 28 years of age. This implies an increased risk of colon cancer in first-degree relatives. Screening for family members should be instituted.

British Society of Gastroenterology (BSG) guidelines recommend that patients who have one first-degree relative diagnosed with colon cancer <45 years of age should have a full colonoscopy at the time of consultation for an indicative family history, or at 35–40 years of age, whichever is later. Further surveillance is guided by findings at the initial colonoscopy. If the first colonoscopy is normal, a second colonoscopy is recommended at 55 years of age.

American Gastroenterology Association (AGA) guidelines recommend that first-degree relatives of patients diagnosed with colorectal cancer at <60 years of age should have colonoscopy performed every 5 years, starting at 40 years of age or at an age 10 years younger than the index case. Our patient was 28 years old at the time of diagnosis. AGA guidelines imply initiation of screening colonoscopy in first-degree relatives at 18 years of age, and every 5 years thereafter, which many healthcare systems would feel too burdensome for the diagnostic return. Testing of the tumour for microsatellite instability with MSI analysis or loss of a mismatch repair gene is appropriate when colorectal cancer is diagnosed in young patients (see Case 17).

Further reading

Crosland A, Jones R (1995). Rectal bleeding: prevalence and consultation behaviour. *BMJ*; **311**: 486–8.

Dunlop MG (2002). Guidelines on large bowel surveillance for people with two first degree relatives with colorectal cancer or one first degree relative diagnosed with colorectal cancer at <45 years. *Gut*; **51**(Suppl. V): v17–v20.

Levin B, Lieberman DA, McFarland B *et al.* (2008). American Cancer Society Colorectal Cancer Advisory Group; US Multi-Society Task Force; American College of Radiology Colon Cancer Committee. Screening and surveillance for the early detection of colorectal cancer and adenomatous polyps, 2008: a joint guideline from the American

Cancer Society, the US Multi-Society Task Force on Colorectal Cancer, and the American College of Radiology. *Gastroenterology*; **134**: 1570–95.

Spinzi G, Dal Fante M, Masci E *et al.* (2007). Lack of colonic neoplastic lesions in patients under 50yr of age with hematochezia: a multicentre prospective study. *Am J Gastroenterol*; **102**: 2011–15.

Wolpin BM, Mayer RJ (2008). Systemic treatment of colorectal cancer. *Gastroenterology*: **134**; 1296–1310.

Case 35

A 19-year-old pharmacy student presented with perianal pain, diarrhoea, 7kg weight loss, nausea, and vomiting over a 4-month period. He had travelled to Pakistan to see relatives 5 years previously, but had otherwise been born and brought up in the UK.

He had a perianal abscess, which was drained under anaesthetic and a flexible sigmoidoscopy was carried out. This showed rectal ulceration. Biopsies were consistent with Crohn's disease; Ziehl–Nielsen stain and a gamma-interferon release assay QuantiFERON®-TB Gold were negative. He was treated with corticosteroids and antibiotics after drainage of the abscess, with a good response. Azathioprine was started as primary prophylaxis against relapse.

Two weeks after discharge from hospital he was re-admitted with diarrhoea for 48 hours, fever (39.4°C), chills, rigors, and arthralgia.

Investigations showed:

- Hb 12.3g/L, WCC 20.6 x 10^9/L, platelets 544 x 10^9/L
- CRP >160mg/dL
- Bilirubin 16μmol/L, ALT 38 IU/L, ALP 257 IU, albumin 42g/dL
- Chest radiograph: normal
- MRI abdomen and pelvis: normal.

Questions

35a) What is the most likely diagnosis?

35b) What is the best management on admission?

35c) What are the treatment options on recovery?

35d) What are the treatment-related risks of lymphoma?

Answers

35a) **What is the most likely diagnosis?**

The most likely diagnosis is **azathioprine toxicity**. The most common symptoms of intolerance, which affect up to 20% of patients, are flu-like symptoms (myalgia, headache, diarrhoea) that characteristically occur after 2–3 weeks and cease rapidly once the drug is withdrawn. Profound leucopenia can develop suddenly and unpredictably, in between blood tests, although it is very rare within a month of starting therapy (<0.3%) and also rare at any stage during therapy (approximately 3%). Hepatotoxicity and pancreatitis are uncommon (<5%).

A **recurrent abscess** complicating Crohn's disease is unlikely in view of the normal MRI. A **new infection** needs to be considered, for example CMV or EBV, but it is too early for azathioprine to have caused appreciable immunosuppression. It is possible that this could still have been a missed diagnosis of **tuberculosis** (see Case 26). This had been considered and a QuantiFERON®-TB had been performed and was negative.

There are two new techniques of interferon-γ release assays that target two specific proteins of *Mycobacterium tuberculosis* (ESAT-6 and CFP-10). These are not affected by BCG-vaccination or environmental mycobacterial exposure, and are commercially available (ELISPOT or QuantiFERON®-TB). Multiple studies, including immunocompromised patients, have demonstrated that interferon-γ release assays are more sensitive and specific than a standard tuberculin skin test, although they have not been validated in patients with inflammatory bowel disease. The problem is that sensitivity may still be appreciably less than 100%, so gastroenterologists (and others) should beware the false sense of security of a negative ELISPOT or QuantiFERON®-TB result.

35b) **What is the best management on admission?**

The best management is to **stop azathioprine** immediately. Although it is likely that this is azathioprine toxicity, investigation and treatment of other possibilities should be undertaken until a diagnosis is established. These include blood cultures, intravenous corticosteroids and empirical antibiotics. In this case, the patient made a rapid and full recovery consistent with azathioprine toxicity.

35c) **What are the treatment options on recovery?**

This patient has multiple poor prognostic factors including young age, perianal disease and corticosteroid treatment at diagnosis. The best treatment for this patient includes immunomodulator therapy, because it has potential for modifying the future course of the disease. Mercaptopurine is inappropriate since there was hyper-acute intolerance of azathioprine. Mercaptopurine has a role in subacute intolerance, characterized by nausea and flu-like symptoms, but without hepatitis, pancreatitis, or fever. Up to 70% of patients with this pattern of intolerance to azathioprine can tolerate mercaptopurine, but patients should be warned that a third cannot tolerate mercaptopurine: this is evident after a dose or two of mercaptopurine. Mercaptopurine should then be stopped and further advice sought.

Methotrexate should be considered. Intramuscular methotrexate 25mg/week has been compared with azathioprine 2mg/kg/day in 54 patients with corticosteroid-dependent active Crohn's disease, and no difference in this under-powered study was found between the two medications, either for effect or speed of response. Unlike azathioprine, methotrexate has been subject to properly powered randomized controlled trials for induction and maintenance of remission in corticosteroid-dependent Crohn's disease. Variable absorption of oral methotrexate has been demonstrated compared with subcutaneous administration, but for practical reasons oral dosing is more convenient and preferred by patients. If methotrexate is used, concurrent administration of folic acid once a week is advisable (the alliteration **M**ethotrexate on **M**onday, **F**olic acid on **F**riday is often helpful). **Biological therapy** should also be considered. Specialist advice from a gastroenterologist specializing in inflammatory bowel disease is generally appropriate for managing Crohn's disease refractory to one immunomodulator, so that the strategy and timing of biological therapy can be planned.

35d) **What are the treatment-related risks of lymphoma?**

There is about a four-fold increased risk of lymphoma in patients treated with azathioprine or mercaptopurine relative to the lymphoma rate expected in the general population. As azathioprine and mercaptopurine tend to be used in more severe cases of inflammatory bowel disease, the increased risk of lymphoma could be a consequence of the medication, the severity of the underlying disease, or a combination of the two. It is unclear how the risk of lymphoma changes when therapy is discontinued and whether the risk is dose related. Even if the increased risk is attributable to the medication, it is unlikely to outweigh the potential benefits of these medications for most patients. Prospective evidence from a large French (CESAME) study suggests a two-fold increase; this means that the number-needed-to-harm by lymphoma from azathioprine/mercaptopurine is between 4500 and 11500 at 20–30 years of age. This puts the absolute risk in perspective.

It is also important to consider that inflammation is an independent risk factor for colorectal neoplasia in inflammatory bowel disease. Further data from the CESAME study, a cross-sectional IBD French cohort designed to determine prospectively the risk of cancers associated with the use of immunosuppressive therapy, has shown a 3-fold *decreased* risk of advanced colorectal neoplasia in patients with Crohn's disease or ulcerative colitis on thiopurine therapy. This raises the possibility that the anti-inflammatory effect of thiopurines on the colonic mucosa carries a greater benefit on the risk of colorectal neoplasia than a deleterious effect through drug-induced immunosuppression.

Further reading

Beaugerie L, Seksik P, Carrat F, for the CESAME Study Group (2009). Thiopurine therapy is associated with a three-fold decrease in the incidence of advanced colorectal neoplasia in IBD patients with long-standing extensive colitis: the CESAME prospective data. *J Crohn's & Colitis*; **3**: S5.

Kandiel A, Fraser AG, Korelitz BI, Brensinger C, Lewis JD (2005). Increased risk of lymphoma among inflammatory bowel disease patients treated with azathioprine and 6-mercaptopurine. *Gut*; **54**: 1121–5.

McGovern DPB, Travis SPL (2006). 6-mercaptopurine or azathioprine? In: Irving P, Rampton DS, Shanahan F (Eds). *Clinical Dilemmas in IBD*. Blackwell Publishing: Oxford, **Chapter 13**: 45–7.

Case 36

A 55-year-old woman who worked as a publisher presented with an 8-week history of diarrhoea. She reported up to 12 bowel movements in 24 hours with nocturnal waking to open her bowels. Stools were loose, but contained no macroscopic blood. She experienced lower abdominal cramps and urgency before having to pass stool, and this was especially prominent after a meal. She had no fever or chills but had lost weight. Symptoms started after a course of Co-amoxiclav, which was prescribed for a chest infection. The diarrhoea was having an appreciable impact on her quality of life, interfering with normal daily excursions for fear of not being near a toilet. She had chronic backache, suffered from depression, and was hypothyroid. She was receiving fluoxetine, thyroxine, and had been taking diclofenac for years.

Investigations showed:

- Hb 14.1g/dL, WCC 8.13 x 10^9/L, platelets 320 x 10^9/L
- ESR 8mm/hour
- CRP 45mg/L
- EMA negative
- TSH 2.63mU/L
- Faecal elastase >500μg/g, no excess faecal fat
- Stool culture negative, stool *C. difficile* toxin negative.

Questions

36a) Discuss the differential diagnosis.

36b) What further investigations are appropriate?

36c) What are the characteristics of this condition?

36d) What are the aetiology and the mechanisms of diarrhoea?

36e) How would you manage this patient and what is the long-term outlook?

Answers

36a) **Discuss the differential diagnosis.**

The clinical problem is **chronic diarrhoea** (diarrhoea persisting for >3 weeks). It is important to distinguish **functional diarrhoea** (IBS, see Case 32) from that resulting from an **organic** cause. Clear indicators of an organic cause are a history of nocturnal diarrhoea and weight loss, as in this patient. **Colorectal cancer** is possible, but unlikely, since it generally causes a gradual change in bowel pattern with an increase in stool frequency to a few times a day, rather than diarrhoea a dozen times a day. An elevated CRP suggests underlying **inflammation**. Although the diarrhoea was of sudden onset, there were no other symptoms of infection (no fever or chills), no risk factors for infection (travel history), and stool culture was negative. The onset of diarrhoea after a course of Co-amoxiclav, raises the possibility of **antibiotic-associated diarrhoea** (see Case 22). A test for *Clostridium difficile* toxin in a stool sample was negative. The clavulanic acid in Co-amoxiclav can act to stimulate bowel motility, and penicillin has rarely been described to cause colitis. Antibiotic-associated diarrhoea in the absence of *C. difficile* generally remits after withdrawing the offending drug.

Other common conditions need to be excluded. Our patient was hypothyroid and was taking thyroxine. **Overtreatment** was excluded by a normal TSH. **Coeliac disease** was effectively excluded with a negative endomysial antibody test (see Case 38) in the presence of a normal IgA concentration. New onset ulcerative colitis is highly unlikely in the absence of visible blood in the stool. **Crohn's disease** is possible, because of an elevated CRP, and most patients with Crohn's colitis have non-bloody diarrhoea. There was no history of steatorrhoea and no risk factors for **chronic pancreatitis**, but in view of the weight loss, pancreatic function tests were requested. The faecal elastase was normal, reliably excluding exocrine pancreatic insufficiency. **Bacterial overgrowth** is unlikely in an otherwise healthy person at this age, since it is usually associated with anatomic alteration in the small bowel, by jejunal diverticulosis (see Case 10), or surgery. Clues to the aetiology were the patient's age, female gender, and the fact that she was taking diclofenac. Diclofenac may cause **NSAID-induced enteropathy** or **microscopic colitis**.

36b) **What further investigations are appropriate?**

Colonoscopy is the investigation of choice to obtain mucosal biopsies throughout the colon (see discussion on colonic imaging, Case 34).

Mucosal biopsies are essential in a patient with diarrhoea even if the colonic mucosa looks normal, as in this case. There is rectal sparing in 10–40% of patients with microscopic colitis, which is confined to the right side of the colon in 10%. Consequently full colonoscopy is optimal, but a flexible sigmoidoscopy and biopsies from the left colon will secure the diagnosis in 90%. The choice of investigation depends on availability, but full colonic imaging is mandatory, so colonoscopy was requested.

In this patient, the histopathology of the terminal ileum, rectum and sigmoid mucosal biopsies was normal. Biopsies of the ascending colon, transverse colon, and descending colon showed an increase in chronic inflammatory cells in the lamina propria and intraepithelial lymphocytosis, consistent with **lymphocytic colitis**, one of the types of microscopic colitis (Fig. 36.1 in central colour section).

36c) **What are the characteristics of this condition?**

Microscopic colitis is a condition causing watery diarrhoea in which the colonic mucosa looks normal (or near normal) at colonoscopy, but biopsies show a chronic inflammatory infiltrate in the lamina propria. There are two commonly recognized variants: **lymphocytic colitis** and **collagenous colitis**, but some authorities further subclassify to include 'microscopic colitis not-otherwise-classified', or 'microscopic colitis with giant cells'. Microscopic colitis of any type may be accompanied by weight loss or abdominal discomfort, and patients may have nausea, or suffer faecal incontinence. There is a female predominance, which is more pronounced in people with collagenous colitis, which has a female to male ratio of 7:1. The female to male ratio in lymphocytic colitis is 2.4:1. The peak incidence is at the age of 65 years, but the disease can occur at all ages.

Associated autoimmune conditions include **thyroid disease** (as in our patient), **coeliac disease**, **diabetes mellitus**, **rheumatoid arthritis**, and **asthma**. Certain **drugs** are implicated in the development of microscopic colitis, including NSAIDs, proton pump inhibitors, statins, serotonin-reuptake inhibitors, ranitidine, aspirin, acarbose, lisinopril, ticlopidine, carbamazepine and flutamide. The rectal mucosa is more commonly spared in collagenous colitis (40%) than lymphocytic colitis (10%). Lymphocytic colitis is characterized by >20 intraepithelial lymphocytes per 100 surface cells, and a normal basement membrane. Collagenous colitis is diagnosed on finding a subepithelial collagen band thickened to 10μm (the normal basement membrane is 3μm). The crypt architecture is normal in microscopic colitis. The variants of microscopic colitis are

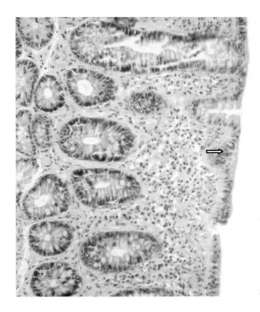

Fig. 36.1 (see colour plate 17) Photomicrograph showing chronic inflammatory cells in the lamina propria, and intraepithelial lymphocytosis (arrow), consistent with lymphocytic colitis.

not exclusive: patients have been reported who have, at different times, three of the subtypes (lymphocytic colitis, collagenous colitis, and not-otherwise-classified).

36d) **What are the aetiology and mechanism of the diarrhoea?**

The cause of microscopic colitis is not known. The hypothesis that an unidentified luminal antigen elicits an unregulated epithelial immune response in a genetically susceptible individual is supported by the observation that diversion of the faecal stream leads to regression of inflammation, which returns once bowel continuity is re-established. This hypothesis is further strengthened by the response of microscopic colitis to an elemental diet. Familial occurrence of microscopic colitis and lymphocytic colitis has been reported. Patients with lymphocytic colitis seem to be more likely to have a family history of coeliac disease, inflammatory bowel disease, and collagenous colitis. Familial cases may also result from shared environmental exposure. Infectious agents including *Yersinia enterocolitica*, *Campylobacter jejuni*, and *C. difficile* have been reported in association with microscopic colitis, and a seasonal pattern of lymphocytic colitis has been suggested, but studies are inconclusive. Stool culture is (by definition) negative at diagnosis.

Many drugs have been associated with microscopic colitis, but causality is not necessarily proven. The association with autoimmune diseases raises the possibility of autoimmune aetiology, but no known antibody or serum marker exists. The mechanism of the diarrhoea is not known precisely, but there is a secretory component with reduced net absorption of Na^+ and Cl^-. Nitric oxide is greatly increased in the colon, in proportion to the inflammation. Nitric oxide synthesis is induced by NF_KB, which is activated in the epithelium of patients with collagenous colitis. Epithelial damage and possibly a barrier to diffusion created by the collagen layer in collagenous colitis may contribute. On the other hand, fasting reduces diarrhoea and indicates an *osmotic* component. Bile acid malabsorption may coexist and worsen diarrhoea.

36e) **How would you manage this patient and what is the long-term outlook?**

Specific therapy includes **withdrawing offending drugs** and prescribing a corticosteroid with low systemic bioavailability, assuming that the diarrhoea is interfering with lifestyle, as it was in our patient. Diclofenac was the likely cause in our patient and she was advised to stop this and substitute paracetamol, augmented by a trial of acupuncture and physiotherapy for her back pain.

Budesonide is the drug of choice. Budesonide 9mg/day for 6–8 weeks has been shown to be effective in collagenous colitis for symptom resolution and improvement of histology. It is then tapered to 6mg and then 3mg for respective 4 week periods, but lower doses may be effective. This is also effective in >90% of patients with lymphocytic colitis. Corticosteroids are not popular with patients, so care should be taken to discuss the reasons for using a corticosteroid that has a topical action on the colon and a low incidence of systemic side effects. The rapid resolution of diarrhoea within days is usually greatly appreciated.

Dietary factors which may exacerbate diarrhoea need to be excluded, including excessive alcohol intake and caffeine consumption. A dairy-free diet is rarely worthwhile. Concomitant diseases including hyperthyroidism and coeliac disease should be excluded. Drugs other than corticosteroids are not often effective. Mild diarrhoea may be treated with colestyramine, a resin that binds bile acids, at 4g 1–3 times/day. Colesevelam is an alternative that is often more palatable. Loperamide has often already been tried by the patient to little effect. Mesalazine can be tried and benefits about half, but less frequently induces remission. There have been no adequate controlled trials.

Relapse occurs in two thirds if an offending agent cannot be identified or stopped. Intermittent or even long-term treatment with budesonide at the lowest effective dose may be required, although there is no trial to support this. In these circumstances calcium and vitamin D supplementation should be considered (although treatment with budesonide for 2 years has not been associated with significant loss of bone density). Azathioprine has been tried in corticosteroid-dependent microscopic colitis, although no controlled data have been published. The long-term outlook is good, with 60–80% in long-term remission without medication, and normalization of histology after 3 years. A very small number of patients may have such refractory disease that requires surgical intervention, including split ileostomy or colectomy. There is no increased risk of colorectal cancer with respect to the general population.

Further reading

Bartlett JG (2002). Antibiotic-associated diarrhoea. *N Engl J Med*; **346**: 334–9.

Chande N, MacDonald JK, McDonald JW (2009). Interventions for treating microscopic colitis: a Cochrane Inflammatory Bowel Disease and Functional Bowel Disorders Review Group systematic review of randomized trials. *Am J Gastroenterol*; **104**: 235–41.

Tysk C, Bohr J, Nyhlin N, Wickbom A, Eriksson S (2008). Diagnosis and management of microscopic colitis. *World J Gastroenterol*; **14**: 7280–8.

Case 37

A 19-year-old first-year university student was transferred to the emergency department shortly after the start of her second term, bedridden for a week, and with a history of anorexia nervosa.

On examination, she weighed 28.8kg (BMI 10.9kg/m²), had a bradycardia (pulse 46bpm), a temperature of 35.6°C, and blood pressure 94/57mmHg.

Investigations showed:

- Hb 17.5g/L, WCC 9.0 x 10⁹/L, platelets 79 x 10⁹/L
- Na 140mmol/L, K 3.6mmol/L, creatinine 84μmol/L
- Phosphate 0.33mmol/L, magnesium 0.92mmol/L
- Bilirubin 58μmol/L, ALT 540 IU, ALP 570 IU, albumin 39g/dL
- CRP normal

Over the next 2 days, her blood results changed (Table 37.1).

Table 37.1 Change in blood results

Day	Na	K	Cr	Ca	P	Mg	Bil	ALT	ALP	Alb	Hb	Pl
1	140	2.8	73	2.35	0.72	0.83	67	586	628	35	14.3	45
2	139	3.6	70	2.25	0.65	0.84	68	601	681	36	15.2	33

Questions

37a) What is the most likely cause of hypothermia, bradycardia, and thrombocytopenia with abnormal liver function tests in this patient?

37b) What other diagnoses should be considered in a patient with anorexia nervosa?

37c) How is the patient's condition best treated?

37d) What is the legal context in which treatment is conducted?

37e) What is the short-term and long-term prognosis?

Answers

37a) **What is the most likely cause of hypothermia, bradycardia, and thrombocytopenia with abnormal liver function tests in this patient?**

Anorexia nervosa is the likely cause of all of this patient's medical problems. Virtually all organ systems are disrupted through starvation, characterized by anorexia nervosa. This patient is critically ill and needs admission for emergency medical care. The most striking feature is the BMI of 10.9kg/m². Thrombocytopenia and abnormal liver function tests occur at a very late, pre-terminal stage of starvation.

Anorexia nervosa is a complex psychiatric illness with potentially severe medical consequences. Patients in the pre-terminal phase commonly have bradycardia, hypotension, and dehydration; amenorrhoea and leucopenia occur at an earlier stage. Delayed gastric emptying, hair loss, and the presence of lanugo (a fine hair pattern on the face, neck, and trunk) are also associated with severe anorexia nervosa. Anaemia should not be attributed to anorexia nervosa without further investigation (below). Of particular concern for adolescents is the potential for delayed onset of puberty and growth. Malnutrition and hormonal dysfunction may contribute to bone loss.

Functional and structural brain abnormalities may also occur in individuals with anorexia nervosa, including enlarged ventricles and decreased grey matter or cognitive deficits in problem solving, attention, memory, and verbal or visuospatial processing. This leads to disorders of executive functioning, so that rational decision making is impaired. This needs to be understood by the general medical team, who are otherwise inclined to dismiss such patients as 'mad'. The attitude that such patients have a self-inflicted injury and must accept the consequences, because they 'do not know what is good for them' is a complete failure to understand the **cognitive consequences of starvation**.

Electrolyte disturbances may be exacerbated by purging or induced vomiting. Elevated hepatic transaminases and renal insufficiency are warning signs of impending death. Cardiac arrhythmias (including a prolonged QT interval) with sudden death are the consequence of hypokalaemia, hypomagnesaemia, or hypophosphataemia.

37b) **What other diagnoses should be considered in a patient with anorexia nervosa?**

Other diagnoses that should be considered include:

- **Coeliac disease**: an anti-endomysial antibody should be checked as part of this patient's workup

- **Crohn's disease**: a high CRP, anaemia, or thrombocytosis should always raise the possibility of Crohn's disease, which can present with anorexia, weight loss, and no pain or diarrhoea. Sadly there is a substantial literature on Crohn's disease misdiagnosed as anorexia nervosa

- **Addison's disease** (or pituitary failure) should be considered if there is a low Na with a normal or relatively high K. Very readily overlooked

- **Paracetamol** (or other drug) **overdose** may account for the abnormal liver function tests and needs to be considered in the context of acute deterioration in any patient with anorexia nervosa

- Always beware a diagnosis of anorexia nervosa if the individual does not have the disturbed body image that characterizes the condition.

37c) **How is the patient's condition best treated?**

The metabolic mayhem must be recognized as an emergency, but careful re-feeding will reverse the abnormalities. The major adverse consequence of medical treatment of patients with anorexia nervosa is the **refeeding syndrome** (see Case 49), which is potentially life threatening. The principal biochemical features of this syndrome are hypophosphataemia, hypomagnesaemia, hypokalaemia, fluid retention, and thiamine deficiency. This causes peripheral oedema (a useful clinical sign of pre-terminal anorexia), congestive heart failure, cardiac dysrrhythmias, skeletal muscle weakness, respiratory failure, metabolic acidosis, ataxia, seizures, or encephalopathy and death.

When a patient with anorexia nervosa has hypokalaemia, hypophosphataemia, elevated transaminases, bradycardia, or thrombocytopenia, urgent intravenous treatment is necessary.

Initial management

Intravenous fluids are required to correct dehydration.

Electrolyte (K, Mg and P) replacement: the patient should be monitored twice daily until stable, which is usually within 72–76 hours (refeeding guidelines: see Case 49).

Intravenous vitamins are required, including thiamine (e.g. Pabrinex 2 vials, for 3 days).

Monitoring: pulse rate, blood pressure and temperature should be monitored every 6 hours. Patients with heart rates <50 beats/min or orthostatic hypotension should be on bed rest.

Psychiatric asessment (see below), almost invariably requiring detention under the Mental Health Act or equivalent, is required to ensure compliance with controlled refeeding.

Controlled refeeding: oral refeeding is the best approach to weight restoration, but patients who are critically ill with electrolyte disturbance require controlled nasogastric feeding. Such patients are archetypal manipulators, encouraging doctors and nurses to believe that such an invasive approach is unnecessary, that they have learned a lesson, and that oral refeeding is possible. When life is threatened by transaminitis, electrolyte disturbance, or bradycardia, do not believe it. It is important to liaise with the consultant psychiatrist, but the cognitive impairment associated with starvation precludes rational behaviour. Such patients create havoc on a general ward, preventing controlled refeeding and calling on staff out of hours to change their treatment. Although nasogastric feeding can be viewed as coercive by patients, in retrospect, most patients and families consider nasogastric feeding to have been helpful in recovery. It helps to have defined protocols for management and (as importantly) to stick to agreed treatment plans.

Dietitian: a weight gain of 0.2kg/day is a reasonable goal. The dietitian is best placed to be the single person who governs the refeeding regimen, and without whose sanction no treatment is ever changed. This appears unduly dogmatic, but without a single person responsible for controlled refeeding, the regimen is always manipulated and changed, usually by appeal to doctors on call or nurses unfamiliar with the treatment plan. It should be emphasized that the dogmatic approach to controlled refeeding only applies to the stage of biochemical disturbance, since this is a life-threatening event. Once refeeding has been accomplished, a cooperative consensual approach is (inevitably) more productive.

Continuous supervision: a framework for managing patients with life-threatening anorexia nervosa is best established in advance. In practice, patients with biochemical disturbance requiring nasogastric refeeding should have 1:1 care with a psychiatric nurse or assistant. This may seem an impossible goal, but without continuous attention, the patient will interrupt feeding (pull out the tube, tip the feed down the sink), march up and down the ward to burn energy, or binge on carbohydrates rather than follow a controlled eating schedule. This then defeats the object. Since the mortality of severe anorexia nervosa is 30%, any other condition with this mortality would merit special nursing care.

Consistent nursing instructions: so challenging to general medical and nursing staff are these patients that a protocol agreed in advance (between general physician, psychiatrist and appropriate specialist colleagues) is the only way to ensure consistent care.

Distinguish between the medical emergency of the refeeding phase for biochemical disturbance, and the psychiatric phase for addressing the psychological disturbance that has lead to anorexia nervosa.

Long-term management

Medical hospitalization is often brief and does not allow adequate time for psychiatric intervention. Liaison with a psychiatrist with a special interest in eating disorders is a crucial part of continuing management and care.

37d) **What is the legal context in which treatment is conducted?**

A key concept in the ethical and legal analysis relating to compulsory treatment is that of the **capacity to consent** to, or refuse, treatment. An adult patient with such capacity has the right to refuse any, even life-saving, treatment. On this account, compulsory treatment is only justified if the patient lacks capacity. Most mental health statutes internationally allow mental health professionals to detain and treat patients with a psychiatric disorder who are at risk to themselves or others, without consideration of whether or not the patient lacks capacity. There are exceptions to this, since the question of capacity is the key factor in the compulsory treatment of anorexia nervosa.

Treatment without consent and the management of treatment refusal is particularly contentious in the context of anorexia nervosa. The dilemma is that it is very difficult to engage patients in psychological therapies if treatment is compulsory. Furthermore, refeeding unwilling patients may lead to short-term weight gain, but be ineffective in the long run.

Outcome studies suggest that the **long-term prognosis** following compulsory treatment is poor. Even if compulsory treatment were shown to be effective, there remains an ethical debate about the circumstances in which compulsory treatment is justifiable. Anorexia nervosa at a pre-terminal phase often involves implementing a refeeding programme that requires the use of strict supervision, enforcement of specific dietary plans, prevention of exercising or purging, and nasogastric feeding. Recommendations will vary according to the jurisdiction, but it behoves any doctor or carer to make themselves aware of the legal constraints that govern practice.

37e) **What is the short-term and long-term prognosis?**

Although weight-restoration therapy is reliably helpful in the short-term management of anorexia nervosa, the long-term benefit remains unclear. Even after successful completion of structured behavioural programmes, attitudes about weight and eating behaviour remain abnormal. As a result, relapse rates are high. For inpatient treatment programmes, nearly 50% with anorexia nervosa who undergo weight-restoration therapy have a relapse during the first year after hospitalization.

After weight restoration, outpatient treatment specifically aims to prevent relapse. Patients and families are informed about the need for vigilance regarding eating behaviour and weight. The specific type of relapse prevention is selected on the basis of the patient's previous therapy and success with initial attempts at weight maintenance.

Estimates of long-term full recovery for adolescents with anorexia nervosa range from 33% to 57%, so relapse is common. There are few controlled studies on the efficacy of **relapse-prevention** strategies. Antidepressant medication appears to be of limited value, although cognitive behavioral therapy may help some patients. Additional studies are needed to identify the essential components of care for patients with anorexia nervosa, as well as relapse-prevention strategies.

People with anorexia nervosa have a 6–7-fold increase in mortality (including natural and unnatural causes of death). Anorexia nervosa itself has a **standardized mortality ratio** of 650. Suicide accounts for 20–30% of deaths in anorexia nervosa. Factors associated with an increase in fatal outcome include:

- Older age at first admission (>20 years of age)
- Repeated admissions
- Hospitalization for other psychiatric and somatic disorders.

Further reading

Attia E, Walsh BT (2008). Behavioral management for anorexia nervosa. *New Engl J Med*; **360**: 500–6.

Papadopoulos FC, Ekbom A, Brandt L, Ekelius L (2009). Excess mortality, cause of death and prognostic factors in anorexia nervosa. *Br J Psychiatry*; **194**: 10–17.

Sylvester C, Forman S (2008). Clinical practice guidelines for treating restrictive eating disorder patients during medical hospitalisation. *Curr Opin Paed*; **20**: 390–97.

Tan JOA, Hope T, Stewart A, Fitzpatrick R (2006). Competence to make treatment decisions in anorexia nervosa: thinking processes and values. *Philos Psychiatry Psychol*; **13**: 267–82.

Case 38

A 38-year-old Asian pharmacist was referred from the endocrinology clinic for a gastroenterology opinion. She had been treated for hypothyroidism for 12 years, but she remained persistently tired, despite adequate thyroid replacement therapy.

She reported a long history of tiredness, accompanied by headaches, joint pains, blisters on her face, and occasional mouth ulcers. Gastrointestinal symptoms included abdominal bloating and occasional vomiting. She was taking thyroxine, alfacalcidol, potassium, zinc, magnesium, selenium, and vitamin C supplements. She had had a thyroidectomy and parathyroidectomy 3 years before. She was a non-smoker and drank alcohol infrequently. Her mother had diabetes mellitus, and her father and grandfather both had bowel cancer in their sixties. Physical examination was unremarkable.

Investigations showed:

- Hb 12.4g/dL, WCC 6.1 x 10^9/L, platelets 279 x 10^9/L, MCV 86fL
- Ferritin 6μg/L, folate 2.9μg/L, vitamin B_{12} 1815ng/L
- TSH 0.28mU/L, free-T_4 13.0pmol/L
- Albumin 47g/L, Ca 2.31mmol/L, glucose 6.4mmol/L
- LFTs normal
- Endomysial antibody: negative
- IgA <0.05g/L
- HLA DQB1 0201 (DQ2), HLA DQB1 0302/11 (DQ8).

Questions

38a) What is the likely diagnosis and most appropriate investigation?

38b) What is the significance of the IgA concentration?

38c) What is the significance of the HLA typing?

38d) Name other disease associations.

38e) How should this patient be managed?

38f) What if the patient does not respond to standard management?

Answers

38a) What is the likely diagnosis and most appropriate investigation?

- The likely diagnosis is coeliac disease.
- An upper gastrointestinal endoscopy and distal duodenal biopsy should be carried out.

The **definitive investigation** for coeliac disease is an upper gastrointestinal endoscopy and distal duodenal biopsy. The likely diagnosis of coeliac disease is suggested by the low iron and folate, both of which are absorbed in the proximal small bowel, which is primarily involved in coeliac disease. A biopsy should always be recommended, even if endomysial antibody positive, because of the implications of a life-long gluten-free diet (below).

- Endoscopy: scalloped and fissured duodenal mucosa (Fig. 38.1 in central coloured section)
- Histology: subtotal villous atrophy, crypt hyperplasia and a significant increase in intraepithelial lymphocytes (Fig. 38.2 in central colour section).

The diagnosis of coeliac disease in this patient was based on the clinical symptoms (fatigue, mouth ulcers), iron and folate deficiency, and histopathology. The endomysial antibodies were negative, because the patient has IgA deficiency (below). The HLA typing is characteristic of coeliac disease, although this is generally only performed when there is diagnostic doubt (below). **Villous atrophy** on its own is not specific for coeliac disease. Improvement of histological grade on a gluten-free diet confirms the diagnosis although, if there is a clinical response, endoscopy is not routinely repeated. Other conditions associated with villous atrophy in the small bowel include giardiasis, NSAID ingestion, Crohn's disease, Whipple's disease, common variable immune deficiency, radiation enteropathy, HIV infection, tuberculosis, and tropical sprue (which has almost disappeared from clinical practice).

Coeliac disease in adults now most commonly presents with iron deficiency anaemia, but may present with non-specific gastrointestinal symptoms such as anorexia, abdominal pain, vomiting and diarrhoea, or less commonly constipation. The patient may report weight loss or failure to gain weight. It may also cause arthralgia, alopecia, dermatitis herpetiformis, oral ulcers, abnormal liver functions (transaminitis), or neurological manifestations (migraine, cerebellar ataxia, or peripheral neuropathy).

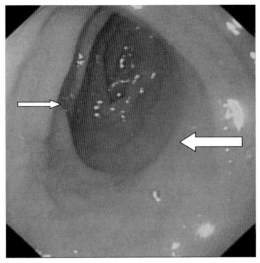

Fig. 38.1 (see colour plate 18) An endoscopic photograph of this patient's duodenum, showing a paucity of folds (large arrow) with fissuring (small arrow), although endoscopy in coeliac disease is commonly normal.

Coeliac disease has a worldwide distribution and all races are affected. Prevalence data from southern Asia and Africa are scant. The true incidence in countries where rice, rather than wheat is the staple may be underestimated. The prevalence in Western Europe and North America is 1:100 to 1:300 people.

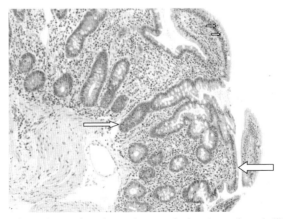

Fig. 38.2 (see colour plate 19) A photomicrograph showing subtotal villous atrophy, with blunting of the villi (large arrow), crypt hyperplasia (small arrow), and increased intraepithelial lymphocytes (tiny arrows).

38b) **What is the significance of the IgA concentration?**

This patient has **isolated IgA deficiency**. Isolated IgA deficiency is the most common primary deficiency of humoral immunity. Low serum IgA renders the endomysial antibody test unreliable for the exclusion of coeliac disease. If the diagnosis is strongly suspected (such as in someone with unexplained iron deficiency, or a family history of coeliac disease), then small bowel (distal duodenal) biopsies need to be obtained. Antibodies to tissue transglutaminase are of the IgG subclass and are both sensitive for the diagnosis of coeliac disease in patients with IgA deficiency, but may be positive in patients with other autoimmune disorders. People with IgA deficiency may have antibodies to IgA, which may predispose to transfusion reactions. Selective IgA deficiency is more common in patients with coeliac disease than in the general population, with 1 case in 40, compared with 1 in 400. There is no specific therapy. IgA deficiency is thought to be associated with a higher incidence of autoimmune disease, atopy, and infections.

38c) **What is the significance of the HLA typing?**

The HLA typing is consistent with coeliac disease. The main value of HLA typing is to *exclude*, rather than confirm the diagnosis. Not all people with either HLA DQ2 or HLA DQ8 have coeliac disease, but the disease does not occur in patients without either of these alleles. Therefore, the absence of both of these alleles has a **high negative predictive value**. This is useful in cases where endomysial antibodies are negative and distal duodenal biopsies are inconclusive. Subtle histopathological signs may be difficult to interpret, and improvement on a gluten-free diet difficult to determine if the index biopsy showed minor changes, such as an increase in intraepithelial lymphocytes without villous atrophy. Our patient had both susceptibility alleles.

38d) **Name other disease associations**

Conditions associated with coeliac disease include:

- Autoimmune disorders
- Malignancy
- Chromosomal disorders.

Coeliac disease is associated with **autoimmune disorders** (autoimmune thyroid disease, Addison's disease, hypoparathyroidism, pernicious anaemia, and Type 1 diabetes mellitus). Patients have an increased risk of developing **malignancy**, including intestinal (enteropathy-associated

T-cell) lymphoma and extraintestinal lymphoma, oropharyngeal and oesophageal adenocarcinoma, cancers of the small and large bowel, hepatobiliary system, and pancreas. The risk of breast cancer appears to be reduced. An increased frequency of coeliac disease has been reported in patients with **chromosomal disorders** such as Turner's syndrome, Down's syndrome and William syndrome, but it is difficult to determine whether this reflects reporting bias.

38e) **How should this patient be managed?**

Management of coeliac disease includes:

- Lifelong gluten-free diet
- Screening for vitamin and mineral deficiencies
- Screening for osteoporosis.

The only accepted therapy for coeliac disease is the **life-long exclusion of gluten** from the diet. This implies elimination of wheat, barley and rye. Rice, corn and oats are gluten free, but oats may be contaminated with gluten during growing or processing. An experienced dietitian should be asked to give detailed advice about gluten-free sources of starch that can be used as flour alternatives for baking. Gluten-free products, including bread, can be obtained on prescription in the UK, for patients with a diagnosis confirmed by biopsy.

Patient support organizations are available and patients are advised to join a local organization such as **Coeliac UK** in the UK (www.coeliac.org.uk). Newly diagnosed patients with coeliac disease should be screened for deficiencies of vitamins and minerals, including iron, calcium, vitamin B12 and folate. Any deficiencies should be treated. All patients should also be screened for osteoporosis, which is prevalent; adherence to a gluten-free diet is associated with improvement in bone mineral density, although calcium supplements are commonly needed. The dietitian should estimate dietary calcium intake.

Endomysial antibodies may be repeated after several months on a gluten-free diet; a persistently positive test suggests poor compliance with a gluten-free diet, and is an indication for repeat endoscopy and biopsy to assess the histological response. A negative test does not necessarily imply dietary compliance, which is best assessed by a specialist dietitian. Antibodies of the IgG subclass are not reliable for follow up of dietary compliance, since these remain positive. A poor clinical response is also an indication for repeat endoscopy and biopsy, although other diagnoses should be considered.

38f) **What if the patient does not respond to standard management?**

Causes of management failure in coeliac disease include:

- Dietary non-compliance
- Wrong diagnosis
- Associated condition
- Progression to a complication.

The intentional or unintentional ingestion of gluten is the usual cause of a poor therapeutic response or recurrent symptoms. Much depends on the symptoms. The first thing to do is to ask a dietitian to make a formal reassessment of **dietary compliance**. The next step is to consider the symptoms: persistent diarrhoea may result from associated microscopic colitis (remember that coeliac disease rarely causes diarrhoea without weight loss), hypolactasia, bacterial overgrowth, thyrotoxicosis, inflammatory bowel disease, or pancreatic insufficiency. Persistent fatigue may be due to Addison's disease, hypothyroidism, or nutritional deficiency (iron, magnesium, zinc). When there is loss of an initially good response, progression to a complication should be considered.

Serious **complications of coeliac disease** are rare, but include refractory sprue, ulcerative jejunitis, enteropathy-associated T-cell lymphoma, or intestinal adenocarcinoma. Repeat endoscopy with a request to the histopathologist for immunohistochemistry to exclude clonal expansion of T-cells is important, as well as cross-sectional (CT) imaging to look for lymphadenopathy. Double-balloon enteroscopy to obtain tissue is appropriate if a lesion is identified; the alternative is a laparoscopic full thickness intestinal biopsy. Strict compliance with a gluten-free diet reduces the risk of these complications if maintained over the long term.

Further reading

Cataldo F, Lio D, Marino V, Picarelli A *et al.* (2000). IgG1 antiendomysium and IgG antitissue transglutaminase (anti-tTG) antibodies in coeliac patients with selective IgA deficiency. *Gut*; **47**: 366–9.

Catassi C, Fasano A (2008). Celiac disease. *Curr Opin Gastroenterol*; **24**: 687–91.

Haines ML, Anderson RP, Gibson PR (2008). Systematic review: The evidence base for long-term management of coeliac disease. *Aliment Pharmacol Ther*; **28**: 1042–66.

Heap GA, van Heel DA (2009). Genetics and pathogenesis of coeliac disease. *Semin Immunol* **May 13**. [Epub ahead of print].

Case 39

A 76-year-old non-English speaking woman presented to the gastroenterology outpatient department with a 4-month history (through an interpreter) of nausea, decreased appetite, early satiety, and 3kg weight loss. She had mild abdominal discomfort and pancreatic surgery 25 years previously for a pancreatic abscess, but no history of diabetes or steatorrhoea. She had atrial fibrillation, for which she was on warfarin.

On examination, her pulse rate was 76 and irregular, consistent with atrial fibrillation, blood pressure 125/86mmHg, and she was afebrile. No abdominal masses were palpable.

Investigations showed:

- Hb 11.5g/dL, WCC 5.6 x 10^9/L, platelets 165 x 10^9/L
- Na 130mmol/L, K 4.1mmol/L, creatinine 85μmol/L
- Bilirubin 20μmol/L, AST 25 IU/L, ALT 35 IU/L, ALP 60 IU/L, GGT 70 IU/L.

In view of the anaemia and symptoms, she had a gastroscopy. This did not reveal any mucosal lesions, and the stomach inflated well, but there was an impression of extrinsic compression of the stomach. A CT of the abdomen was carried out (Figs 39.1 and 39.2).

Questions

39a) Explain the CT appearance and the differential diagnosis.

39b) Explain the management options for this patient and the pros and cons of each option.

39c) What are the complications of the above management strategies?

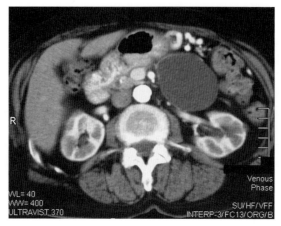

Fig. 39.1 CT scan.

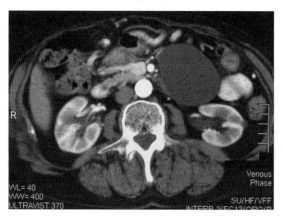

Fig. 39.2 CT scan.

Answers

39a) **Explain the CT appearance and the differential diagnosis**

The CT shows a **pancreatic pseudocyst**. There is a low attenuation, unilocular cyst, with accompanying signs of an atrophic pancreas. If this were a complex pseudocyst, the density of the fluid would be higher than in an uncomplicated pseudocyst, owing to the presence of haemorrhage or gas that develops because of bacterial infection. The precise relationship to the stomach can be seen. There is no associated calcification or pancreatic duct dilatation.

Pancreatic pseudocysts need to be distinguished from pancreatic cystic neoplasms (see Case 29), acute fluid collections, organized pancreatic necrosis, pancreatic abscess, pseudoaneuryms, and duplication cysts.

Pseudocysts result from pancreatic inflammation or trauma leading to pancreatic duct disruption and the accumulation of fluid in the lesser sac. They are usually anechoic on ultrasound and unilocular. They generally contain thin brown fluid, rich in amylase and inflammatory cells, but no mucin (see Table 29.1). They are not lined by a true epithelium (hence the term pseudo-) and therefore have no malignant potential. Instead, they have a thick wall of granulation tissue that takes approximately 4–6 weeks to develop after an episode of acute pancreatitis. The incidence is 10–20% after acute pancreatitis and 20–40% in chronic pancreatitis. Most pseudocysts regress within 6 weeks

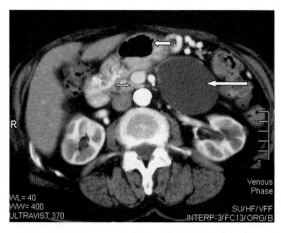

Fig. 39.1 CT scan showing a low attenuation, unilocular cyst (long arrow), with accompanying signs of an atrophic pancreas (short arrow), in the lesser sac (stomach shown by medium arrow).

of diagnosis, and an expectant management is appropriate in the first instance. Chronic pseudocysts are more commonly associated with chronic pancreatitis.

39b) **Explain the main management decisions for this patient and the pros and cons of each option.**

The main management decision is whether to be **conservative** (no drainage) or **interventional** (drainage). The size of pseudocyst is not itself an indication for drainage. Patients with a stable pseudocyst do not require therapy unless they have symptoms. Pseudocyst drainage should be considered in the following circumstances:

- Abdominal pain
- Gastric outlet obstruction
- Early satiety
- Weight loss
- Jaundice
- Suspected infection of the cyst
- Increasing size of the cyst.

The patient had abdominal discomfort, early satiety, and weight loss. There was no evidence of gastric outlet obstruction or jaundice. In view of the history of pancreatic surgery and the atrophic pancreas, it was assumed to be a chronic pseudocyst. Comorbidity had to be considered in the management. The patient was on warfarin for atrial fibrillation, which would need to be stopped before drainage.

Drainage can be achieved by:

- Surgery (cystogastrostomy)
- Percutaneous insertion of catheter under radiological guidance
- Endoscopic drainage guided by endoscopic ultrasound. This is possible in 90% of cases, either through the wall of the stomach or duodenum, with the insertion of a flanged stent.

There are no prospective studies that compare endoscopic drainage to conservative management, percutaneous or surgical drainage. Nevertheless, endoscopic drainage is probably the treatment of choice since it is less interventional than surgery and does not involve an external drain that is prone to infection. It may not be possible if the cyst contents are thick, or the cyst is multilocular.

39c) **What are the complications of the above management strategies?**

The complications of conservative management are that the patient's symptoms are unlikely to resolve and may deteriorate.

Surgical management carries appreciable morbidity (6–37%) and mortality (1–16%), with a cyst recurrence rate of up to 20%. **Percutaneous drainage** has a high recurrence rate (up to 70%). Although continuous percutaneous drainage with an indwelling catheter decreases recurrence, the complication rate is 5–60%, including infection, bleeding, and fistula formation. **Endoscopic drainage** has a morbidity of 9–25%, resulting from complications such as bleeding from penetration of adjacent vessels or varices, perforation, infection, pancreatitis, stent migration or occlusion, and pancreatic duct damage. Infection of a pseudocyst usually indicates inadequate drainage of fluid. The mortality is 0–1%. Definitive treatment is possible in up to 75%, and recurrence rates as low as 5% have been reported. However, endoscopic drainage of pseudocysts should be carried out only with interventional radiology support and surgical back up.

Our patient underwent endoscopic drainage under endoscopic ultrasound guidance and had two transmural stents inserted. Her symptoms resolved. After stenting, it was decided to discontinue her warfarin, since it had only been given for atrial fibrillation and there was no evidence of mural thrombus or history of a cerebrovascular event.

Further reading

AGSE guideline (2005). The role of endoscopy in the diagnosis and the management of cystic lesions and inflammatory fluid collections of the pancreas. *Gastrointest Endosc*; **61**: 363–70.

Brugge WR, Lauwers GY, Sahani D, Fernandez-del Castillo C, Warshaw AL (2004). Cystic neoplasms of the pancreas. *N Engl J Med*; **351**: 1218–26.

Vignesh S, Brugge WR (2008). Endoscopic diagnosis and treatment of pancreatic cysts. *J Clin Gastroenterology*; **42**: 493–506.

Case 40

A 42-year-old shop assistant with hypertension and obesity had a routine blood test, which showed a raised ALP. She was asymptomatic. She was on ramipril 5mg/day and a combined oral contraceptive pill. She had lost 10kg in 5 months, but attributed this to a diet. She did not smoke or drink. Examination, including breast and rectal examinations, was normal.

Investigations showed:

- Hb 12.3g/dL, WCC 10.19 x10^9/L, platelets 405 x 10^9/L, MCV 86fL
- Electrolytes and renal function normal
- Bilirubin 5μmol/L, ALT 16 IU/L, ALP 527 IU/L, albumin 48g/L
- AFP 3.0 IU/mL, CEA 0.5μg/L, CA125 7 IU/L, CA 19-9 <1 IU/L
- Ultrasound scan: multiple liver lesions, consistent with metastases
- MRI: multiple large, irregular, enhancing lesions occupying about a third of the liver. Normal spleen, kidneys, adrenals, pancreas (Fig. 40.1)

Questions

40a) Discuss the clinical dilemma and differential diagnosis in this patient.

40b) How would you investigate the problem?

40c) Discuss the diagnosis.

40d) How should the condition be managed?

40e) What other advice might you offer?

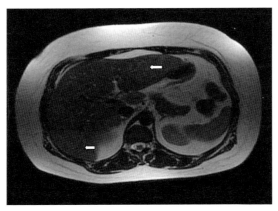

Fig. 40.1 Multiple focal liver lesions with irregular enhancement.

Answers

40a) **Discuss the clinical dilemma and differential diagnosis in this patient.**

The dilemma is that the patient is young, asymptomatic, and has multiple focal hepatic lesions suggestive of metastasis. There is a disparity between the lack of symptoms and the extent of liver involvement. Since there is no evidence of a primary tumour, it is tempting to take the imaging report at face value and diagnose a carcinoma of unknown primary. Her weight loss, which she had attributed to a diet, might conceivably have had a more sinister cause. A diagnosis of malignancy, however, should not be assumed without confirmatory histopathology. It is possible that these are multiple benign lesions. Benign lesions of the liver in a young woman include **hepatic haemangiomas, focal nodular hyperplasia,** and **hepatic adenomas,** in decreasing order of prevalence.

Hepatic haemanigiomas are the most common benign solid lesions of the liver, found in up to 20% of the population. They are three times more common and often larger or multiple in women than in men, typically presenting in the 4th and 5th decades of life. Size may vary from a few millimetres to more than 20cm. Most haemangiomas are asymptomatic and discovered incidentally. Large lesions may cause symptoms because of a mass effect, with pain resulting from distension of the hepatic (Glissen`s) capsule, or a feeling of fullness, early satiety, nausea and vomiting because of compression of adjacent vicera. Both dynamic contrast-enhanced CT and MRI are used to diagnose haemangiomas when lesions have been detected by ultrasound. They rarely require resection.

Focal nodular hyperplasia is the second most common solid lesion of the liver, with a prevalence of up to 8%. They are eight times more common in women than in men and may be multiple in 20% of cases. The lesions are rarely symptomatic and are usually identified incidentally during ultrasound examination of non-specific symptoms in 75% of cases. Abdominal pain is unusual. Infarction, haemorrhage and necrosis are rare in these lesions. Malignant transformation is not known to occur. A characteristic central scar is typically seen on radiological imaging (CT or MRI).

Hepatic adenomas are usually found in women in their reproductive years and are clearly associated with oral contraceptive drugs. They exhibit some radiographic features (well circumscribed hyperintense lesions in T1 weighted MRI, or isointense on CT with peripheral enhancement), but are often difficult to characterize by imaging alone.

They can increase in size and number in pregnancy or if the oral contraceptive pill is continued.

40b) **How would you investigate the problem?**

The most common malignancies that spread to the liver in women are primary tumours of the breast, lung, and colon. These three sites represent >50% of primary tumours in women. A history should identify whether a young woman is at risk of a cancer family syndrome (see Case 17). Our patient had no significant family history and had never smoked.

Apart from a thorough clinical examination including examination of the breasts and a digital rectal examination, imaging should include a chest radiograph. Cross-sectional imaging of the abdomen and pelvis (CT and MRI) is appropriate if not already performed. In our patient, no primary tumour had been found. Tumour markers are of limited value as diagnostic tests, with the exception of α-fetoprotein (AFP). The role of CA 19-9, CEA, or CA 125 is in the follow-up of proven malignancy of the pancreas, colon and ovaries respectively, after diagnosis. They perform poorly as diagnostic tests, because they are non-specific, with a high false-positive rate that is misleading and distressing for the patient. A liver biopsy is appropriate when there is diagnostic doubt about a liver lesion, but the risk of tumour tracking along the biopsy site and the option of surgical resection if the lesion is isolated, should be considered (see Case 14). The liver biopsy was consistent with a **hepatic adenoma**. There was no evidence of malignancy.

40c) **Discuss the diagnosis.**

Hepatic adenomas are uncommon in woman who do not take oral contraceptive drugs, with an incidence of 1/million in this group. Among women taking contraceptives the incidence is estimated at 40/million. The incidence has consequently risen since the 1960s, when oral contraceptives became available. Adenomas of the liver are common in glycogen storage disease types I and III, when they occur in young males (< 20 years of age).

The diagnosis is usually coincidental, since pain occurs in only a quarter of individuals. Severe pain may follow necrosis of the adenoma, haemorrage into the lesion or rupture with haemorrhage into the peritoneum. All these consequences are exceptional, but the risk is increased when there are multiple or large lesions, subcapsular location, continued use of oral contraceptives, and in pregnancy. Liver function tests are usually normal, but may be abnormal after haemorrhage or with multiple lesions. Malignant transformation to hepatocellular carcinoma is reported to occur in cross-sectional studies in 10% of cases but there are no prospective studies. Liver biopsy is unnecessary when an adenoma can be diagnosed on radiological grounds in the appropriate clinical setting.

Molecular studies have attempted to classify hepatic adenomas in an attempt to identify subtypes that may be at risk of malignant transformation, but have been inconclusive. Asymptomatic hepatic adenomas do not need resection.

40d) **How should the condition be managed?**

The oral contraceptive should be stopped. Repeat imaging after an interval of 6–12 months is often appropriate to reassure both patient and physician. Shrinkage usually occurs when oral contraceptives have been stopped, but this is not universal. Surgery should be considered for symptomatic, large (>5cm), single lesions. Resection of an uncomplicated adenoma has a mortality of <1%, but up to 8% if emergency resection is required for haemorrhage. Haemorrhage into the peritoneal cavity has a mortality of 7% and may be managed by selective embolization of the hepatic artery. Orthotopic liver transplantation has been carried out in patients with multiple adenomas or those associated with glycogen storage disease.

Since our patient had no symptoms, she was followed up with repeat imaging after stopping oral contraceptives. The largest lesion (7cm) had shrunk to 5cm 10 months later.

40e) **What other advice might you offer this patient?**

The patient should be advised that lesions may enlarge if she became pregnant. She should also be aware of the uncertain risk of malignant transformation.

This patient subsequently had an uncomplicated pregnancy.

Further reading

Bahirwani R, Reddy KR (2008). Review article: the evaluation of solitary liver masses. *Aliment Pharmacol Ther*; **28**: 953–65.

Lim KH, Ward SC, Roayaie S *et al.* (2008). Multiple inflammatory and serum amyloid A positive telangiectatic hepatic adenomas with glycogenated nuclei arising in a background of nonalcoholic steatohepatitis. *Semin Liver Dis*; **28**: 434–9.

Rebouissou S, Bioulac-Sage P, Zucman-Rossi J (2008). Molecular pathogenesis of focal nodular hyperplasia and hepatocellular adenoma. *J Hepatol*; **48**: 163–70.

Vetcläinen R, Erdogan D, de Graaf W *et al.* (2008) Liver adenomatosis: re-evaluation of aetiology and management. *Liver Int*; **28**: 499–508.

Viale G, Mastropasqua MG (2006). Diagnostic and therapeutic management of carcinoma of unknown primary: histopathological and molecular diagnosis. *Ann Oncol*; **17**(Suppl 10): x163–x167.

Case 41

A 23-year-old female architecture student presented to the emergency department with a 2-week history of bloody diarrhoea and abdominal discomfort, but no pain. She had returned from a field trip with colleagues in India a month previously, but her colleagues had remained well. She reported passing up to 10 loose bowel motions per day with bleeding, and had several episodes of nocturnal diarrhoea. She was a vegetarian and her only medical history was presumed infectious diarrhoea 3 years previously. Her cousin had Crohn's disease, but there was no illness in immediate family members.

On examination, she appeared dehydrated and had a temperature of 38.2°C, with a tachycardia (pulse 104bpm) and blood pressure 90/50mmHg. There was no abdominal distension, but there was mild generalized tenderness.

Investigations showed:

- Hb 12.5g/L, WCC 14.5 x 10^9/L, platelets 600 x 10^9/L
- Na 130mmol/L, K 3.2mmol/L, creatinine 75μmol/L, urea 15mmol/L
- ESR 65mm/hour
- CRP 87mg/L
- Plain abdominal radiograph as shown in Fig. 41.1.

Questions

41a) What is the differential diagnosis?

41b) What treatment should be instituted?

41c) What investigations should be carried out?

41d) There was a limited response to treatment after 3 days; the patient still had eight bloody bowel motions per day and a CRP of 50mg/L, although she was apyrexial and had a pulse rate of 72bpm. How does this change management?

41e) What is the natural history of this condition?

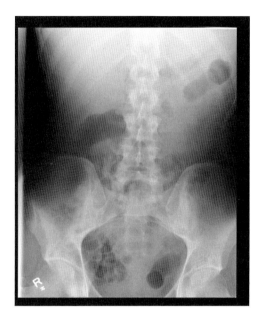

Fig. 41.1

Answers

41a) **What is the differential diagnosis?**

Given the acute history, the major differential diagnosis is between **infective colitis** and **acute severe ulcerative colitis**. Crohn's colitis is unlikely, since it usually causes diarrhoea, severe abdominal pain, and weight loss, but not bloody diarrhoea. The most common organisms causing **infective colitis** with bloody diarrhoea are *Shigella* spp, *Campylobacter* spp, *Entamoeba histolytica*, *Escherichia coli* 0157 H7, *Clostridium difficile*, and *Yersinia* spp. *Salmonella* spp and *Giardia lamblia* do *not* cause bloody diarrhoea. Clinical clues for an infective cause are the recent onset and travel to India. None of her contacts, however, had diarrhoea, and she had little abdominal pain, which characterizes *Campylobacter* and *Shigella* spp. **Amoebiasis** is certainly possible. A history of travel to an endemic area and fever should raise suspicion. *E. coli* and *C. difficile* are much less likely in the absence of a recent history of eating meat from a questionable source, or antibiotic therapy. This patient also fits the criteria for **acute severe ulcerative colitis**, which is defined by the Truelove and Witts' criteria of ≥6 bloody bowel motions per day plus one or more of the following: pulse >90bpm, temperature >37.8°C, Hb<10.5g/dL, or ESR >30mm/hour.

41b) **What treatment should be instituted?**

Treatment must cover BOTH **infective colitis** and **acute severe colitis**. It is better to treat both rather than either alone, and it is potentially dangerous to treat for infection alone while awaiting other investigations. Intravenous corticosteroids will not put the patient at risk if the diagnosis turns out to be infection. An appropriate treatment regimen would be:

- Intravenous hydrocortisone 100mg four times/day
- **Rectal hydrocortisone** 100mg in 100ml 0.9% saline twice daily
- **Subcutaneous heparin** once daily to reduce the chance of the patient developing a deep venous thrombosis
- **3L of fluid/day** (2L 0.9% saline and 1L 5% dextrose), with 60–80mmol KCl/day. Such patients always become hypokalaemic
- **Antibiotics** to cover the possibility of infective colitis, because this is the first attack and there has been recent overseas travel: intravenous metronidazole 500mg three times/day and oral ciprofloxacin 500mg twice daily are appropriate, although antibiotics do not alter the outcome of acute severe inflammatory colitis

- Ask the nurses to **monitor stool frequency** and the pulse and temperature four times/day. This helps objective decision-making
- If **pain relief** is needed in acute colitis, it may indicate impending perforation. It is best to avoid opioids and hyoscine butyl bromide (Buscopan) because these can promote dilatation, and avoid NSAIDS since these can exacerbate colitis. Paracetamol is safe. If pain persists, the plain abdominal radiograph should be repeated that day.

41c) **What investigations should be carried out?**

The following investigations should be carried out on admission.

Abdominal radiograph is required in any patient with diarrhoea severe enough to need admission. The mucosal appearance of the colon looks oedematous in acute colitis (unlike the crisp outline to the haustral folds in a normal colon), the wall is thickened, and mucosal islands may be present, which indicate residual rests of mucosa surrounded by ulceration. The colon may also be dilated (>5.5cm), which then represents toxic megacolon that needs urgent specialist gastroenterology and surgical opinions (see Case 22).

Three stool cultures for *C. difficile* toxin assay, microscopy culture and sensitivity, and ova cysts and parasites are required. With the current history of travel to India, it is advisable to send a hot stool to the laboratory for immediate microscopy to exclude amoebic colitis.

Monitor blood tests: FBC, U&E daily and a CRP on days 3 and 5 are required. Repeat the abdominal radiograph after 24hr if there is established or incipient colonic dilatation (diameter >5.5cm).

41d) **There was a limited response to treatment after 3 days. The patient still had eight bloody bowel motions per day and a CRP of 50mg/L, although she was apyrexial and had a pulse rate of 72bpm. How does this change management?**

The patient has had a poor response to intensive treatment. This is defined on day 3 of intensive treatment as a stool frequency >8/day, or a CRP>45mg/L, and frequency 3–8/day. This is associated with a high risk (85%) of colectomy on that admission. Treatment needs to be changed as a consequence and specialist advice sought urgently. Options for medical rescue therapy include intravenous ciclosporin 2mg/kg once daily (if serum cholesterol >3mmol/L and magnesium >0.5mmol/L) OR infliximab 5mg/kg infusion. This is a specialist decision, but should not be delayed: if local advice is unavailable, a regional specialist should be contacted. Contingency plans in case surgery is necessary should also be started: better to introduce a surgeon (as 'probably unnecessary') at this

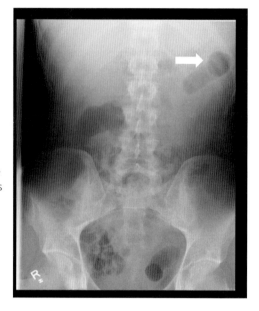

Fig. 41.1 Abdominal radiograph in acute severe colitis showing oedematous colonic mucosa without visible haustra and a thickened wall (arrow). The absence of any faecal residue is consistent with a pancolitis. The colonic diameter is 4.5cm.

stage, than a day or two later (as 'unfortunately essential'). This is one of the reasons for specialist input. This patient was given infliximab (5mg/kg infusion) and responded well.

41e) **What is the natural history of this condition?**

Improvement in the management of acute severe ulcerative colitis has improved mortality from severe attacks of ulcerative colitis from 75% in 1933, 24% in 1955 to <1% in specialist centres today. This can be attributed to intravenous corticosteroids and early surgery for lack of response. Nevertheless, the colectomy rate for acute severe colitis (29%) has remained stable over the past 30 years. Ciclosporin or infliximab appear to defer, rather than prevent colectomy, although further trials are in progress.

Further reading

Brown S, George B, Blakeborough A, Haboubi N, Travis SPL (2008). ACPGBI Position statement on the management of acute severe colitis. *Colorectal Dis*; **10**(Suppl 3): 8–29.

Stange EF, Travis SPL, Vermeire S *et al.* for the European Crohn's and Colitis Organisation (ECCO) (2008). European Consensus on the diagnosis and management of ulcerative colitis: definitions and diagnosis. *J Crohn's & Colitis*; **2**: 1–4.

Jacobovits S, Travis SPL (2006). The management of acute severe colitis. *Br Med Bull*; **75–76**: 131–44.

Case 42

A 35-year-old single mother from a remote part of South Africa was referred from the neurology unit for evaluation of abnormal liver enzymes. She had presented initially with transverse myelitis. She was on antihypertensive medication and had had a Caesarian section 6 years before. Apart from the weakness in her lower limbs and dysuria, she volunteered no other symptoms.

On clinical examination, her pulse rate was 84bpm, and blood pressure 130/80mmHg. She was pale, but anicteric. There was no palpable lymphadenopathy, finger clubbing, or oedema. She had oral thrush. The cardiorespiratory examination was unremarkable. Abdominal examination was normal, without organomegaly. She had no signs of chronic liver disease.

Investigations showed:

- Hb 11.4g/dL, WCC 3.3 x 10^9/L, platelets 200 x 10^9/L
- ESR >90mm/hour
- INR 1.0
- Bilirubin 13μmol/L, ALT 76 IU/L, ALP 632 IU/L, GGT 682 IU/L, albumin 36g/L
- HbsAg negative, anti-HCV negative
- HIV positive
- CD4 count 7 cells/uL.

Questions

42a) Discuss the clinical problem and differential diagnosis.

42b) How would you proceed with investigation?

42c) How would you manage this patient?

42d) Discuss liver involvement in HIV in the context of highly active antiretroviral therapy (HAART).

Answers

42a) **Discuss the clinical problem and differential diagnosis.**

The two considerations in our patients are:

- The level of immune deficiency
- The pattern of liver function tests derangement.

Apart from transverse myelitis, this young woman presents with **abnormal liver function tests (LFTs)** and evidence of **impaired cell mediated immunity**. Serology for HIV was positive and a CD4 cell count of 7 cells/μl confirmed **advanced immune deficiency**. Her HIV infection was newly diagnosed and she had never received any antiretroviral medication.

The pattern of LFT derangement is predominantly that of **cholestasis** (ALP three times the upper limit, with a raised GGT). This indicates either diffuse infiltration of the liver (see Case 48), space-occupying lesions, or biliary tract disease. Infiltration or space-occupying lesions of the liver result from:

- Malignancy
- Disseminated infection involving the liver.

Malignancies involving the liver in HIV may occur at any level of immune deficiency, but become more common as immune deficiency progresses. In HIV, **non-Hodgkin's lymphoma** usually presents in extranodal sites, with up to 16% of cases involving the liver. Imaging of the liver usually reveals mass lesions. **Kaposi's sarcoma** of the liver is usually not clinically evident, but has been found in up to 50% of autopsies, in series from the pre-HAART era. It has been more commonly found in homosexual men and is caused by infection with human herpesvirus 8 (HHV 8).

Opportunistic infections are much more likely in the absence of HAART with a **CD4 cell count** <200 cells/μl and often involve the liver. **Tuberculosis** is the most common concern. At CD4 counts >200 cells/μl, tuberculosis is usually confined to the lungs, presenting with clinical and radiological characteristics similar to those in the immune competent host. Once the CD4 count drops to <200 cells/μl, atypical presentations are more frequent. The typical apical distribution reactivated (secondary) tuberculosis (see chest radiograph, Case 26) is not seen in advanced immune deficiency. Appearances on the chest radiograph resemble those seen in primary tuberculosis, with alveolar infiltrates, air-bronchograms,

basal infiltrates, mediastinal lymphadenopathy, and miliary shadowing. Dissemination with involvement of multiple organs is frequent.

In contrast to *Mycobacterium tuberculosis*, ***Mycobacterium avium* complex** infection occurs in advanced HIV and is purely opportunistic. It is more frequently documented in cohorts from developed countries. *Mycobacterium avium* complex infection rarely occurs at CD4 counts >50 cells/µl. Liver infection is usually clinically silent, with systemic symptoms of fever, night sweats and weight loss. Systemic **cytomegalovirus** infection may involve the liver and occurs in advanced immune deficiency. Again symptoms are predominantly systemic. **Fungal infections** also occur late. Hepatomegaly is common in systemic histoplasmosis, which usually occurs in endemic areas such as the mid-West of the USA. Apart from *Histoplasma capsulatum*, other opportunistic fungal infections include *Cryptococcus neoformans*, coccidioidomycosis, and blastomycosis, all of which may involve the liver in disseminated disease. *Pneumocystis jiroveci* has also been reported to involve the liver.

Biliary tract involvement infection in HIV is well recognized: cryptosporidia leads to an **AIDS cholangiopathy**. It is characterized by irregular intrahepatic and extrahepatic bile ducts resembling primary sclerosing cholangitis (see Case 50), but the associated papillary stenosis is considered specific. Large duct biliary obstruction unrelated to HIV, including gallstone disease, may occur in patients with HIV, so commonplace disorders should not be overlooked!

42b) **How would you proceed with investigation?**

An **opportunistic infection** was the most likely cause, and since these are usually disseminated in advanced HIV, they may be diagnosed in any accessible organ. The patient's chest radiograph showed basal infiltrates, giving a differential diagnosis of *Pneumocystis jiroveci* (formerly *carinii*) pneumonia, tuberculosis, *Mycobacterium avium* complex infection, histoplasmosis, or malignancy. Tuberculosis, was by far the most likely diagnosis, but difficult to confirm in the absence of sputum production. *Mycobacterium avium* complex and disseminated fungal infection remained possible. Our patient had no respiratory symptoms so *Pneumocystis jiroveci* pneumonia was unlikely. Histopathology is often the simplest (and quickest) way to diagnose infection and exclude malignancy; bronchoscopy would be reasonable, but depends on local expertise and liver biopsy is often more accessible (See Figs 42.1a and 42.1b).

Further investigation showed:

- Ultrasound of the liver showed no evidence of biliary duct dilation or gallstones. Normal appearances of liver parynchyma.
- MRCP: normal appearances of the intrahepatic and extrahepatic biliary tree.

This effectively excluded biliary tract disease, and the normal scan indicates that diffuse hepatic infiltration is the cause of the liver dysfunction.

- Liver biopsy showed multiple non-caseating granulomas (Figs 42.1a and 42.1b in the central colour section).

The differential diagnosis of **granulomatous hepatitis** in HIV-postive patients includes:

- Tuberculosis
- *Mycobacterium avium* complex infection
- Histoplasmosis.

Disseminated tuberculosis is still by far the most likely cause, despite the lack of caseation or organisms on Ziehl–Neilsen staining. In series from developing countries tuberculosis causes most cases of granulomatous hepatitis in patients with HIV. A microbiological diagnosis is often difficult, because these patients are usually sputum negative, and treatment has to be based on the clinical picture in an area of high prevalence.

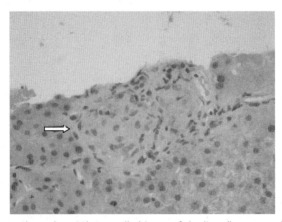

Fig. 42.1a (see colour plate 20) A needle biopsy of the liver (haematoxylin and eosin stain) showing a granuloma (arrow).

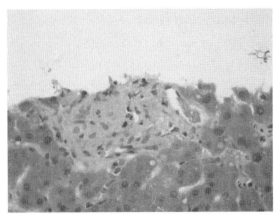

Fig. 42.1b (see colour plate 21) The same biopsy using a Periodic Acid Schiff stain. The granuloma does not contain stored glycogen, so is PAS-negative.

42c) **How would you manage this patient?**

- Treatment of the presumed tuberculosis
- Institution of HAART.

The treatment of tuberculosis in a patient with HIV is generally the same as for HIV-negative patients (see Case 26). Medication should, however, always be given **daily** (not twice weekly as in some regimens) and in cases of poor response, therapy may be prolonged by 3 months (i.e. extension of the continuation phase from 4 months to 7 months). Treatment of tuberculosis always precedes the institution of HAART. This is to ensure that antituberculous drugs are tolerated and to reduce the possibility of immune reconstitution syndrome.

42d) **Discuss liver involvement in HIV disease in the context of highly active antiretroviral therapy (HAART)**

In the pre-HAART era, liver involvement in patients with HIV was mainly because of opportunistic infection. Although coinfection with HBV and HCV was well recognized in view of similar modes of transmission, coinfections had little impact on outcomes. The outcome was determined by the natural history of the underlying HIV disease. With the institution of HAART, the natural history of HIV infection was altered dramatically. As a consequence, coinfection with hepatotropic viruses has become significant, because patients survive long enough to develop endstage liver disease. In the past decade liver disease has become an important cause of death in HIV-positive patients, accounting for

15% of deaths. For this reason HIV-positive patients in developed countries may now be considered for liver transplantation in the same way as HIV-negative patients with endstage liver disease.

Active **HBV infection** occurs in up to 10% of HIV-positive patients. The course of HBV infection in HIV is more rapid. With the institution of HAART in a patient with HBV coinfection, recovery of the immune system may lead to a flare of the hepatitis with fulminant liver failure. For this reason the HAART regimen needs to contain antiretroviral agents with efficacy against both HIV and HBV. Lamivudine is effective, but when used as the sole agent, rapidly results in HBV resistance. Tenofovir or entecovir are also effective against both viral infections when used in combination with lamivudine. For a three-drug HAART regimen, two of the three drugs should be active against HBV for patients with HIV-HBV coinfection.

Coinfection with HCV occurs in 13–80% of HIV-positive patients, being most common in intravenous drug users. HCV infection in the context of HIV is associated with higher viral loads, the rapid development of fibrosis, and rapid progression to cirrhosis (which may develop within 10 years in these patients). Toxicity from HAART is also higher in patients with HCV coinfection. Despite this, HAART probably reduces liver-related mortality in these patients. Pegylated interferon and ribavirin remain the therapy of choice for HCV-HIV infection. Unfortunately a sustained virological response is less common for all HCV genotypes in patients who also have HIV. Therapy for HCV is best delayed until immune reconstitution has occurred on HAART.

Drug-related liver toxicity on HAART occurs in about 10%. In patients with hepatotoxicity the mortality is 3%. Risk factors for hepatotoxicity include

- The use of ritonavir
- Baseline elevated transaminases
- HCV coinfection
- Underlying liver disease with advanced fibrosis.

A lactic acidosis syndrome with progressive microvesicular steatosis of the liver is specifically associated with nucleoside reverse transcriptase inhibitors, including zidovudine, didanosine, and stavudine. This syndrome may be fatal if not recognized. Hepatotoxicity from antituberculous therapy has been discussed (see Case 1).

Further reading

Ocama P, Katwere M, Piloya T *et al.* (2008). The spectrum of liver diseases in HIV infected individuals at an HIV treatment clinic in Kampala, Uganda. *Afr Health Sci*; **8**: 8–12.

Sharma SK, Mohan A, Kadhiravan T (2005). HIV-TB co-infection: Epidemiology, diagnosis & management. *Indian J Med Res*; **121**: 550–67.

Terzic D, Brambolic B, Singer D *et al.* (2008). Liver enlargement associated with opportunistic infections in patients with human immunodeficiency virus infection. *J Gastrointest Liver Dis*; **17**: 401–4.

Wilcox CM, Saag MS (2008). Gastrointestinal complications of HIV infection: changing priorities in the HAART era. *Gut*; **57**: 861–70.

Case 43

A 42-year-old male caretaker had abnormal liver function tests when he went to see his family practitioner about back pain and fatigue. He remembered being jaundiced for 2 weeks when he was 18 years of age, but this was never investigated. He drank 2–3 cans of beer each week. He had not been tested for hepatitis C, but he had used intravenous drugs from 17 years of age until he was 24 years. There was no family history of liver disease or autoimmune disease. He was a non-smoker and not on any regular medication. He had been diagnosed with depression in the past and had taken fluoxetine 2 years ago.

On examination, there were multiple spider naevi, but no evidence of hepatosplenomegaly, ascites, or encephalopathy.

Investigations showed:

- Hb 15.2g/dL; WCC 5.6 x 10^9/L; platelets 126 x 10^9/L
- Prothrombin time 13.2 sec
- Bilirubin 30μmol/L; ALT 122 IU; ALP 205 IU; albumin 43g/L
- AFP 5 IU/mL
- HCV antibody positive
- HCV RNA 2,016,074 IU/mL
- HBsAb positive and HBcAb positive
- Ultrasound abdomen revealed a coarse liver texture, and an enlarged spleen (15cm)

Questions

43a) What is the most likely reason for jaundice when the patient was 18 years old?

43b) How severe is the patient's liver disease and what is his prognosis?

43c) Outline the advice that should be given to the patient regarding transmission.

43d) What further investigations are needed and what is the best treatment?

43e) What are the contraindications and possible complications of treatment?

Answers

43a) **What is the most likely reason for jaundice when the patient was 18 years old?**

Acute presentation of hepatitis C with jaundice is very rare and most individuals present in the chronic phase with abnormal liver function tests. About 20–30% will spontaneously clear hepatitis C infection, which probably occurs within 6 months of acute infection. This cohort will have hepatitis C antibodies, but undetectable HCV RNA in the serum. Such people do not need follow-up and should be considered as uninfected. HCV RNA is therefore an important confirmatory test for hepatitis C infection, since treatment cannot be based on the detection of antibodies alone. In this man, jaundice almost certainly resulted from **acute hepatitis B** infection, which is cleared in 90% of adults who become infected. This is consistent with the detection of hepatitis B core and surface antibodies.

43b) **How severe is the patient's liver disease and what is his prognosis?**

The presence of thrombocytopenia and splenomegaly in a patient with chronic liver disease is highly suggestive of **cirrhosis**, which was subsequently confirmed by liver biopsy. About 10% of people with hepatitis C will progress to cirrhosis within 20 years. Risk factors for progression are coexistent heavy alcohol intake, immunosuppression such as HIV, or organ transplantation, age >40 years at infection, and male gender. Once cirrhosis develops, 25% will develop complications (such as ascites) by 10 years. There is a 1% per year risk of primary liver cell cancer once cirrhosis develops. The degree of elevation of ALT is unrelated to the extent of liver fibrosis although those with persistently normal liver function tests tend to have less fibrosis and progress more slowly. In contrast to HIV, HCV viral load is not a prognostic indicator and is mainly used to evaluate the response to therapy.

43c) **Outline the advice that should be given to the patient regarding transmission.**

Transmission of HCV is either percutaneous (blood transfusion or needle-stick injury) or non-percutaneous (sexual contact, perinatal exposure). After the introduction of anti-HCV screening of blood donors in 1991, the rate of transfusion-related cases of HCV declined significantly in the UK. Intravenous drug use is now the most common risk factor in the UK. Sexual transmission is rare, but has been reported in homosexuals. Hepatitis C is more prevalent in southern Europe and the

Indian subcontinent, where inadequate cleaning of needles used for vaccination has been a prevalent iatrogenic cause in the past. There is no effective vaccine and no effective post-exposure prophylaxis against HCV. Emphasis should be placed on counselling HCV-infected patients and those at risk of infection.

The patient should be advised to avoid sharing razors or toothbrushes and to cover any open wound. Safe sexual practice, such as the use of condoms, should be encouraged in patients with multiple sexual partners, although this is not recommended for people involved in long-term monogamous relationships. HCV-infected patients who are users of intravenous drugs should be vaccinated against HBV if not immune.

43c) **What further investigations are needed and what is the best treatment?**

An **endoscopy** to screen for varices, **hepatic ultrasound**, and measurement of **AFP** every 6 months, to screen for hepatocellular carcinoma (see Case 14), are appropriate. The viral **genotype** and **viral load** should be measured.

The goal of therapy in hepatitis C infection is a **sustained virological response**, defined as undetectable HCV RNA in peripheral blood 24 weeks after antiviral treatment has stopped. **Standard treatment** for hepatitis C consists of pegylated interferon-α given once weekly, together with oral ribavirin. Overall cure rates are 50%, but this depends on the viral genotype. Only 45% with genotype 1 (the most common type in the UK) are cured after a 12-month course of therapy, compared with 60–70% for genotype 3, and 90% with genotype 2. Only 6 months' therapy is needed for genotype 2. Cure rates are lower in cirrhosis or coinfection with HIV.

43d) **What are the contraindications and possible side effects of treatment?**

Ribavirin may cause a 3–4g/dL drop in haemoglobin. A substantial side effect of interferon is psychological depression, fatigue, or irritability. Relative **contraindications** to therapy include a myocardial infarction within 6 months or severe cardiac failure, haemoglobinopathies, renal failure (since ribavirin is excreted by the kidneys), decompensated liver disease, immunosuppression (such as transplant patients), uncontrolled thyroid disease, pregnancy, and male partners of pregnant women.

Potential **side effects** of combined therapy include:

• Flu-like symptoms (to be expected with interferon)
• Diarrhoea

- Fatigue
- Skin rashes
- Increased susceptibility to infection
- Thyroid dysfunction
- Psychiatric disturbance
- Bone marrow suppression
- Local reactions at injection sites.

Side effects frequently necessitate interruption of treatment and dose reduction. Severe or life-threatening side effects are infrequent but do occur. A good **predictor of treatment response** is loss of detectable HCV RNA within 4 weeks of starting therapy.

This patient was treated with pegylated interferon and ribavirin for 12 months. He needed antidepressants during therapy and had to stop work as a consequence. He returned to work a month after stopping therapy. His HCV RNA at 4 weeks dropped to 1540 IU/ml and was undetectable at week 12. Six months after stopping therapy his liver function was normal and HCV PCR remained negative, consistent with cure.

Further reading

Bruno S, Facciotto C (2008). The natural course of HCV infection and the need for treatment. *Ann Hepatol*; **7**: 114–9.

Baldo V, Baldovin T, Trivello R, Floreani A (2008). Epidemiology of HCV infection. *Curr Pharmac Design*; **14**(17): 1646–54.

Blonski W, Reddy KR (2008). Hepatitis C virus infection and hepatocellular carcinoma. *Clin Liver Dis*; **12**: 61–74.

Fabris P, Fleming VM, Giordani MT, Barnes E (2008). Acute hepatitis C: clinical aspects, diagnosis, and outcome of acute HCV infection. *Curr Pharmac Design*; **14**: 1661–5.

Santantonio T, Fasano M (2008). Therapy of acute hepatitis C: a review of literature. *Curr Pharmac Design*; **14**: 1686–9.

Case 44

A 27-year-old Chinese woman was referred for assessment of chronic hepatitis B infection. A raised ALT 600 IU/L had been found when travelling abroad. On return to the UK, she was seen for right upper quadrant pain and found to have hepatitis B. Her main complaint at presentation was fatigue in addition to the pain. She had never used intravenous drugs and had no history of blood transfusion, tattoos, or jaundice. She had undergone a laparoscopic cholecystectomy 7 years previously, but this had not relieved the pain. On examination, she had no evidence of chronic liver disease or portal hypertension.

Investigations showed:

- Hb 12.5g/dL, WCC 8.7 x 10^9/L, platelets 251 x 10^9/L
- Bilirubin 13μmol/L, ALT 32 IU/L, ALP 162 IU/L, albumin 41g/L
- Viral markers: HBsAg positive, HBeAg positive, anti-HBe negative, anti-HBc IgM negative, HBV DNA 67.8 million IU/mL, HCV antibody negative
- Liver screen (see Case 1) otherwise negative
- Ultrasound scan of the abdomen: increased echogenicity in the liver
- CT and MRI of the abdomen: cholecystectomy noted, otherwise unremarkable
- Liver biopsy: chronic hepatitis with minimal activity and mild fibrosis.

Questions

44a) Interpret the serology.

44b) Discuss the mode of transmission.

44c) Discuss the management options.

44d) What is the long-term prognosis?

44e) What is the significance of the abdominal pain and fatigue?

Answers

44a) **Interpret the serology.**

Our patient has serological evidence of **HBeAg-positive chronic hepatitis B. Chronic infection** is defined by positive HBsAg serology for >6 months. She is likely to be in the **immunotolerant phase** of hepatitis B, usually seen in young people and characterized by high levels of viral replication. This is indicated by an HBV DNA >10^7 copies/mL (1 IU = 2.5–5 copies) with normal liver function tests. This phase may last decades before progressing to active disease. A normal ALT on one occasion does *not* imply immunotolerance, since the ALT should be shown to be normal over time.

Progression to **active disease** is recognized by a rise in the ALT and may lead to loss of HBeAg and seroconversion. This in turn may lead to the expression of anti-HBe antibodies, suppression of viral replication, and normalization of ALT with inactive liver histology and minimal fibrosis. This is termed the **inactive carrier state**. Our patient has already had a single flare when her ALT rose to 600 IU/mL, but this failed to clear the virus. If she has repeated flares of hepatitis, detected by an elevated ALT and this still fails to clear the virus, it is likely that she will develop fibrosis.

44b) **Discuss the mode of transmission.**

The time of transmission in this patient is unclear, although probably occurred at birth or in childhood. Hepatitis B is **parenterally transmitted** through contact with contaminated body fluids, either sexually, intravenous drug use and sharing of needles, transfusion of contaminated blood products, body piercing or tattoos, or vertically transmitted from mother to child. Transmission of hepatitis B in Asia is often **vertical** from mother to baby in the perinatal period. Perinatal transmission leads to chronic hepatitis in 90% of affected individuals in the absence of hepatitis B immunoglobulin and vaccination at birth. **Horizontal transmission** during childhood carries a 20–30% risk of chronic infection. In contrast, <1% of people who contract hepatitis B in adulthood develop chronic hepatitis B.

Our patient had no history of any risk factors that could have lead to her contracting a blood-borne illness. Her husband tested negative for hepatitis B.

44c) **Discuss the management options.**

Treatment options for chronic hepatitis B include **no treatment**, **treatment for a finite period** with the aim of precipitating HBeAg seroconversion and sustained post-treatment viral suppression, or **long-term treatment** to suppress viral replication. Treatment aims to delay or arrest progression to cirrhosis, hepatic decompensation, and endstage liver disease, as well as reducing the risk of hepatocellular carcinoma.

Treatment of finite duration involves pegylated interferon-α2a, 180µg/week. This is indicated in those with HBeAg-positive chronic hepatitis (with an elevated ALT). These regimens lead to HBeAg seroconversion to HBeAb-positive (the primary endpoint of clinical trials and treatment) in about a third of patients. The response is durable in up to 90% of responders followed for 7 years. Interferon therapy usually has side effects: flu-like symptoms, fatigue, weight loss, alopecia, bone marrow suppression, and alterations of mood with depression (see Case 43). Treatment is contraindicated in decompensated liver disease, and used with caution in cirrhosis.

Long-term therapy is required for patients with HBeAg-positive chronic hepatitis B who do not seroconvert with interferon, or those with HBeAg-negative chronic hepatitis B (Table 44.1). In some chronic hepatitis B carriers (HBsAg-positive, HBeAb-positive with a normal ALT) the virus mutates, leading to a rise in viral load, abnormal liver blood tests, and liver damage known as **HBeAg-negative chronic hepatitis B**. Several nucleoside or nucleotide analogues suppress HBV. They are given as monotherapy, unlike treatment of HIV or HCV. Drugs include **lamivudine**, **adefovir**, **tenofovir**, and **entecavir**. The latter two are particularly resistant to viral mutation even after continuous monotherapy for 3 years. Life-long treatment is likely to be necessary.

Since our patient had normal ALT she was unlikely to benefit from interferon therapy. She only had mild fibrosis and minimal activity on liver histology. Long-term viral suppression was unlikely to be beneficial and risks provoking viral resistance, making subsequent therapy more difficult. We therefore followed her up with ALT measurements every 3 months. The plan was to **identify a two-fold increase in ALT**, which would prompt a finite course of interferon therapy, hoping to provoke seroconversion. Loss of HBsAg and viral eradication is uncommon. The patient's husband and children tested negative for HBsAg, and immunization to hepatitis B was recommended. During follow up, she had a flare of ALT to 102 IU/L. She was given a course of therapy with pegylated interferon-α2a, although unfortunately this did not lead to seroconversion on this occasion.

Table 44.1 The natural history of hepatitis B

Phase	Serum ALT	HBe Ag	Anti-HBe	HBV-DNA		
				Level	Copies/mL	IU/mL
Immune tolerance	Normal or minimally elevated	Positive	Negative	Very high	10^8–10^{12}	20m–20bn
HBeAg-positive chronic hepatitis	Persistently elevated	Positive	Negative	High	10^6–10^{10}	200k–2bn
HBeAg-negative chronic hepatitis	Elevated and often fluctuating	Negative	Positive	Moderate, fluctuating	10^4–10^8	2k–20m
Inactive carrier	Normal	Negative	Positive	Low or not detectable	$<10^4$	<2k

44d) What is the long-term outlook?

The **natural history** of chronic hepatitis B infection is variable. Adverse outcomes include liver cirrhosis, hepatic decompensation, endstage liver disease, and the development of hepatocellular carcinoma. **Risk factors for cirrhosis** in chronic hepatitis B are similar to those for HCV (see Case 43), and include age >40 years at diagnosis, male gender, severe fibrosis at presentation, recurrent flares of hepatitis, high levels of HBV replication, HBV genotype C, mutant strains of virus, coinfection with HDV, HIV or HCV, and heavy alcohol consumption. Once cirrhosis is established the risk of hepatocellular carcinoma increases. Older age is probably a surrogate marker of longer duration of infection, as is Asian ethnicity, since infection is usually acquired early in life. Of particular relevance to our patient is that repeated flares without viral clearance, increases the risk of progression to cirrhosis. The risk of developing cirrhosis over a 5-year period in a patient of East Asian origin, with HBeAg-positive chronic hepatitis B is 8%. The risk of hepatocellular carcinoma is 0.01–0.1%/year in patients with chronic hepatitis B without cirrhosis, and 1–3%/year in the presence of cirrhosis.

44e) What is the significance of the abdominal pain and fatigue?

Neither abdominal pain nor fatigue is attributable to chronic hepatitis B infection. The patient had had right upper quadrant pain for at least 7 years. Biliary type pain, in the absence of gallstones often results from **sphincter of Oddi dysfunction** (often known as SOD, by name and nature!).

In sphincter of Oddi dysfunction, biliary-type pain recurs or persists after cholecystectomy. It is sometimes referred to as post-cholecystectomy syndrome. Residual gallstones, tumours, or common bile duct strictures should first be excluded.

Sphincter of Oddi dysfunction presents as pain, commonly with fatigue, sometimes with abnormal liver function tests, and occasionally a dilated common bile duct or pancreatic duct. Sphincter of Oddi dysfunction is classified on the basis of whether or not there is a dilated common bile duct or raised alkaline phosphatase during pain attacks.

Type 1 is defined as a dilated common bile duct and a two-fold elevation in ALP on two occasions, which responds best to treatment with endoscopic sphincterotomy. Type 2 is defined as an elevated ALP or dilated CBD and responds to sphincterotomy in less than two-thirds of cases. Type 3 is characterized by biliary type pain with a normal CBD and without a rise in ALP. Type 3 is most difficult to treat and the risks (pancreatitis and mortality) associated with intervention by sphincterotomy cannot be justified. Patients should be treated medically, often with a low dose of a tricyclic as in irritable bowel syndrome (see Case 32). Our patient had type 3 sphincter of Oddi dysfunction unrelated to her liver disease and she responded to amitriptyline 10–25mg at night.

Further reading

Corazziari E (2003). Sphincter of Oddi dysfunction. *Dig Liver Dis*; **35**(Suppl. 3): S26–S29.

Dusheiko G, Antonakopoulos N (2008). Current treatment of hepatitis B. *Gut*; **57**: 105–24.

Fattovich G, Bortolotti F, Donato F (2008). Natural history of chronic hepatitis B: Special emphasis on disease progression and prognostic factors. *J Hepatol*; **48**: 335–52.

Papatheodoridis GV, Manolakopoulos S, Dusheiko G, Archimandritis AJ (2008). Therapeutic strategies in the management of patients with chronic hepatitis B virus infection. *Lancet Infect Dis*; **8**: 167–78.

Case 45

A 47-year-old woman presented with a 2-week history of abdominal distension. She had an 18-year history of type 2 diabetes, now controlled with insulin. She also had peripheral vascular disease with a left, below-knee amputation. There was no history of myocardial infarction, neuropathy, or retinal disease. Current medications were enalapril, atenolol, aspirin, amlodipine, and insulin. She drank <10 units/week of alcohol and denied ever having been a heavy drinker.

On examination, her pulse was 80bpm, blood pressure 150/80mmHg, and she was apyrexial. There were no stigmata of chronic liver disease. Ascites was present and there was pitting oedema to the sacrum. Her BMI prior to the ascites was 31kg/m².

Investigations showed:

- Hb 12.5g/dL, WCC 10.1 x 10⁹/L, platelets 100 x 10⁹/L
- Na 132mmol/L, K 3.5mmol/L, urea 6.3mmol/L, creatinine 87μmol/L
- Random blood glucose 8.7mmol/L
- Bilirubin 4μmol/L, AST 95 IU/L, ALT 70 IU/L, ALP 434 IU/L, GGT 40 IU/L, albumin 26g/L
- Ferritin 440μg/L
- Prothrombin time 14.0 sec
- Abdominal ultrasound: coarse liver texture, ascites, normal sized spleen
- Ascitic fluid analysis: albumin 4g/L, WCC <250 cells/mL, no malignant cells
- CA125 1052 IU/ml (normal range 0–30)
- CT of the abdomen: enlarged irregular liver, splenomegaly, patent portal vein.

Questions

45a) What is the differential diagnosis and what other serological blood tests are appropriate?

45b) What should be the next investigation?

45c) What is the natural history of this condition?

45d) Which patients should have a liver biopsy?

45e) How could the patient's liver disease have been prevented?

Answers

45a) **What is the differential diagnosis and what other serological blood tests are appropriate?**

The differential diagnosis of ascites in this patient includes:

- Cirrhosis
  - Non-alcoholic fatty liver disease (NAFLD)
  - Alcoholic liver disease
  - Haemochromatosis
  - Autoimmune liver disease
  - Chronic viral hepatitis (B or C, see Cases 43 and 44)
  - Cryptogenic cirrhosis
- Right heart failure
- Ovarian cancer with peritoneal metastases.

This patient is likely to have **cirrhosis**, because there is thrombocytopaenia, hypoalbuminaemia, an elevated prothrombin time, and an abnormal appearance of the liver on both ultrasound and CT scan. The sensitivity and specificity, however, of ultrasound or CT for the diagnosis of cirrhosis is low. The patient is at particular risk of NAFLD because she has type 2 diabetes, obesity, and hyperlipidaemia. NAFLD is, however, a clinico-pathological diagnosis that is made after the exclusion of other liver disorders.

The following aetiologies need to be excluded:

- Significant alcohol consumption (>20g/day ethanol)
- Haemochromatosis (although an elevated ferritin, usually <1000µg/L, is common in NAFLD)
- Chronic viral hepatitis
- Alpha-1 antitrypsin deficiency
- Autoimmune liver disease.

In NAFLD, it is the ALT and GT that are commonly abnormal, although a third of patients have cholestatic liver function tests with an elevated ALP and GT. The ALT is characteristically higher than the AST, in contrast to alcoholic liver disease. A high ALT/AST ratio reverses in the presence of cirrhosis. A low platelet count is common in cirrhosis.

It is important to exclude **right heart failure** as a cause of ascites, by examination (elevated jugular venous pressure, pulsatile liver), and by echocardiogram. Our patient had no clinical signs of right heart failure and the echocardiogram was normal. It is also prudent to check that the hypoalbuminaemia is not caused by nephrotic syndrome. The patient's 24-hour urinary protein was <1g.

An elevated CA125 can occur in cirrhosis, although it is important to exclude **ovarian cancer**. No malignant cells were seen in the ascitic fluid (sensitivity 60–70%). The coarse liver texture on ultrasound and CT, the splenomegaly and low protein ascites with a serum ascites albumin gradient >11g/L, is characteristic of cirrhosis.

45b) **What should be the next investigation?**

This patient needs a **liver biopsy** (Figs 45.1 and 45.2 in the central colour section). Since the patient had ascites and a BMI >30kg/m^2, this was carried out via the transjugular route. Transjugular liver biopsy is appropriate in the presence of ascites, coagulopathy (PT prolonged >5 sec above the normal upper range) or platelets <60 x 10^9/L. Liver biopsy helps confirm the stage of cirrhosis and establishes the aetiology. The histological features of NAFLD associated with cirrhosis are those of non-alcoholic steatohepatitis (NASH). These include Mallory's hyaline, macrovesicular fat, and a chronic inflammatory portal infiltrate with interface hepatitis and a varying degree of fibrosis. The amount of fat in hepatocytes often declines as cirrhosis develops. The histopathological features are indistinguishable from alcoholic liver disease, so a clinical history is needed to differentiate the two conditions. Many cases of cryptogenic cirrhosis (i.e. unknown cause) are attributable to non-alcoholic fatty liver disease.

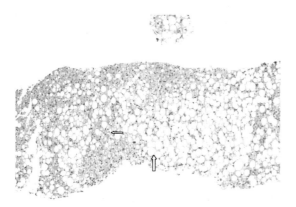

Fig. 45.1 (see colour plate 22) Liver biopsy in non-alcoholic fatty liver disease (low power) showing steatosis (large arrow) and interface hepatitis (small arrow).

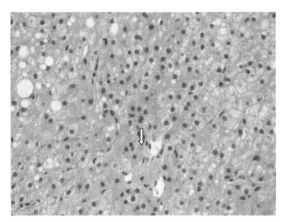

Fig. 45.2 (see colour plate 23) Liver biopsy in non-alcoholic fatty liver disease (high power) showing Mallory's hyaline (arrow).

45c) **What is the natural history of this condition?**

NAFLD can be separated on histopathology into simple steatosis and **non-alcoholic steatohepatitis** (NASH). Only NASH is associated with fibrosis and progression to cirrhosis. It typically presents with asymptomatic abnormal liver function tests. The prevalence of NAFLD is 3–7%. About a third of those with NASH will develop cirrhosis, although this may take several decades. NASH is associated with increased liver-related mortality.

Factors associated with more severe disease include:

- Obesity
- Type 2 diabetes
- Age >45 years
- Hypertriglyceridaemia
- The role of gender is contentious. Some studies suggest that female gender is an independent risk factor for more severe disease.

45d) **Which patients should have a liver biopsy?**

Patients who present with **cirrhosis of unknown cause** should have a liver biopsy. When a patient presents with abnormal liver function tests and NAFLD is suspected, a period of lifestyle modification is generally appropriate before biopsy. This means weight reduction for 3–6 months.

Biopsy is required for patients:

- in whom liver tests fail to correct after lifestyle modification
- >45 years of age

- with a BMI $>30kg/m^2$
- with type 2 diabetes
- with features suggestive of cirrhosis
- if ALT levels remain persistently above twice the upper level of normal.

45e) **How could the patient's liver disease have been prevented?**

This patient was always at high risk of NAFLD, because she had type 2 diabetes, obesity, and hypercholesterolaemia. She now presents with evidence of decompensated cirrhosis. If NASH had been diagnosed at an earlier stage, progression to cirrhosis would probably have been delayed by:

- **Improved diabetic control**: she is already on insulin and her control should be optimized. Although there is no evidence of a beneficial effect of metformin on hepatic fibrosis, it can be given in the presence of cirrhosis. The thiazolidinediones (such as pioglitazone) act on peroxisome proliferator-activated receptor gamma (PPARγ) to increase insulin receptor expression in adipocytes and hepatocytes. This can improve LFTs but can also increase body weight.
- **Weight loss**, which improves liver fibrosis even when severe.
  - Exercise (difficult in this particular case because of below-knee amputation and peripheral vascular disease)
  - Gastric banding has been shown to improve liver disease.
- **Abstinence** from alcohol, because alcohol aggravates steatosis and contributes to cellular damage.

Further reading

Ali R, Cusi K (2009). New diagnostic and treatment approaches in non-alcoholic fatty liver disease (NAFLD). *Ann Med*; **41**: 265–78.

Dixon JB, Bhathal PS, Hughes NR, O' PE (2004). Non alcoholic fatty liver disease: improvement in liver histological analysis with weight loss. *Hepatology*; **39**: 1647–54.

Garcia-Compean D, Jaquez-Quintana JO, Gonzalez-Gonzalez JA, Maldonado-Garza H (2009). Liver cirrhosis and diabetes: risk factors, pathophysiology, clinical implications and management. *World J Gastroenterol*; **15**: 280–8.

Case 46

A 68-year-old woman presented with a 10-day history of a flu-like illness followed by a week of jaundice. She complained of lethargy, myalgia, and nausea, but no vomiting. She had lost no weight. She lived on a small holding with her husband and kept livestock, including sheep and goats. She had epilepsy for which she was taking carbamazepine.

On examination, she looked ill. Her Glasgow Coma Score was 15, but she was dehydrated and jaundiced. Her pulse was 110bpm and blood pressure 90/60mmHg. Her temperature was 38°C. Examination of the abdomen was unremarkable.

Investigations showed:

- Hb 10.6g/dL, WCC 12 x 10^9/L, neutrophils 10 x 10^9/L, platelets 27 x 10^9/L
- Blood film: left shift of myeloid cells, peripheral plasma cells
- Prothrombin time 18 sec
- Haptoglobin 1.9g/L
- Na 123mmol/L, K 3.0mmol/L, urea 31mmol/L, creatinine 280μmol/L
- Bilirubin 208μmol/L, ALT 24 IU/L, ALP 279 IU/L, albumin 32g/L
- CRP 133g/L
- Abdominal ultrasound showed a large stone in the gallbladder, with prominent intrahepatic bile ducts, but normal extrahepatic ducts. Normal spleen and kidneys.

Questions

46a) Describe how you would establish a diagnosis.

46b) What is particularly notable in the history?

46c) How do we treat this condition?

46d) What are the complications and outcomes of this condition?

Answers

46a) **Describe how you would establish a diagnosis.**

Presentation with flu-like symptoms, fever, and jaundice suggests an infectious cause. This is supported by the markedly elevated CRP and leucocytosis with prominent neutrophilia and left shift. **Bacterial infections with septicaemia** should first be considered, including ascending cholangitis, pneumonia, or urinary tract infections. A raised ALP is common with systemic bacterial infection, but cholangitis can also occur with only mildly elevated ALP. Blood cultures are mandatory and should be followed by empiric therapy with broad-spectrum antibiotics.

Acute viral hepatitis may present with a similar syndrome, but the ALT was normal in this case. Hepatitis A (see Case 16), hepatitis B, and hepatitis E commonly present with acute hepatitis. Epstein–Barr virus infection may cause jaundice in 10% of cases but is usually contracted in childhood or early adulthood. There were no risk factors for parenterally or enterically transmitted hepatitis. There is also a marked disparity between the renal impairment and severity of liver dysfunction, since the prothrombin time was only mildly prolonged. Renal impairment is only associated with severe hepatitis.

A travel history is important, because other infections should be considered, including malaria and rickettsial infection. Our patient had not recently travelled, but she had been in contact with animals.

46b) **What in the history is specifically significant?**

The close contact with farm animals is relevant. **Brucellosis** has to be considered since the patient kept sheep and goats. *Brucella melitensis* is associated with goats and *B. ovis* with sheep. Either is acquired from contact, including unpasteurized milk, and present with an acute febrile illness (*B. melitensis* is named after David Bruce, who identified this organism as the cause of Malta Fever). When severe the illness may be associated with jaundice, but the ALP is usually raised since brucellosis causes granulomatous hepatitis (see Case 42).

The most likely diagnosis was **leptospirosis**. This characteristically causes a disproportionately high bilirubin compared with the ALT and ALP. Where there are farms there are rats and the ubiquitous spirochete, *Leptospira interrogans*, is specifically associated with rats. A wide range of mammals may harbour the organism in the renal tubules, including cattle, dogs (which become severely ill), pigs, and all kinds of rodents.

Rodents are the most important vector. The organism is transmitted through direct contact with infected urine, or indirectly through contact with contaminated water or soil. Leptospira survive in the environment for long periods if conditions are wet. Occupational exposure occurs in vets, farmers, rat catchers, sewage or slaughterhouse workers, and recreational exposure occurs during immersion in contaminated rivers or lakes.

The diagnosis is made through **dark field microscopy** or **culture** of urine. In the first (leptospiraemic) phase of the illness, blood cultures may be positive and in the second (immune) phase urine culture may be positive. The diagnosis is frequently considered late in the illness. A serological agglutination test is the reference method, but requires a 4-fold rise in titres to be diagnostic, so two samples separated by an interval of 10 days are needed. Recent seroconversion may be demonstrated by ELISA methods that detect IgM antibodies.

Investigations showed:

- Leptospira ELISA IgM positive 1:2560
- Leptospira microscopic agglutination test positive at 1:2560
- Blood cultures were negative, probably because they were taken in the second phase of the illness.

46c) **How do we treat this condition?**

Leptospira spp. are sensitive to most antibiotics, with the exception of chloramphenicol. Mild illness may be treated with oral doxycycline. Severe illness should be treated intravenously with either **penicillin G** 1.5 million units 6-hourly, or **ampicillin** 1g 6-hourly if the diagnosis is established. In the absence of an established diagnosis, a broad-spectrum antibiotic should be used. A third-generation cephalosporin was a reasonable choice in our patient.

This patient was started on intravenous fluids and cefotaxime 1g 3 times a day IVI on admission, following appropriate procurement of blood cultures and before serology results were known. Improvement in all respects occurred over the following 3 days, and she survived the illness without permanent sequelae.

46d) **What are the complications and outcomes of this condition?**

Leptospirosis classically has **two phases**. The **leptospiraemic phase** follows direct exposure, commonly through intact skin, after a 7–14-day incubation period. Blood cultures may be positive, and it characteristically causes a flu-like illness, with fever, intense myalgia, headache, anorexia, nausea, vomiting, lymphadenopathy and conjunctival injection. Conjunctival injection is an important clue, as it is particularly characteristic. Myalgia is frequently severe, especially with *L. hajji* caught from cattle, particularly affecting the calves, back and abdominal muscles. This is followed by a period of up to 3 days when the fever subsides, before the onset of the **immune phase**. Organisms may then be present in the urine, but leptospiraemia is over. A second clinical phase does not occur in mild cases, but when it does there is **hepatorenal** and **pulmonary** symptoms. **Weil's disease** is the combination of jaundice, splenomegaly, and renal failure in a patient with leptospirosis (classically *L. icterohaemorrhagiae*). Pulmonary involvement is indicated by a nonspecific cough and dyspnoea, but severe pulmonary haemorrhage can occur that may be fatal.

Leptospirosis needs to be differentiated from viral haemorrhagic fever (Lassa, Marburg, and Ebola) when the illness presents with petichiae, purpura and epistaxis, but the travel history is usually then the clue to diagnosis. Severe gastrointestinal and intracranial haemorrhage, haemolysis, cardiac involvement, ARDS, rhabdomyolysis, and pancreatitis have been described but are rare.

Ninety percent of symptomatic disease is mild, but severe cases may be associated with a mortality of 40%. **Poor prognostic markers** include hypotension, oliguria, hyperkalaemia, metabolic acidosis, dyspnoea, cough, haemoptysis, alveolar lung infiltrates, WCC >12.9 x 10^9/L, and thrombocytopenia. Liver failure is usually not the cause of death. Patients who survive make a full recovery of liver and renal function, although residual hypertension has been reported.

Further reading

Ahmad SN, Shah S, Ahmad FMH (2005). Laboratory diagnosis of Leptospirosis. *J Postgrad Med*; **51**: 195–200.

Bal AM (2005). Unusual clinical manifestations of Leptospirosis. *J Postgrad Med*; **51**: 179–83.

Kaul DR, Flanders SA, Saint S (2005). Clinical problem-solving. Clear as mud. *N Engl J Med*; **352**: 1914–18.

Vijayachari P, Suqunan AP, Shriram AN (2008). Leptospirosis: an emerging global health problem. *J Biosci*; **33**: 557–69.

Case 47

A 20-year-old woman presented with a 3-day history of jaundice, nausea, and abdominal discomfort. She had noticed dark urine, but had normal stool and no itch. She was born in Poland and had been for a 2-week holiday to Thailand, returning 2 weeks ago. She had previously been fit and well, and was on no medication. She drank <10 units/week. Examination was normal apart from jaundice.

Investigations showed:

- Hb 9.5g/dL, WCC 14 x 10^9/L (10.5 neutrophils), platelets 171 x 10^9/L
- Na 133mmol/L, K 3.7mmol/L, urea 4.2mmol/L, creatinine 98μmol/L
- Bilirubin 377μmol/l, AST 43 IU/L, ALT 69 IU/L, ALP 130 IU/L, albumin 28g/L
- CRP normal
- Prothrombin time 26 sec.

On examination the following day, she looked well, apart from deep jaundice. There was no encephalopathy. Urine output was <30ml/hour.

Further investigations:

- Hb 7.0g/dL, WCC 21.8 x 10^9/L, platelets 144 x 10^9/L
- Blood film: polychromasia, burr cells, microspherocytes; no fragmented cells
- Reticulocytes 6.7% (normal range <2%)
- Prothrombin time 30 sec
- Na 134mmol/L; K 4.8mmol/L; creatinine 164μmol/L
- Bilirubin 489μmol/L; AST 59 IU/L, ALT 42 IU/L, ALP 69 IU/L, albumin 23g/L
- Abdominal ultrasound: no comment on liver texture, splenomegaly (14cm).

Questions

47a) What is the diagnosis?

47b) How is the condition usually diagnosed?

47c) What is the treatment?

47d) What other symptoms can this disorder present with?

47e) Should siblings be screened and if so how?

Answers

47a) **What is the diagnosis?**

The diagnosis is acute liver failure due to **Wilson's disease**. All other causes of acute liver failure should be considered (see Case 1) and a full liver screen should be carried out, but the haemolysis is characteristic of Wilson's disease. Wilson's disease is a rare autosomal recessive disorder of copper metabolism. The major physiological aberration is excessive absorption of copper from the small intestine and decreased excretion of copper by the liver. The **genetic defect**, localized to chromosome 13q, affects the copper-transporting adenosine triphosphatase gene (ATP7B) in the liver. The process of incorporating copper into caeruloplasmin and excretion of excess copper into bile is impaired in Wilson's disease. As liver copper levels increase, copper is released into the circulation and deposited in other organs.

Symptoms generally present from 6 years to 40 years of age. Hepatic dysfunction is the presenting feature in more than half of patients. The three major patterns of hepatic involvement are:

- Chronic hepatitis (elevated transaminases)
- Cirrhosis (the most common initial presentation)
- Acute hepatic failure.

This case presented with acute hepatic failure and severe coagulopathy; encephalopathy can occur. Acute intravascular haemolysis and early renal failure are clues to the diagnosis. **Haemolysis** is due to rapid release of copper into the circulation, which also causes acute renal tubular dysfunction. Acute viral hepatitis is usually the working diagnosis, because the patient is not suspected of having underlying liver disease. An important clue to Wilson's disease is the **disproportionately low serum AST** (usually much less than 1500 IU/L), which would be exceptional in acute viral hepatitis. The ALP is usually in the normal range or even low for age, and the serum **bilirubin is disproportionately elevated** because of haemolysis. However, biochemical indices are not specific. The acute presentation of Wilson's disease is more common in women than in men (4:1 ratio).

47b) **How is the condition usually diagnosed?**

The diagnosis is confirmed by measurement of serum caeruloplasmin, urinary copper excretion, hepatic copper content, and the detection of Kayser–Fleischer rings. A patient with the classic combination of chronic liver disease, tremor or dystonia, and Kayser–Fleischer rings is readily diagnosed, but such patients are exceptional. There are two major disturbances of copper deposition in Wilson's disease: a reduction in the rate of incorporation of copper into caeruloplasmin, and a decrease in the biliary excretion of copper. Table 47.1 shows typical levels in a patient with Wilson's disease compared with the normal reference ranges.

Serum caeruloplasmin: many patients with Wilson's disease have a caeruloplasmin within the normal range. Caeruloplasmin is an acute phase protein, and increases in response to inflammation, pregnancy, oestrogen use, or any infection. Falsely low caeruloplasmin concentrations may occur in any protein deficiency state, including nephrotic syndrome, malabsorption and protein-losing enteropathy. Caeruloplasmin levels may also be low in 10–20% of heterozygotes for the Wilson's disease gene, but who do not develop the disease and do not require treatment.

Serum copper concentration is low, in parallel with the low serum caeruloplasmin, in most patients with Wilson's disease. Very high levels are detected in acute liver failure, because of rapid release of copper from the liver.

Urinary copper excretion rate is >100µg/d (reference range, <40µg/d) in most patients with symptomatic Wilson's disease. The rate may also be elevated in other cholestatic liver diseases. Both the sensitivity and the specificity of this test are insufficient for it to be used as a screening test, but it usefully confirms the diagnosis and helps to evaluate response to chelation therapy. A provocative test of urinary copper excretion in which penicillamine (500mg orally every 12 hours) is given while a 24-hour urinary collection is obtained sometimes provides useful information: a normal person excretes as much as 20 times the baseline level

Table 47.1 Copper measurements in Wilson's disease and normal individuals

Measurement	Wilson's disease	Normal adults
Serum caeruloplasmin	0–200	200–350
Serum copper (µg/L)	190–640	700–1520
(µmol/L)	3–10	11–24
Urinary copper (µg/day)	100–1000	<40
(µmol/day)	>1.6	<0.6
Liver copper (µg/g dry weight)	>200	20–50

after penicillamine, but a urinary excretion of >25µmol of copper 24 hours after penicillamine is diagnostic of Wilson's disease.

Hepatic copper concentration is the gold standard for diagnosis of Wilson's disease. A liver biopsy with sufficient tissue reveals levels >250µg/g of dry weight, even in asymptomatic patients. This assumes the absence of cholestatic liver disease, which leads to reduced biliary secretion and copper accumulation in the liver. A normal hepatic copper concentration (reference range 15–55µg/g) effectively excludes the diagnosis of untreated Wilson's disease.

Kayser–Fleischer rings: slit-lamp examination may reveal Kayser–Fleischer rings. These are found at the limbus and are caused by copper deposition in Descemet's membrane in the cornea. A careful slit-lamp examination is mandatory and can be the most rapid way of making the diagnosis: it is only visible on direct inspection when iris pigmentation is light and copper deposition is heavy. Kayser–Fleischer rings are observed in up to 90% of individuals with symptomatic Wilson's disease, and are almost invariably present in patients with neurological manifestations. Kayser–Flesicher rings may be absent in 10–50% of patients with exclusively hepatic involvement, and in presymptomatic patients. Consequently, the absence of Kayser–Flesicher rings does not exclude the diagnosis, and are no longer considered pathognomonic of Wilson's disease unless accompanied by neurological manifestations. They have been observed in patients with chronic cholestatic disorders, such as partial biliary atresia, primary biliary cirrhosis, and primary sclerosing cholangitis.

47c) **What is the treatment of this condition?**

Patients with **fulminant hepatic failure** from Wilson's disease need immediate referral for **liver transplantation**, because such patients do not respond well to chelation treatment.

Patients with a prognostic index (Table 47.2) of >7 should be considered for liver transplantation. Our patient had a score of 8. Most patients who exceed a score of 7 die within 2 months of diagnosis unless they have a liver transplant. Prognosis after liver transplantation is good. In a study of 55 patients with Wilson's disease who underwent transplantation, the 1-year survival rate was 79%, and overall survival rate was 72% 20 years after transplantation.

The mainstay of therapy for Wilson's disease is the use of **chelating agents** and medications that block copper absorption from the gastrointestinal tract (Table 47.3). There are three recognized treatments:

Table 47.2 Prognostic index in fulminant Wilson's disease

Score	0	1	2	3	4
Serum bilirubin (mmol/L)	<100	100–150	151–200	201–300	>300
Serum AST (IU/L)	<100	100–150	151–200	201–300	>300
Prolongation of prothrombin time (seconds)	<4	4–8	9–12	13–20	>30

- Penicillamine
- Trien (trientine)
- Zinc.

With effective chelation therapy, most patients live normal, healthy lives. Early treatment is critical, and outcome is best for patients in whom the disease is diagnosed and treatment initiated before the disease causes symptoms. There is a potential role for gene transfer therapy in the future.

47d) **What other symptoms can this disorder present with?**

Neuropsychiatric: most patients who have neuropsychiatric manifestations also have cirrhosis. The most common neurological feature

Table 47.3 Medical treatment of Wilson's disease

Drug	Mechanism	Dose	Monitoring for efficacy	Monitoring for side effects
Penicillamine	Increases urinary excretion of copper	Initially 1–1.5g/d, Maintenance: 1g/day	Urinary copper excretion 500–800µg/d. Estimated non-caeruloplasmin-bound copper <100µg/L	Full blood count (thrombocytopenia, leucopenia, aplastic anemia). Urinalysis (proteinuria). Examine skin for rashes
Trientene	Increases urinary excretion of copper. May impair intestinal absorption of copper	1–1.2g/day	As with penicillamine	Full blood count. Iron studies
Zinc	Interferes with copper absorption, increases copper excretion in stools	Initially 50mg three times/day. Maintenance: titrate against efficacy	24-hour urinary copper 200–400µg/day. Estimated non-caeruloplasmin bound copper <100µg/L	Serum Zn

is **asymmetric tremor**, occurring in half of individuals with Wilson's disease. The character of the tremor is variable and may be predominantly resting, postural, or kinetic. Frequent early symptoms include difficulty speaking, excessive salivation, ataxia, mask-like facies, clumsiness, and personality changes. Late manifestations (now rare because of earlier diagnosis and treatment) include dystonia, spasticity, grand mal seizures, rigidity, and flexion contractures. Psychiatric features include emotional lability, impulsiveness, disinhibition, and self-injurious behaviour. About 10–20% of patients present with psychiatric symptoms and the cause may be overlooked.

Musculoskeletal: osteopenia is common in Wilson's disease. An **arthropathy** resembling premature osteoarthritis generally involves the spine and large appendicular joints, such as knees, wrists, and hips. Symptomatic joint disease occurs in 20–50%, usually late in the course of the disease and frequently > 20 years of age. Osteochondritis dissecans, chondromalacia patellae, and chondrocalcinosis have also been described.

Haematological: haemolytic anaemia is a rare (10–15%) but characteristic complication of the disease, usually in conjunction with acute hepatic presentations.

Renal: the gene is expressed in kidney tissue, so any renal manifestations may be primary or secondary to release of copper from the liver. Patients resemble those with Fanconi's syndrome, with defective renal acidification and excess **renal losses of amino acids**, glucose, fructose, galactose, pentose, uric acid, phosphate, and calcium. Urolithiasis, found in up to 16% of patients, may result from hypercalciuria or poor acidification. Haematuria and nephrocalcinosis are reported, as are proteinuria and peptiduria. Both can occur as part of the disease process or after therapy as an adverse effects of penicillamine.

47e) **Should siblings be screened and if so how?**

More than 300 mutations in the ATP7B gene for Wilson's disease have been detected. Genetic markers that closely flank the gene are used for pre-symptomatic diagnosis of siblings of a known patient, when the patient and parents are available for testing. Overt symptoms of Wilson's disease have not been reported in heterozygotes. In the absence of marker analysis, screening should include a physical examination, liver biochemical tests, serum copper and caeruloplasmin levels, 24-hour urinary copper measurement, and careful slit-lamp examination.

Further reading

Perri RE, Hahn SH, Ferber MJ (2005). Wilson Disease – keeping the bar for diagnosis raised. *Hepatology*; **42**: 974.

Roberts EA, Schilsky ML (2008). American Association for Study of Liver Diseases. Diagnosis and treatment of Wilson disease: an update. *Hepatology*; **47**: 2089–111.

Schilsky ML (2005). Wilson disease: new insights into pathogenesis, diagnosis, and future therapy. *Curr Gastroenterol Rep*; **7**: 26–31.

Case 48

A 75-year-old retired truck driver was referred for evaluation of abnormal liver function tests, which had been found at a routine check-up. He was asymptomatic. Prior medical history included a myocardial infarction 4 years before, benign prostatic hypertrophy, and jaundice at 17 years of age. He had never had a tattoo, drank very little, but had had blood transfusions following a prostatectomy in 2001. He had not recently travelled and was a non-smoker.

On examination, his pulse rate was 69bpm with frequent extrasystoles, and blood pressure was 145/80mmHg. He was apyrexial. There was no jaundice, pallor, lymphadenopathy, or oedema. Cardiovascular examination was unremarkable and his chest was clear. A liver edge was palpable 8cm below the costal margin, but percussion indicated a liver span of 15cm, which is only slightly enlarged. The spleen was clearly palpable, but did not cross the midline. There were no signs of chronic liver disease or portal hypertension.

Investigations showed:

- Hb 13.4g/dL, WCC 7.66 x 10^9/L, platelets 96 x 10^9/L
- INR 1.2
- Bilirubin 22μmol/L ALT 78 IU/L, ALP 1269 IU/L, GGT 1017 IU/L, albumin 36g/L
- Blood film: platelets reduced on film. No platelet clumps seen. Howell–Jolly bodies seen.
- Ultrasound of the abdomen: the liver was diffusely heterogeneous and coarse in texture. The portal venous flows were normal. There was marked splenomegaly and the spleen had a bipolar length of 18cm. It, like the liver, had a very coarse, heterogeneous internal architecture.

Questions

48a) Discuss the differential diagnosis in this patient.

48b) What are Howell–Jolly bodies and why are they significant?

48c) What further investigations would you plan?

48d) Discuss this condition.

Answers

48a) **What is the differential diagnosis in this patient?**

Splenomegaly may be caused by congestion, infiltration, immune activation or expansion of haematopoietic cell lines and reticuloendothelial cells within the organ. Clinical examination should include a search for chronic liver disease with portal hypertension (**congestive splenomegaly**), signs of haemolysis and anaemia (**extramedullary haematopoiesis** and expansion of reticuloendothelial cells), signs of chronic inflammatory disease or infections (**immune activation**), and signs of haematological **malignancy** (such as lymphoma or leukaemia) or any other **infiltrative** condition (such as amyloid). Hepatomegaly associated with splenomegaly may result from liver disease causing portal hypertension, extramedullary haematopoiesis, or infiltration by the same condition.

The presence of a high ALP with a raised GT suggests hepatic infiltration. Our patient had no signs of haemolysis and was not anaemic. There was no evidence of chronic liver disease or portal hypertension, nor was there any sign of a chronic inflammatory disorder.

Malignant infiltration is likely, most commonly a **lymphoma**. Even though the patient had no peripheral lymphadenopathy, axial lymph nodes may be present and would favour Hodgkin's disease. **Leukaemia** and **myeloproliferative** conditions may also enlarge liver and spleen. Primary **angiosarcoma** may originate in the spleen or metastasize from the liver to the spleen. Other **solid tumours** rarely metastasize to the spleen, but melanoma can (and does!). There was no evidence of previous or concurrent melanoma in or patient.

Non-malignant infiltration may result from extracellular depositions such as **amyloidosis**, **sarcoidosis**, or **tuberculosis** (associated with immune hyperplasia). Lipid **storage diseases** (e.g. Gaucher's disease) will not present at this age.

Our patient had a very, but not 'massively', enlarged spleen. Massive enlargement is defined as a spleen palpable >8cm below the costal margin. Some consider a spleen that crosses the midline as massively enlarged. Massive enlargement is caused by non-Hodgkin's lymphoma, chronic myeloid leukaemia, chronic lymphatic leukaemia, hairy cell leukaemia, myelofibrosis, and sarcoidosis.

48b) **What are Howell–Jolly bodies and why are they significant?**

Howell–Jolly bodies are remnants of the nucleus of red blood cells from their immature stages, which are then detected in mature erythrocytes on a peripheral blood film. Such remnants are usually removed by the spleen, so the presence of Howell–Jolly bodies implies either absence of the spleen (e.g. splenectomy) or functional hyposplenism. Our patient clearly has a spleen that does not function. Diseases that are associated with impaired splenic function with an intact spleen include coeliac disease, sickle cell disease (splenic infarction), systemic lupus erythematosis, rheumatoid arthritis, Grave's disease, Sjögren's syndrome, chronic liver disease, alcoholism, inflammatory bowel disease, and Whipple's disease. Amyloidosis and sarcoidosis may also cause functional hyposplenism.

As a marker of hyposplenism, Howell–Jolly bodies are insensitive, but specific. They do not occur in mild hyposplenism. Their presence implies a level of functional hyposplenism thought to put the patient at risk of **overwhelming postsplenectomy infection**. Such infections are often cryptic with a short prodrome. Encapsulated organisms are usually responsible (*Streptococcus pneumoniae*, *Haemophylus influenzae*, or *Neisseria meningitidis*). Massive bacteraemia causes septic shock and disseminated intravascular coagulation. The mortality is up to 80% and death may occur within 24–48 hours.

48c) **What further investigation would you plan in this patient?**

A **CT scan** of the chest, abdomen, and pelvis would identify any lymphadenopathy in the chest or abdomen, a primary malignancy, or metastases. **Tissue** is needed to make a diagnosis. Because the liver is affected, a **liver biopsy** is appropriate, although a lymph node biopsy, bone marrow examination, or even a diagnostic splenectomy may be required.

CT of chest and abdomen: the liver has an expanded, rounded and heterogeneous appearance, measuring 14.5 x 10cm on axial section. The prostate is enlarged to 62mm diameter. There are degenerative changes of the spine. There is no suspicious bone lesion, and the lungs clear. The kidneys, adrenals, and pancreas are all normal. There is no gross lymphadenopathy, although there are some small mesenteric nodes and general streaking of the intra-abdominal fat (Fig. 48.1).

Liver biopsy shows **angiosarcoma** (Fig. 48.2 in central colour section).

48d) **Discuss this condition**

Angiosarcoma is a rare vascular tumour, accounting for 2% of all primary liver tumours. Primary angiosarcoma of the liver has a strong male predominance, with a 4:1 ratio of males to females. Individuals are usually > 60 years of age. Metastases to the lung, spleen and bones may occur

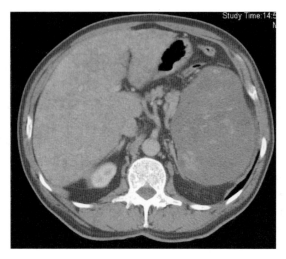

Fig. 48.1 CT scan showing enlargement of liver and spleen, with a heterogenous parynchymal appearance in both organs.

in descending order of frequency. It is strongly associated with environmental or occupational exposure to carcinogens, including colloidal **thorium dioxide**, arsenic compounds, **polyvinyl chloride**, inorganic copper, radiation exposure, and anabolic steroids. A history of exposure is not commonly identified, however, as was the case with our patient. Nevertheless, because of the implications it is important that the patient is asked carefully about all their jobs and recreational activities.

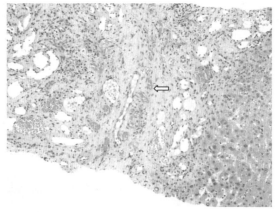

Fig. 48.2 (see colour plate 26) Angiosarcoma of the liver. Vascular channels are identifiable (arrow), but not the characteristic spindle-shaped cells at this magnification.

An angiosarcoma shows areas of necrosis and haemorrhage with one of four different growth patterns: multiple nodules, a large dominant mass, a mixture of these, or (unusually) a diffuse infiltrating tumour, which was the case in our patient. Histopathology shows spindle-shaped cells, which may form vascular channels and are positive for vascular endothelial cell markers (CD31 and CD34) on immunohistochemistry (Fig. 48.2).

No effective therapy exists. Neither excision of a localized tumour nor chemotherapy alters the outcome. Cases of angiosarcoma diagnosed incidentally on liver transplantation for another indication show rapid recurrence and have a poor prognosis. Liver transplantation is therefore contraindicated. Survival from the time of diagnosis is <1 year in most instances, regardless of therapy. Management is palliative.

Thorium dioxide (Thorotrast, Th^{232}) was used worldwide as a radiographic contrast medium between 1928 and 1955, in a 25% colloidal solution. It is taken up by the reticuloendothelial cells. Th^{232} is radioactive, emitting α and β particles and γ rays. It lingers in the body and may be seen on CT scan 50 years after administration. It can be responsible for hyposplenism, bone marrow failure, and is associated with angiosarcoma of the liver. Our patient had neither a history of Thorotrast administration, nor any sign of residual Thorotrast on CT imaging.

Exposure to **arsenic** comes from contamination of drinking water (India), burning of arsenic coal (China), or medicinal administration (Fowler's solution, used worldwide for chronic myeloid leukaemia 1931–1953). The polymerization of **vinyl chloride** in the polyvinyl chloride (PVC) industry since the mid 1930s lead to high levels of exposure among workers in the industry. The first case of angiosarcoma because of this occupational exposure was identified in 1974. Since then tight controls on the work environment have been implemented and cases caused by this exposure now occur rarely, if at all.

Further reading

Kim HR, Rha SY, Cheon SH *et al.* (2009). Clinical features and treatment outcomes of advanced stage primary hepatic angiosarcoma. *Ann Oncol*; **20**: 780–7.

Maluf D, Cotterell A, Clark B *et al.* (2005). Hepatic angiosarcoma and liver transplantation: Case report and literature review. *Transplant Proc*; **37**: 2195–9.

Muller AF, Toghill PJ (1995). Hyposplenism in gastrointestinal disease. *Gut* 1995; **36**: 165–7.

Van Kampen RJW, Erdkamp FLG, Peters FPJ (2007). Thorium dioxide-related haemangiosarcoma of the liver. *Neth J Med*; **65**: 279–82.

Case 49

A 49-year-old female carer developed severe abdominal pain over the course of a fortnight, with diarrhoea, weight loss, and vomiting. She was admitted via the emergency department, where a CT scan showed intestinal obstruction, a stenosing tumour in the transverse colon, and liver metastases. She was taken to theatre, where an extended right hemicolectomy was performed, with resection of a gangrenous loop of small bowel. This was complicated by an anastomotic leak requiring further laparotomy and ileostomy, following which there was wound dehiscence and discharge through two enterocutaneous fistulas. Seventeen days after the initial admission, on a Friday, parenteral nutrition was requested urgently.

On examination, the patient weighed 61kg, had lost 15kg in the previous 4 weeks, and had an output through the wound manager of 1650mL in the past 24 hours.

Investigations showed:

- Hb 10.3g/L, WCC 9.4 x 10^9/L, platelets 100 x 10^9/L
- Bilirubin 45μmol/L, ALT 39 IU, ALP 157 IU
- Albumin 20g/dL, phosphate 0.61mmol/L, magnesium 0.82mmol/L
- CRP >160mg/L.

Questions

49a) Interpret the blood results.

49b) What are the dangers of starting parenteral nutrition immediately?

49c) What is the best advice?

49d) What is the optimal management strategy?

Answers

49a) **Interpret the blood results.**

This patient is dehydrated, evidenced by a disproportionate increase in urea compared with creatinine, in the context of a high stoma output (>1200ml/d) and high potassium (see Case 33). She is almost certainly septic given the low albumin (20g/dL). Sepsis is also consistent with the high CRP (>160mg/L). The anaemia and hyperbilirubinaemia are most probably due to haematoma formation and resorption after two major operations. The thrombocytopenia is likely to be caused by bone marrow suppression from sepsis, which will also be contributing to the anaemia. **Sepsis** and **hypovolaemia** are therefore the key messages in this complex situation: both are surprisingly easy to overlook, because the patient is apyrexial and the stoma output is frequently not measured except on a specialist ward.

49b) **What are the dangers of starting parenteral nutrition immediately?**

This patient is at risk of **refeeding syndrome**, which is defined as severe fluid and electrolyte shifts with related metabolic mayhem in malnourished patients undergoing refeeding (see Case 37). The principal biochemical features of refeeding syndrome are hypophosphataemia, hypomagnesaemia, hypokalaemia, glucose intolerance, fluid overload, and thiamine deficiency. **Clinical consequences** can include congestive heart failure, cardiac arrhythmias, skeletal muscle weakness, respiratory failure, metabolic acidosis, ataxia, seizures, encephalopathy, and death.

Patients at risk include those who have had:

- complete starvation for >7 days
- >20% loss of body weight in <3months
- catabolic state caused by sepsis.

Because this patient has been referred on a Friday afternoon (as so often happens, when the urgency of the situation is recognized before the weekend!), there is greater risk of the clinical consequences of refeeding syndrome if feeding is started immediately, simply because monitoring over the weekend is often suboptimal. Designated central venous access for parenteral nutrition is also a problem, unless insertion has already been organized, or if (improbably) the patient has an untouched central line port. **Parenteral nutrition is never an emergency**: the risk of death from refeeding exceeds the risk of delaying nutrition pending appropriate preparation.

49c) **What is the best advice?**

After explaining the dangers of starting intravenous nutrition immediately and over the weekend to the surgeons looking after her, the ward nurses, the patient, and her family, preparation includes **rehydration, electrolyte *and* vitamin replacement**, with daily monitoring according to refeeding guidelines below. This is enough to keep the team looking after the patient occupied over the weekend, knowing that they are doing the best thing for the patient.

Electrolyte replacement: electrolytes need immediate replacement if the potassium is <2.5mmol/L, magnesium <0.5mmol/L, or phosphate <0.3mmol/L.

- **Low potassium (<2.5mmol)**: **intravenous potassium** is always more appropriate than oral potassium pending parenteral nutrition. A carefully monitored infusion pump should be used to administer 120mmol/L through a central line over 12 hours. Oral potassium usually tastes disgusting. Remember that for the commonly prescribed Sando K, one tablet contains 12mmol, so 5 tablets/day (=60mmol) only meet (and do not exceed) ordinary daily requirements.

- **Low phosphate (<0.3mmol/L)**: **intravenous Addiphos**™ 20ml vial) in 500ml normal saline should be administered over 6 hours. Shake the bag well. One vial of Addiphos™ contains phosphate 40mmol, potassium 30mmol, and sodium 30mmol. Oral phosphate causes diarrhoea and should therefore be avoided.

- **Low magnesium (<0.5mmol/L)**: 50% **magnesium sulphate 6g** (=24mmol, or 12ml) in 500ml normal saline should be given over 6–12 hours. The maximum infusion rate is 4mmol/hour of Mg. Oral magnesium causes diarrhoea.

- **Low calcium**: in practice, calcium is not too much of a problem. If it is low, it is likely to be secondary to magnesium or phosphate deficiency; when these are replaced, the calcium usually returns to normal. If necessary, intravenous calcium gluconate can be given.

In practice, any electrolyte concentration below the normal range (K <3.5mmol/L, P <0.6mmol/L, Mg <0.7mmol/L) merits proactive replacement during the weekend, or 48 hours before parenteral nutrition is started. This is because the refeeding syndrome is characterized by further electrolyte depletion, owing to intracellular shifts of electrolytes.

Intravenous vitamins: thiamine is required. **Pabrinex**™ 1 pair of ampoules (= 250mg thiamine) should be given in 50–100ml normal saline over 30 minutes, daily for 3 days.

Insertion of a designated central venous line ONLY to be used for intravenous feeding: this can be done after the weekend, ideally as a peripherally inserted central catheter (PICC).

Commence intravenous feeding after the weekend, after all the above has been done: if all biochemistry is normal, start feeding. Ensure that the intravenous vitamins are given at least 30 minutes before feeding starts. Start feeding at 20kcal/kg for the first 24 hours, then **increase gradually within the first week** to full feeding, with daily monitoring of electrolytes, magnesium, and phosphate (too frequently forgotten), and further electrolyte replacement for the first 2 weeks.

49d) **What is the optimal management strategy?**

The optimal management strategy is to ask for help from a team experienced in the management of intestinal failure.

Be guided by the **SNAP acronym**:

S: Sepsis (drain abscess, treat infection)

N: Nutrition (establish appropriate route and type of nutritional support)

A: Anatomy (use contrast radiology and cross-sectional imaging to define anatomy when the first two steps have been addressed)

P: Procedure (timely surgery, often many months down the line).

When managing patients with intestinal failure, it is important to **manage expectations**. Patients want a rapid resolution of appalling complications, but precipitate re-operation to restore continuity and repair of enterocutaneous fistulae simply leads to further wound break down, fistulation, and loss of bowel. That way lays dependency on intravenous nutrition and the law courts for inappropriate management. Consequently, these complex patients are best managed in a specialist unit with access to multidisciplinary care.

Patients need to understand that short cuts (such as surgery within weeks) carries high risks, and that patience, months of nutritional support, and timely re-operation are the quickest way to recovery. It is a sad fact that many surgeons and physicians are simply unaware of the availability of specialist centres dealing with intestinal failure, or feel that their patients are not sick enough to merit transfer. The least that can be done is to discuss management with appropriate specialists.

Further reading

Lal S, Teubner A, Shaffer JL. Review article: intestinal failure. *Aliment Pharmacol Ther* 2006; **24**: 19–31.

Mehanna HM, Moledina J, Travis J (2008). Refeeding syndrome: what it is, and how to prevent and treat it. *BMJ*; **336**: 1495–8.

Stanga Z, Brunner A, Leuenberger M *et al.* (2008). Nutrition in clinical practice: the refeeding syndrome: illustrative cases and guidelines for management and treatment. *Eur J Clin Nutr*; **62**: 687–94.

Case 50

A 60-year-old Dutch woman with a history of colitis for 20 years presented to the emergency department with central abdominal pain and vomiting. Symptoms had started an hour after taking bowel preparation for colonoscopy.

In the preceding month, she had lost 9kg in weight, with loss of appetite and borborygmi. Her bowels opened once or twice a day, with no diarrhoea. She had previously had a deep vein thrombosis but no other medical history. She did not smoke, and drank alcohol infrequently.

On examination, her pulse rate was 112bpm and blood pressure 130/80mmHg. She was not pale, or jaundiced. The abdomen was soft and non-tender, without palpable masses or organs.

Investigations showed:

- Hb 13.5g/dL, WCC 13.7 x 10^9/L, platelets 545 x 10^9/L, MCV 96fL
- CRP 19mg/L
- U&E, LFT, and amylase normal
- Abdominal radiograph: prominent small bowel loops scattered throughout the abdomen; no colonic dilatation
- Small bowel enema (performed subsequently): delayed small bowel transit
- CT of the abdomen: segmental colitis with inflammation of terminal ileum; biliary dilatation in the right lobe of the liver
- MRCP: shown in Fig. 50.1.

Questions

50a) What do the patient's symptoms suggest?

50b) The MRCP is diagnostic: what does it show?

50c) Discuss the relationship between this condition and inflammatory bowel disease.

50d) How is this condition managed?

50e) What complications can occur with this condition?

50f) The patient did not respond to medical therapy. A repeat CT scan was carried out (Figs 50.2a and 50.2b). Describe the findings.

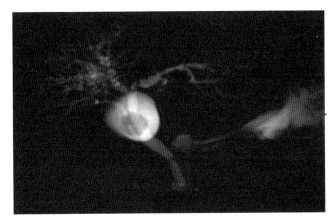

Fig. 50.1

Answers

50a) **What do the patient's symptoms suggest?**

The clinical picture indicates **partial small bowel obstruction**. The abdominal radiograph showed prominent small bowel loops, with no evidence of colonic dilatation. The most likely causes are stricturing small bowel disease or a carcinoma obstructing the ileocaecal valve. Adhesions are a common cause, but the patient had not previously had abdominal surgery. The initial CT scan suggested terminal ileal Crohn's disease, although the small bowel radiology did not show diagnostic images.

50b) **The MRCP is diagnostic: what does it show?**

The MRCP shows marked irregularity of the intrahepatic biliary tree, typical of **primary sclerosing cholangitis** (PSC). This is a chronic cholestatic liver disease of the intrahepatic and/or extrahepatic biliary tree, with inflammation and fibrosis, leading to progressive cholestasis and eventually to biliary cirrhosis with endstage liver disease. Most cases are associated with inflammatory bowel disease.

PSC is typically a male-predominant disease, with a 2:1 male to female ratio. Liver function tests are abnormal in 90% of patients at diagnosis, and are the usual reason for investigation (initially by ultrasound, then MRCP) that leads to diagnosis. Endoscopic retrograde cholangiopancreatography (ERCP) used to be used, but MRCP is now the diagnostic test of choice, because it avoids the complications of ERCP. ERCP is reserved for biliary sampling for cytology, or biliary drainage. Liver biopsy is required only if the MRCP looks normal. Liver function tests may occasionally be normal (in about 10%). The diagnosis in this patient was coincidental to presentation with small bowel obstruction.

Both intrahepatic and extrahepatic bile ducts are involved in 69% with PSC, and 25% have isolated intrahepatic PSC, as in our patient. Just 4% have exclusive extrahepatic involvement, and the remaining 2% have typical biochemical and histological features of PSC, but normal cholangiograms. This is termed '**small duct PSC**' and is thought to have a considerably better prognosis than typical PSC. Progression to cirrhosis and endstage liver disease is slower, and cholangiocarcinoma, the most important complication of PSC, does not occur. Nevertheless, a proportion of patients with small duct PSC (20% in one study) progress to typical PSC.

The median time to death or liver transplantation in PSC is 9–18 years after diagnosis. Jaundice usually precedes other features of cirrhosis, such as ascites.

50c) **Discuss the relationship between this condition and inflammatory bowel disease.**

Inflammatory bowel disease, most often pancolitis, is present in 63–90% of patients with PSC in Northern Europe and North America. PSC develops in 2.4–7.5% of patients with ulcerative colitis and in 1.4–3.4% with Crohn's disease, although in a recent study the prevalence of MRCP features of PSC in patients with ulcerative colitis affecting the whole colon was as high as 17%. The diagnosis of inflammatory bowel disease usually precedes that of PSC by several years, reflecting the insidious nature of PSC and the debilitating symptoms of inflammatory bowel disease. PSC may present years after colectomy. However, the diagnosis of PSC can precede that of inflammatory bowel disease: colonoscopy is appropriate if a patient is found to have PSC, even in the apparent absence of bowel symptoms. Ulcerative colitis in such patients exhibits relative rectal sparing. Crohn's disease in patients with PSC always involves the colon, with or without small bowel involvement.

50d) **How is this condition managed?**

PSC is relentlessly progressive and no current medical therapy improves survival. Liver transplantation is the only life-extending therapy. Although PSC is thought to be immunologically mediated, it does not have the characteristics of a typical autoimmune disease: witness the male predominance, no absence of a specific autoantibody, and poor response to immunosuppression. Ursodeoxycholic acid is recommended for treatment. **Ursodeoxycholic acid** is a hydrophilic bile acid that may displace toxic bile acids, be cytoprotective, and promote bile flow. Studies have shown improvement of biochemical, cholangiographic, and histological characteristics. Ursodeoxycholic acid also appears to reduce the risk of colon cancer in patients with PSC and inflammatory bowel disease. The risk of colon cancer in patients with inflammatory bowel disease and PSC is higher than in inflammatory bowel disease alone. Tumours are more often proximal and subject to late diagnosis. Patients with inflammatory bowel disease and PSC should be enrolled in a surveillance programme at diagnosis, with complete colonoscopy on an annual basis.

50e) **What complications can occur with this condition?**

In addition to the typical features of PSC on the MRCP (Fig. 50.1), there was marked dilatation of the right intrahepatic biliary system. No explanation was found, but this asymmetry should raise a concern about **cholangiocarcinoma**. The lifetime risk of cholangiocarcinoma in patients with PSC is about 23%, but only in those with underlying ulcerative colitis, and very rarely (if at all) in Crohn's colitis. A third of patients who develop cholangiocarcinoma do so within a year of diagnosis of PSC. The annual risk is then about 1.5%. Risk factors for cholangiocarcinoma in patients with PSC include older age, longer duration of ulcerative colitis, and smoking.

Therapy for cholangiocarcinoma is usually palliative, since it is considered a contraindication to liver transplantation. When cholangiocarcinoma complicates PSC it has a dismal prognosis, with a median survival from diagnosis of 5–11 months. The diagnosis remains challenging. Once jaundice and weight loss occur, the disease is advanced. The tumour marker CA19-9 is insufficiently sensitive and specific, and may be elevated in cholestasis of any cause. CT scan and MRCP cannot reliably distinguish benign from malignant stenosis. Positron emission tomography (PET) has shown inconsistent results.

The mainstay of diagnosis of cholangiocarcinoma remains **ERCP with endoscopic brush cytology**. The specificity is 89–100% but the sensitivity is only 69–75%. Biliary fluorescence in situ hybridization (F.I.S.H) and digital image analysis are more sensitive. Transpapillary cholangiography

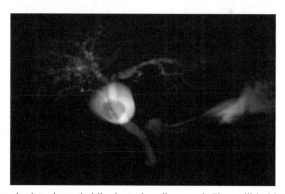

Fig. 50.1 Irregular intrahepatic bile ducts (small arrows). The gallbladder (large arrow) and common bile duct (long arrow) looked normal on this and other images.

with intraductal ultrasonography may help differentiate benign from malignant biliary strictures in the future.

50f) **The patient did not respond to medical therapy. A repeat CT scan was carried out (Figs 50.2a and 50.2b). Describe the findings**

Fig. 50.2a shows wall thickening in the distal transverse colon (arrow) and colonic dilatation, highly suggestive of a carcinoma. Fig. 50.2b shows a mass in the caecum (arrow) highly suggestive of a caecal carcinoma.

An emergency subtotal colectomy was carried out for colonic obstruction. Pathological examination showed synchronous **adenocarcinomas of the colon**, one in the distal transverse colon and one in the caecum. The colon showed chronically active ulcerative colitis. The finding of colon cancer is not surprising, in view of the longstanding colitis, association with PSC (note the proximal cancer), and presentation with bowel obstruction. This case illustrates some of the difficulty in classifying colitis, the indolent nature of PSC, and the complications of longstanding colitis associated with PSC.

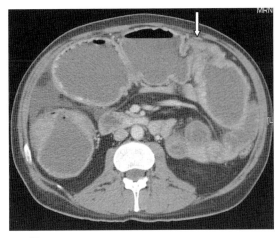

Fig. 50.2a Repeat CT scan.

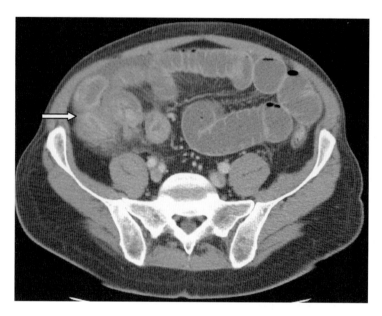

Fig. 50.2b Repeat CT scan (separate level).

Further reading

Bjornsson E, Lindqvist-Ottosson J, Asztely M, Olsson R (2004). Dominant strictures in patients with primary sclerosing cholangitis. *Am J Gastroenterol*; **99**: 502–8.

Björnsson E, Olsson R, Berqquist A *et al.* (2008). The natural history of small-duct primary sclerosing cholangitis. *Gastroenterology*; **134**: 975–80.

Tischendorf JJW, Geier A, Trautwein C (2008). Current diagnosis and management of primary sclerosing cholangitis. *Liver Transpl*; **14**: 735–46.

Tischendorf JJW, Meier PN, Schneider A *et al.* (2007). Transpapillary intraductal ultrasound in the evaluation of dominant bile duct stenoses in patients with primary sclerosing cholangitis. *Scand J Gastroenterol*; **42**: 1011–17.

Loftus EV, Harewood GC, Loftus CG *et al.* (2005). PSC-IBD: a unique form of inflammatory bowel disease associated with primary sclerosing cholangitis. *Gut*; **54**: 91–6.

List of cases by diagnosis

Case 1: Acute liver failure due to isoniazid

Case 2: Autoimmune hepatitis

Case 3: Intrahepatic cholestasis of pregnancy

Case 4: Primary biliary cirrhosis

Case 5: Variceal bleeding

Case 6: Haemochromatosis

Case 7: HIV-associated diarrhoea

Case 8: Ascites

Case 9: Ampullary carcinoma

Case 10: Small bowel bacterial overgrowth

Case 11: Hepatorenal syndrome

Case 12: Pancreatic insufficiency

Case 13: Autoimmune pancreatitis

Case 14: Hepatocellular carcinoma

Case 15: Functional outlet obstruction

Case 16: Hepatitis A

Case 17: Hereditary non-polyposis colon cancer

Case 18: Crohn's disease

Case 19: Perianal Crohns's disease

Case 20: Dyspepsia

Case 21: Portal vein thrombosis

Case 22: *Clostridium difficile*-associated diarrhoea

Case 23: Pregnancy in inflammatory bowel disease

Case 24: Abdominal lymphoma

Case 25: Hepatic encephalopathy

Case 26: Intestinal tuberculosis

Case 27: Eosinophilc oesophagitis

Case 28: Peptic ulcer disease

Case 29: Intrapapillary mucinous neoplasm

Case 30: Pernicious anaemia

Case 31: Cytomegalovirus colitis

List of cases by principal clinical features at diagnosis

Abdominal pain *2, 13, 19, 21, 26, 28, 39, 50*

Abnormal LFTs: *1, 3, 4, 5, 6, 25, 40, 42, 43, 44, 45, 47, 48*

Anaemia: *10, 18, 30, 39, 47*

Ascites: *8, 11, 24, 25, 45*

Vomiting *16, 50*

Constipation *15*

Diarrhoea *7, 10, 12, 18, 22, 31, 32, 33, 35, 36, 41*

Dysphagia: *27*

Encephalopathy *1, 11, 25, 47*

Family history: *17, 21, 27*

Gastrointestinal bleeding *5, 34*

Jaundice: *1, 2, 3, 9, 11, 13, 46 47*

Pruritus: *3, 4*

Weight loss *9, 10, 12, 13, 18, 29, 30, 37, 39, 49, 50*

Other: *14, 33*

List of cases by aetiological mechanisms

Autoimmune conditions: *3, 4, 13, 30*

Drug induced: *1, 35*

Infectious disease: *2, 7, 11, 16, 22, 26, 28, 31, 32, 42, 43, 44, 46*

Inflammatory: *18, 19, 23, 27, 36, 39, 41, 50*

Inherited conditions: *6, 8, 17, 21, 47*

Malignancy: *9, 14, 17, 24, 29, 34, 40, 48*

Physiological: *15, 33, 49*

Psychological: *32, 37*

Toxic: *5, 25*

Other: *10, 12, 45*

Index

Bold indicates the diagnosis of the case discussed within the page range.